Trauma and Cognitive Science: A Meeting of Minds, Science, and Human Experience

T0256229

Trauma and Cognitive Science: A Meeting of Minds, Science, and Human Experience has been co-published simultaneously as *Journal of Aggression, Maltreatment & Trauma*, Volume 4, Number 2 (#8) 2001.

Trauma and Cognitive Science: A Meeting of Minds, Science, and Human Experience

Jennifer J. Freyd, PhD
Anne P. DePrince, PhD
Editors

Trauma and Cognitive Science: A Meeting of Minds, Science, and Human Experience has been co-published simultaneously as *Journal of Aggression, Maltreatment & Trauma*, Volume 4, Number 2 (#8) 2001.

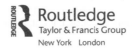

Routledge
Taylor & Francis Group
New York   London

First published by

The Haworth Maltreatment & Trauma Press®, 10 Alice Street, Binghamton, NY 13904-1580
USA

This edition published 2012 by Routledge

Routledge
Taylor & Francis Group
711 Third Avenue
New York, NY 10017

Routledge
Taylor & Francis Group
2 Park Square, Milton Park
Abingdon, Oxon OX14 4RN

Trauma and Cognitive Science: A Meeting of Minds, Science, and Human Experience has been co-published simultaneously as *Journal of Aggression, Maltreatment & Trauma* ™, Volume 4, Number 2 (#8) 2001.

Cover design by Thomas J. Mayshock Jr.

Library of Congress Cataloging-in-Publication Data

Trauma and cognitive science : a meeting of minds, science, and human experience / Jennifer J. Freyd, Anne P. DePrince.
        p. cm.
        "Co-published simultaneously as Journal of aggression, maltreatment & trauma, volume 4, number 2 (#8) 2001."
        Includes bibliographical references and index.
        ISBN 0-7890-1373-8 (alk. paper)–ISBN 0-7890-1374-6 (alk. paper)
        1. Psychic trauma. 2. Cognitive science. I. Freyd, Jennifer J. II. DePrince, Anne P.
RC552.P67 T735 2001
616.85'21–dc21   2001024427

Trauma and Cognitive Science: A Meeting of Minds, Science, and Human Experience

CONTENTS

ABOUT THE EDITORS

Jennifer J. Freyd, PhD, is Professor of Psychology at the University of Oregon. Dr. Freyd's current research includes experimental and survey investigations of memory for trauma with college student, clinical, community, and child populations. Her book, *Betrayal Trauma: The Logic of Forgetting Childhood Abuse,* was published in the fall of 1996 and was released in paperback in February of 1998. Dr. Freyd has received several prestigious honors for her research in cognitive psychology, including a Presidential Young Investigator Award from the National Science Foundation. She is a Fellow of the American Psychological Association, the American Psychological Society, and the American Association for the Advancement of Science. For *Betrayal Trauma*, Freyd received a 1997 Distinguished Publication Award from the Association for Women in Psychology, and the 1997 Pierre Janet Writing Award from the International Society for the Study of Dissociation.

Anne P. DePrince, PhD, earned her doctorate in clinical psychology at the University of Oregon. Her research examines the relationship between trauma, dissociation, and information processing, as well as how emotion and narrative relate to post-traumatic symptoms.

ABOUT THE CONTRIBUTORS

Robert F. Anda, MD, is Medical Epidemiologist and Co-principal Investigator on the Adverse Childhood Experiences Study at the Centers for Disease Control and Prevention (CDC). He has been an epidemiologist for 17 years, doing work on cardiovascular disease (CVD) risk factors, especially psychosocial determinants of CVD. Since 1990, he has worked on the design, implementation, management, and publication of data from the Adverse Childhood Experiences Study.

Michael C. Anderson, PhD, is Assistant Professor at the Department of Psychology, University of Oregon. His research has focused on the role of inhibitory processes as mechanisms of cognitive control. He is the author of a 1995 *Psychological Review* article, "On the status of inhibitory mechanisms in cognition: Memory retrieval as a model case."

Bernice Andrews, PhD, is Senior Lecturer in Psychology at Royal Holloway, University of London. She has researched and published extensively on childhood and adult abuse, and was a member of the British Psychological Society's Working Party on Recovered Memories. A recent publication appeared in the *British Journal of Psychiatry*, "Characteristics, context and consequences of memory recovery among adults in therapy" (Andrews, Brewin, Ochera, Morton, Bekerian, Davies, & Mollon, 1999).

Laura E. Boeschen, a doctoral student in clinical psychology from the University of Arizona, is currently on internship at the Veterans Affairs Palo Alto Health Care System. Her graduate work has focused on potential mediators of sexual assault and PTSD.

J. Douglas Bremner, MD, is Assistant Professor of Diagnostic Radiology and Psychiatry, Yale University School of Medicine; Research Associate Physician, VA Connecticut Healthcare System; and Director-Trauma Assessment Unit, Yale Psychiatric Institute. He is the Co-editor of *Trauma, Memory and Dissociation*, as well as *Post-Traumatic Stress Disorder: A Comprehensive Text*. Dr. Bremner conducts neuroimaging and neurobiological studies of the consequences of childhood sexual abuse and of posttraumatic stress disorder. He is trained in Psychiatry and Nuclear Medicine, and directs the Yale Trauma Research Program.

Chris R. Brewin, PhD, is Professor of Clinical Psychology at University College, London, and a consultant at the Traumatic Stress Clinic. His research concerns trauma and memory, illustrated by his article, "A dual representation theory of post-traumatic stress disorder" (Brewin, Dalgleish, & Joseph, *Psychological Review*, 1996).

Catherine Classen, PhD, is Research Associate at the Department of Psychiatry and Behavioral Sciences, Stanford University School of Medicine. She is the editor of *Treating Women Molested in Childhood*, published in 1995.

James A. Coan, MA, Department of Psychology, University of Arizona, is author of a 1997 *Ethics and Behavior* article, "Lost in a shopping mall: An experience with controversial research."

Anne P. DePrince, PhD, earned her doctorate in clinical psychology at the University of Oregon. Her research examines the relationship between trauma, dissociation, and information processing, as well as how emotion and narrative relate to post-traumatic symptoms.

Valerie J. Edwards, PhD, is Senior Staff Fellow, Centers for Disease Control and Prevention (CDC). For the past three years, she has worked as a Fellow on the Adverse Childhood Experiences (ACE) study. Her research interests are in the effects of childhood adversity on adult health and well-being.

Vincent J. Felitti, MD, is an internist with Kaiser Permanente in San Diego, where he founded the Department of Preventive Medicine 25 years ago. Originally trained in infectious diseases, he now works extensively with patients suffering from the long-term sequelae of childhood abuse, and those with the common genetic disorder, Hemochromatosis. He is also Associate Clinical Professor of Medicine at the University of California, San Diego.

Aurelio José Figueredo, PhD, is Associate Professor of Psychology; Director, Ethology and Evolutionary Psychology, Department of Psychology, University of Arizona; and first author of "Sex, money, and paternity: The evolutionary psychology of domestic violence," *Ethology and Sociobiology*, 1993.

Robyn Fivush, PhD, is Professor of Psychology at Emory University. Her research focuses on the early development of autobiographical memory for both everyday and stressful events. She is the co-editor of several books, including *Knowing and Remembering in Young Children*, and *The Remembered Self: Accuracy and Construction in the Life Narrative*.

Jennifer J. Freyd, PhD, is Professor of Psychology at the University of Oregon. Dr. Freyd's current research includes experimental and survey investigations of memory for trauma with college student, clinical, community, and child populations. Her book, *Betrayal Trauma: The Logic of Forgetting Childhood Abuse,* was published in the fall of 1996 and was released in paperback in February of 1998. Dr. Freyd has received several prestigious honors for her research in cognitive psychology, including a Presidential Young Investigator Award from the National Science Foundation. She is a Fellow of the American Psychological Association, the American Psychological Society, and the American Association for the Advancement of Science. For *Betrayal Trauma*, Freyd received a 1997 Distinguished Publication Award from the Association for Women in Psychology, and the 1997 Pierre Janet Writing Award from the International Society for the Study of Dissociation.

James W. Hopper, PhD, is Research Associate at the Department of Psychiatry, Boston University School of Medicine and The Trauma Center, Boston, MA. His recent research has focused on measuring changes in traumatic memories associated with effective treatment, and the biology of affect dysregulation in PTSD and Complex PTSD.

Ira E. Hyman, Jr., PhD, is Associate Professor at Western Washington University. He conducts research on human memory. His recent work has focused on false childhood memories, memory for phobia onset, traumatic memory, and unconscious influences on remembering. He teaches courses in human cognition, research design, and statistics.

Terence M. Keane, PhD, is Professor and Vice Chairman of Psychiatry at Boston University School of Medicine; Chief of Psychology at Boston VA Medical Center/Outpatient Clinics; and Director of the National Center for PTSD-Boston. He is Co-editor of *Assessing Psychological Trauma and PTSD,* published in 1997.

Cheryl Koopman, PhD, Associate Professor (Research), Department of Psychiatry and Behavioral Sciences, Stanford University School of Medicine, teaches Sophomore Dialog on Traumatic Stress: Antecedents, Consequences, and Intervention. She is first author of an article in press in the *Journal of Child Sexual Abuse*, "Acute stress reactions to everyday stressful life events among sexual abuse survivors with PTSD."

Mary P. Koss, PhD, is Professor, Public Health, Psychiatry, Family and Community Medicine, and Psychology, Arizona Prevention Center and the Arizona Health Sciences Center, University of Arizona in Tucson. She is co-author of "Traumatic memories: Empirical foundations, forensic and clinical implications," *Clinical Psychology: Science and Practice*, 1995. Dr. Koss has focused her research on sexual assault for the past 25 years. Her empirical work includes epidemiological studies of rape prevalence, characteristics of sexually aggressive men, and the psychological and physical health impact of sexual victimization. Her most recent work has focused on modeling cognitive changes during rape recovery.

Kirsten N. Nevill-Manning, MS, is Project Coordinator, Department of Psychiatry and Behavioral Sciences, Stanford University School of Medicine. She has also worked as a child protection social worker in New Zealand.

Dale F. Nordenberg, MD, is Adjunct Professor at Emory University in the Department of Pediatrics. Dr. Nordenberg is a board certified pediatrician and a CDC trained epidemiologist. He has worked in domestic and international public health for more than 10 years.

Mark A. Oakes graduated from Western Washington University, where he obtained his BA in English and Psychology. He is currently working toward his PhD at the University of Washington, where he is studying social and cognitive psychology. His current research interests emphasize the role of self-concept in memory distortion and implicit attitudes.

Janet E. Osterman, MD, MSc, is Director, Residency Training in Psychiatry, and Assistant Professor of Psychiatry, Boston University School of Medicine. Dr. Osterman's research has focused on the psychological trauma of waking up during general anesthesia, the subsequent development of post-traumatic stress disorder, and factors causing these to be poorly recognized or understood.

Kathy Pezdek, PhD, is Professor of Psychology at Claremont Graduate School, Claremont, California. She received her PhD in cognitive psychology from the University of Massachusetts, Amherst. Her research has focused on the suggestibility of memory, and eyewitness memory.

She has directed the program in Applied Cognitive Psychology at Claremont Graduate School since 1981, and is currently the Editor of *Applied Cognitive Psychology.*

Jonathan W. Schooler, PhD, is Associate Professor of Psychology, and Research Scientist at the Learning Research and Development Center, University of Pittsburgh. He is Co-editor of *Scientific Approaches to Consciousness,* published in 1997.

David Spiegel, MD, is Professor and Associate Chair of Psychiatry and Behavioral Sciences, Director of the Psychosocial Treatment Laboratory, and Medical Director of the Complementary Medicine clinic at Stanford University School of Medicine, where he has been a member of the faculty since 1975. He has published five books and more than 260 journal articles and chapters on psychosocial oncology, hypnosis, acute and post-traumatic stress disorder, and psychotherapy. His research is supported by the National Institute of Mental Health, the National Cancer Institute, the John D. and Catherine T. MacArthur Foundation, the Fetzer Institute, and the Nathan S. Cummings Foundation, among others.

Bessel A. van der Kolk, MD, is Professor of Psychiatry, Boston University School of Medicine; Medical Director, The Trauma Center, Boston, MA; and past President of the International Society for Traumatic Stress Studies. He is the author of over 100 scientific articles on the impact of trauma on the mind, brain, and memory, as well as three books, including *Traumatic Stress: The Effects of Overwhelming Experience on Mind, Body and Society* (with McFarlane and Weisaeth), published in 1996.

death. He continued his story by sharing that the mortar round essentially disintegrated his buddy and that as a result of the explosion he was covered with his friend's remains. Unable to be rescued from the battle scene for hours, Mr. K. remembered vomiting, defecating, and feeling paralyzed by the horror of what he was enduring. Upon inquiry, he stated he had forgotten about the circumstances surrounding his friend's death, had not remembered being covered with his friend's remains, and had not thought about the switching of positions since the day it occurred. When the memory returned it returned completely, in all its horrific detail.

This case was my first exposure to the nuances of traumatic memory. The year was approximately 1979, and our group was in the process of establishing one of the first treatment and research programs for a disorder that was eventually to become known as PTSD. I introduce this volume with this case study for several reasons. First, it is a case that is devoid of many of the political issues and arguments that have surrounded the trauma and memory controversy. The case's protagonist, if you will, is a male, was an adult at the time of the traumatic event, was a decorated military veteran, and had experienced this traumatic event in the context of war. Second, the antagonist, if you will, was the enemy–the North Vietnamese. Third, the treatment that was employed in this case was cognitive-behavioral therapy (CBT), the treatment of choice for PTSD as rated by mental health experts when developing best practice guidelines (Foa, Keane, & Friedman, 2000). Finally, the case demonstrates some of the extraordinary properties of the memory systems when processing traumatic events. The overarching event was recalled (i.e., the assault, his personal injuries, and the death of his best friend), while fundamentally important details were not recalled (i.e., his role in his friend's death over which he felt great conflict, and the horror of being covered with the body parts of a friend).

Clouding the scientific study of the parameters of memory following traumatic events was its placement in the context of childhood sexual abuse. This was, perhaps, not the best venue for the debate. Childhood sexual abuse and incest raise many socio-political issues that remain unresolved and contentious. It raises issues of gender inequality and power differentials; it raises issues antithetical to our conservative notions of family; and it is increasingly being discussed in the context of the adversarial judicial system. Childhood sexual abuse is a topic about which everyone in society feels strongly and the debate about childhood sexual trauma and memory has demonstrated to us all that the interface of science and politics can yield vitriolic debates and irrational, unyielding positions.

Placing the issue of trauma and its impact on memory within the context of war, however, mollifies strident beliefs and opinions, while permitting us to focus on the crucial scientific questions. With centuries of experience and knowledge surrounding war trauma and its impact on individuals and their memories, with a growing empirical data base suggesting that the rates of forgetting childhood sexual abuse are significant, and with substantive personal and professional experiences appearing in the literature, the conference entitled *Trauma and Cognitive Science: A Meeting of Minds, Science, and Human Experience* at the University of Oregon began with the conviction that traumatic events can be processed in fundamentally different ways, and can be forgotten completely, or, as in the introductory example, in fragments. How does this phenomenon occur? Why does it occur? What are the mechanisms involved? What motivates this forgetting? How frequently does this occur? What are the consequences of this forgetting for society? What are the consequences of this forgetting for the individual? What can we do to help individuals to recover from the impact of traumatic events? What role should therapists play in the recovery of memories of traumatic events? And finally, how do therapists optimally manage situations wherein people have recovered memories of traumatic life events? These questions and many more served to intrigue the presenters and the attendees to this conference for three stunningly beautiful summer days in Eugene, Oregon.

Participants in the meeting represented diverse research perspectives. Included were cognitive scientists, developmental scientists, neuroscientists, and still others identified themselves as clinical researchers. This permitted a discussion of the issue at multiple levels of analysis, as it necessarily must. Rarely do researchers from different backgrounds and training assemble in a single place to study and discuss a single problem. The University of Oregon and the Secret Garden Inn offered the diverse participants the opportunity to discuss, debate, and consider the problem of traumatic memory in the most idyllic setting. The meeting began early each morning, continued through meals and breaks in informal ways, and then proceeded through dinner and into the night as the participants learned and exchanged information bearing on the issue. Theories, constructs, methods, and models were presented, evaluated, modified, and ultimately future directions evolved as a function of the dialogue. Additional studies and enduring collaborations followed from the discussions.

Approaching the problem of traumatic forgetting from different levels, models, and methods provides unique opportunities for progress. As traditional academic departments are being reconsidered in light of new scientific advances, bringing the integration of various skills and perspectives to bear on complex societal problems is clearly the wave of future research progress. While the present meeting enjoined cognitive scientists, neuroscientists, and behavioral scientists, perhaps future meetings will also bring cultural anthropologists, sociologists, and molecular (psycho) biologists to the table. Increasing the analysis from the molecular to the physiological, to the cognitive and the behavioral, as well as to the social and cultural levels will bring even more possibilities for scientific advances to the fore. While many of us would like to place the mind at the central level of analysis, considerable knowledge exists about the influence of social and cultural factors on the functioning of the mind. As well, the data on the role of neurotransmitter systems and other biochemical factors on cognition and perception are indisputable, and a comprehensive understanding of trauma's impact on memory will ultimately require input from all levels of scientific analysis.

Rarely do scholars and academic researchers in mental health gather for meetings on such a highly specific topic. The participants owe a special debt of gratitude to Professors Jennifer Freyd and Chris Brewin for their leadership and direction. They conceptualized the conference as one that would bring together diverse research groups, promote integration, and foster collaborations. They were remarkably successful in achieving their goals. It was a meeting we will all remember for the duration of our careers as a highlight: great people, compelling intellects, challenging discussions, delicious food, all in a spectacular setting. Speaking on behalf of all participants, let me express my deepest appreciation to all those who made the meeting possible. The contents of this volume reflect a piece, perhaps only a small piece, of what was produced that weekend. Long lasting professional and personal relationships that transcend the boundaries of time and place are represented here. These will endure far beyond the time we spent in the Secret Garden.

Terence M. Keane

REFERENCE

Foa, E. B., Keane, T. M., & Friedman, M. J. (2000). *Effective Treatments for PTSD*. New York: Guilford Press.

The Meeting of Trauma and Cognitive Science: Facing Challenges and Creating Opportunities at the Crossroads

Anne P. DePrince
Jennifer J. Freyd

SUMMARY. This article argues for the necessity of a multidisciplinary approach to traumatic stress studies. The intersection of cognitive science and trauma offers both challenge and potential. The current article considers these challenges and opportunities in light of lessons learned at the 1998 Meeting on Trauma and Cognitive Science, held at the University of Oregon. The article will discuss the creation of this volume from the 1998 Meeting. *[Article copies available for a fee from The Haworth Document Delivery Service: 1-800-342-9678. E-mail address: <getinfo@haworthpress inc.com> Website: <http://www.HaworthPress.com> © 2001 by The Haworth Press, Inc. All rights reserved.]*

KEYWORDS. Trauma research, cognitive science, multidisciplinary

Trauma research presents a number of challenges to investigators. Some of these challenges lie in larger societal issues, such as denial, while others lie in traditional division of areas within psychology. The intersection of cogni-

Address correspondence to: Anne P. DePrince, Department of Psychology, 1227 University of Oregon, Eugene, OR 97403-1227 (E-mail: adp@dynamic.uoregon.edu).

[Haworth co-indexing entry note]: "The Meeting of Trauma and Cognitive Science: Facing Challenges and Creating Opportunities at the Crossroads." DePrince, Anne P., and Jennifer J. Freyd. Co-published simultaneously in *Journal of Aggression, Maltreatment & Trauma* (The Haworth Maltreatment & Trauma Press, an imprint of The Haworth Press, Inc.) Vol. 4, No. 2 (#8), 2001, pp. 1-8; and: *Trauma and Cognitive Science: A Meeting of Minds, Science, and Human Experience* (ed: Jennifer J. Freyd, and Anne P. DePrince) The Haworth Maltreatment & Trauma Press, an imprint of The Haworth Press, Inc., 2001, pp. 1-8. Single or multiple copies of this article are available for a fee from The Haworth Document Delivery Service [1-800-342-9678, 9:00 a.m. - 5:00 p.m. (EST). E-mail address: getinfo@haworthpressinc.com].

amidst the more traditional divisions in psychology, as they both challenge and seek to work within the current paradigm. However, trauma researchers inevitably find that any one of the traditionally defined areas within psychology does not have adequate scope to address the myriad ways that trauma influences human functioning. We are ultimately ill served by the arbitrary boundaries that implicitly assume human behavior can be divided neatly for the benefit of the researcher. As trauma researchers, we cannot afford to have training in only one particular area and neglect other lines of research that could profoundly inform our study. Most important we cannot train a future generation of trauma researchers without a multidisciplinary approach.

Trauma, therefore, challenges the very divisions on which so much of psychology has been organized. Trauma research requires of us a broad expertise: a willingness to seek out training from our colleagues; openness to new paradigms, methodologies, and analyses. Trauma research often requires a multidisciplinary approach. One such promising approach lies at the intersection of trauma and cognitive science.

1998 Meeting on Trauma and Cognitive Science

In July, 1998, 14 experts whose work employed creative bridges between trauma and information processing came together at the Meeting on Trauma and Cognitive Science at the University of Oregon. The meeting was organized by Jennifer J. Freyd (University of Oregon) and Chris R. Brewin (University of London), with assistance by Anne DePrince and Vonda Evans (University of Oregon). Presenters included Michael Anderson, Bernice Andrews, J. Douglas Bremner, Chris Brewin, Catherine Classen, Robyn Fivush, Jennifer Freyd, Ira Hyman, Terence Keane, Mary Koss, John Morton, Kathy Pezdek, Jonathan Schooler, and Bessel van der Kolk. These participants represented diverse origins within traditional divisions of psychology, including developmental, cognitive, cognitive neuroscience, social, and clinical areas. They were united by common interests in information processing and trauma.

The goal outlined for the meeting was to share knowledge and theory relevant to understanding the way in which trauma interacts with information processing. In particular, the meeting was intended to focus on how traumatic information is encoded, stored, and later retrieved from memory. A number of related topics were considered, including disturbances of consciousness during and after trauma, the accuracy of memory for trauma, the need for multi-level models of memory, the effects of early trauma on subsequent information processing, and inhibitory processes in memory. The intention of the conference was to focus on research while keeping in mind the significant ethical, clinical, and societal implications of trauma work.

The conference opened with a welcome from the University of Oregon research community made by Don Tucker, as well as a special address by University of Oregon President Dave Frohnmayer. Approximately 150 people attended the Meeting presentations on July 17, 18, and 19 on the University of Oregon campus. The audience met the presenters with enthusiastic and challenging questions about empirical data, conceptualizations of trauma and clinical implications of the discussions (see Brewin & Andrews, in this volume, for a report on the question and answer periods). As the conference progressed, each presentation galvanized the next. Presenters incorporated previous comments, occasionally looking up from the prepared talk to expand on thoughts provoked earlier in the day. Last-minute changes inspired by the previous speakers and scribbled in the margins of many presenters' talks testified to the truly collaborative atmosphere created by this group. The talks, discussion, and questioning pushed new conceptualizations and challenged old paradigms. Perhaps most striking was the community that developed quickly between the participants as they debated the latest theories.

In retrospect, the words do not come easily to describe the gathering, except perhaps to note the profound humanity of it: a humanity that reminded each researcher that the topic of discussion was not an impersonal group of subjects somewhere, but real people's pain and triumphs in the face of trauma; a humanity that always kept the ethics and implications of the conclusions drawn from data at the forefront of discussion; and a humanity that joined those who, at times profoundly disagreed, and at other times ardently agreed, in simultaneous roles as colleague, teacher, and student.

Current Volume

Many of the contributions to the current volume came directly from presentations, while other articles represent extensions of material presented during the conference. We hope that the volume conveys to the reader the excitement of the multidisciplinary approach taken during the conference. The ideas represent new and challenging conceptualizations, compromises, and questions. While this volume is a report on where these experts see the field of trauma now, it is perhaps even more an inspiration and challenge for future research.

The ideas in this volume represent a community of researchers coming together to forge a new way of thinking and working. Though the researchers came from different theoretical perspectives, held different personal opinions, and had different training backgrounds, their participation in the conference and this volume bridges one to the other. They have forged a community with diversity and respect. They have, in essence, modeled an alternative to approaches that are grounded in traditional delineation of areas, and have made an important contribution to psychology as a whole. They show us that trauma cannot be taken out of context, and that it cannot belong to any one area of psychology. Rather, working to understand trauma and its effects on the individual, as well as society, is a responsibility we share, and it requires our joint efforts, collaboration, and respect.

Volume Organization

The current volume is organized to preserve the order of presentations from the 1998 Conference. The volume begins with two articles by van der Kolk and colleagues. Much as he did at the conference, van der Kolk and colleagues open by capturing the spirit of the volume in terms of interfacing cognitive and clinical issues. These articles echo that spirit, expanding on two different aspects of the conference presentation. Articles by Pezdek and by Hyman and Oakes take the reader through important considerations of "false memories" and suggestibility. These articles reflect the importance of addressing difficult questions, assumptions, and personal beliefs with regard to this much-politicized area of the field. Hyman (1998) captured the essence of the tensions we must maintain when evaluating work on false memories during the question and answer period at the conference. He noted, "It's a very uncomfortable thing, but I think both as scientists in terms of some of these questions and as individuals in terms of particular abuse histories, sometimes the thing to do is just maintain some uncertainty. It's not a comfortable thing, but that may be really the safest thing to do, rather than to force a conclusion one way or another, which really may not be possible."

Schooler's article brings to the volume an important piece in terms of focusing on individual accounts of memory for trauma in order to push the bounds of current theory, which was very much a critical contribution of his to the conference as well. Schooler offers a refreshing qualitative approach to study in this area, and captures the balance between science and human experience, as he did during the conference. During the question and answer period at the conference, Schooler (1998) noted, "There is a certain gratification and excitement about making progress on scientific issues . . . when your research is looking into other individuals' tragedies, there is this balance that we have to maintain, you have to not confuse the excitement of the research with the really horrendous negativity of the trauma."

The next three articles, authored by Freyd, Bremner and Anderson respectively, take the reader from applying cognitive paradigms to trauma research somewhat broadly, to a narrower cognitive science approach, and then one level deeper to propose a mechanism for retrieval-induced forgetting. Leading off this triumvirate, Freyd and DePrince review their recent research on dissociation and attention, combining the training and paradigms of cognitive psychology with application to theoretical developments in clinical domains. This article reviews a program of research aimed at drawing on multidisciplinary methods and expertise. Following Freyd and DePrince, Bremner complements the contributors who bring cognitive methods to this volume by introducing a cognitive neuroscience viewpoint. In Bremner's article we see the spirit of multidisciplinary approaches as he reviews studies based in cognitive neuroscience with participants from clinical populations. Picking up on the exciting advances in cognitive neuroscience, Anderson's creative article challenges the reader to consider the applications of a model of active forgetting that speaks to mechanisms that may underlie some forms of traumatic forgetting.

The final three content articles are authored by Koss, Fivush, Classen and their colleagues. These articles, together, draw in perspectives on how the narrative of trauma intersects with psychological distress, healing, and therapy. These researchers balance the depths reached when we talk with those who have experienced trauma, and the approaches we take to these issues as scientists. Koss and colleagues report on exciting quantitative and qualitative data that bring in the survivors' voice. This valuing of the survivors' voice in empirical research mirrors the critical and challenging issues (e.g., socialization of women, importance of considering culture) Koss raised during the question and answer period. Discussing a study with women who reported rape and were of Hispanic Catholic background, Koss (1998) noted, "I can just anecdotally tell you, in that group, that there is such a shame attached to this, and such a hesitancy to talk about it, that you even can observe it at the level of not being willing to use language."

Like Koss and her colleagues, Fivush and colleagues report on a large-scale study that makes such an important contribution to the field in terms of reaching broad ranges of people. The article by Fivush and colleagues takes on the important issue of autobiographical memory disturbances in childhood abuse survivors. Fivush and colleagues consider the important question of the impact of trauma on autobiographical memory for mundane events in childhood, not just memory for abuse itself. Classen and colleagues bring many of the issues raised throughout the volume together in reporting on pilot work at Stanford Medical Center looking at treatment for PTSD with women who were abused in childhood. In so doing, Classen and colleagues raise central questions about how interventions should be designed and implemented based on our current understanding of research and politics in traumatic stress studies. Classen (1998) raised a related point during the conference when she asked, "If I said to a client, 'tell me more about that experience,' is that a technique?"

Brewin and Andrews bring together many themes from the full conference in their review of the question and answer periods. In synthesizing the question and answer periods, they offer the reader more insight into the breadth and depth covered during the conference, as well as create a framework by which we can pursue the questions that will challenge the field to continue

ories of subjects with and without current Post-Traumatic Stress Disorder. Our findings suggest the need for more rigorous methods for the assessment of the evolution of traumatic memories. In order to develop a comprehensive and integrated understanding of the nature of traumatic memory, we need to combine careful clinical observations with replicable laboratory methods, including those of cognitive science and neuroscience. *[Article copies available for a fee from The Haworth Document Delivery Service: 1-800-342-9678. E-mail address: <getinfo@haworthpressinc. com> Website: <http://www.HaworthPress.com> © 2001 by The Haworth Press, Inc. All rights reserved.]*

KEYWORDS. Memory, awareness during anesthesia, Post-Traumatic Stress Disorder, traumatic memories

INTRODUCTION

The understanding of how people process traumatic events has, until recently, been entirely within the domain of clinical practice and observation. Traditionally, the fields of clinical psychology and psychiatry on the one hand, and cognitive science and neuroscience on the other, have had such widely divergent samples, methodologies and concepts on which they based their understandings of memory processes, that there has been a veritable confusion of tongues between these disciplines. During the past decade, when the observation that people may lose all memory for sexual abuse experiences and retrieve them at a later time was brought to the public's attention, many cognitive scientists took an incredulous stance. Yet for over a century this observation had been consistently reported in the psychiatric literature on other traumatized populations. Despite dozens of reports, starting with Pierre Janet (1889) in the 1880s, followed by Breuer and Freud (1893), repeated during the first World War (Myers, 1915; Southard, 1919), the second World War (Sargant and Slater, 1941) and the Vietnam War (van der Kolk, 1987), most laboratory scientists disregarded the validity of these observations. In the past decade a small group of cognitive scientists began to take clinical reports seriously (Freyd, 1991, 1994; Morton, 1994; Schooler, 1994). However, because amnesia and delayed recall for traumatic experiences had never been observed in the laboratory, many cognitive scientists adamantly denied that these phenomena existed (e.g., Loftus, 1993; Loftus & Ketcham, 1994), or that retrieved traumatic memories could be accurate (Kihlstrom, 1995).

In both science and therapy we often are confronted with unexpected findings. Whether one is a laboratory scientist or a clinician, such phenomena ideally should provoke new insights and creative theoretical and methodological advances. Laboratory scientists' practice of "controlled" research may render them more prone to observe the phenomena that they set out to measure, while clinicians cannot help but be frequently confronted with unexpected phenomena that don't fit their constructs and models. This often forces them to suspend disbelief and to attend to the unfolding of clinical data for which they have no pre-existing explanations.

Among memory researchers, the issue of whether increased affect enhances or diminishes the accuracy of memory has been hotly debated. The work of Christianson (1992a, 1992b), as well as Yuille and Cutshall (1986), does seem to settle one issue: while there appears to be decreased accuracy for remembering irrelevant details, the central details of stressful events often are remembered with great clarity and accuracy (Loftus, Loftus, & Messo, 1987). However, many traumatized individuals have trouble remembering even the central details of their experience for some period of time (for a comprehensive review, see Brown, Scheflin & Hammond, 1998).

In order to sharpen any discussion on how trauma affects memory we first need to define what is meant by "traumatic memory." The *Diagnostic and Statistical Manual of Mental Disorders, Fourth Edition* (DSM-IV; APA, 1994), definition for Posttraumatic Stress Disorder (PTSD) defines a traumatic memory as a memory of a personally traumatic event. The first DSM-IV criterion for PTSD stipulates that (1) "the person experienced, witnessed or was confronted with an event or events that involved actual or threatened death or serious injury, or a threat to the physical integrity of self or others," and (2) "the person's experience involved intense fear, helplessness, or horror" (APA, 1994, pp. 427 & 431). The second component of traumatic memory is that the memory is experienced as if the event and one's responses to it–sensory, cognitive, emotional and physiological–were happening all over again. Most typically, intense flashbacks and nightmares force traumatized people to cope with constant recurrences of memories without the prospect of relief. The recurrent intrusive recollections and the nightmares themselves become new triggers of panic, which may evoke a variety of avoidance and numbing maneuvers that help dissociate the affective intensity of the experience.

Despite the power of these clinical observations, these phenomena have not been systematically studied in the laboratory. The problem is *not* that laboratory science cannot study traumatic memories, but that laboratory science cannot study traumatic memories under conditions in which *the memories studied are for events that take place in the laboratory.* The event encoded into memory simply cannot be a "controlled" variable in the laboratory science sense, as in landmark work of Loftus and her colleagues with systematically altered films of car accidents (Loftus, 1975, 1979). This is so because, for *ethical* reasons, not scientific ones, the extreme terror and help-lessness that precede the development of PTSD simply cannot be replicated in such a setting. Roger Pitman (personal communication, July 1996) at-tempted to simulate a truly traumatic stressor by having college students watch "The Faces of Death," a film consisting of actual footage of deaths and mutilations of people and animals, in the laboratory. Even this stimulus, which is probably as extreme as any institutional review board would allow, failed to precipitate PTSD symptoms in these normal volunteers.

Hence it appears inescapable that to study the nature of traumatic memo-ries one must study the memories of people who have actually been trauma-tized. Ideally, one's sample would consist of people who had experienced a trauma that was videotaped, and their memories would be assessed immedi-ately after the event. Studies of flashbulb memories (Brown & Kulik, 1977) have come close to this, but the events were not sufficiently traumatic to produce the extremes of terror, helplessness and horror associated with being a direct victim of domestic violence, rape, a major car accident, etc. Less ideal but still quite good is to recruit crime victims, patients in emergency rooms, or other victims of recent trauma and follow the progression of their recollection of the traumatic events. Even studying witnesses of crimes that can be reconstructed very reliably (Yuille & Cutshall, 1986), however, may involve subjects insufficiently traumatized to develop PTSD.

In clinical practice, one often has an opportunity to witness the evolution of traumatic memories beginning shortly after the actual occurrence of the event. It is not unusual for traumatized children (including those who have been raped or witnessed a parent's murder) to initially give a seemingly accurate account of what has happened, but, a year later, to deny that the event occurred and that they have any memory of it. This common clinical observation was supported by Burgess and colleagues' (1995) systematic prospective study of 34 severely abused children. They found that both narrative and implicit memories (behavioral re-enactments) persisted for some time after the abuse, but that the narrative memory was relatively incomplete and fragmented for 41% of the children. Five to ten years after the abuse, many of the children had lost the narrative memory of the abuse, but all of them showed clear signs of implicit, behavioral memories, which mani-fested themselves as somatic complaints, flashbacks, and behavioral reenact-ments of abuse-related scenarios that had previously been reported.

There have been very few systematic studies of the memory processes of acutely traumatized adults. Harvey, Bryant and Dang (1998) assessed motor vehicle accident victims' ability to recall specific traumatic memories in response to cue words within one week of the trauma, and severity of PTSD symptoms 6 months later. They found that poor recall of specific trauma memories within the first week predicted 25% of the variance in PTSD severity at follow-up. Mechanic, Resick and Griffin (1998), studying memory in 92 rape victims, found that within two weeks following the rape there was significant amnesia in a third (37%) of the victims. At a 3-month follow-up, only about one sixth (16%) of the completing subjects had significant amnesia. The rape victims' memory deficits were trauma specific; they did not suffer from generalized memory deficits. Based on all the findings of this study, Mechanic et al. (1998) concluded that (1) following rape there is a high incidence of recovered memory, (2) amnesia and recovered memory occur more often in response to victimization by known perpetrators, which is congruent with Freyd's (1996) theory of betrayal trauma, and (3) dissociation but not ordinary memory processes like forgetting seems to play a primary role in the encoding, storage, and retrieval of traumatic memories.

THE DEVELOPMENT
OF THE TRAUMATIC MEMORY INVENTORY

Shobe and Kihlstrom (1997) recently published an article claiming that traumatic memories are qualitatively not any different from memories of ordinary events. Without actually having studied the memories of traumatized individuals themselves, they dismissed all existing observational studies of the memories of individuals with PTSD out of hand. Their rationale for doing so is found in the article's final section, "Clinical lore and scientific evidence."

> Although their ideas about the underlying mechanisms are different, Terr, van der Kolk and Whitfield all agree on the outcome: Memories of trauma, or at least of certain forms of trauma, are encoded by processes, such as repression and dissociation, that make them difficult to retrieve as coherent verbal narratives. The result is that traumatic memories are primarily available as isolated, nonverbal, sensory, motor, and emotional fragments. If this conclusion were valid. . . . (1997, p. 74)

Shobe and Kihlstrom have reversed the order of things. First, clinicians working with traumatized individuals found themselves confronted with unexpected observations: incoherent memories of "isolated, nonverbal, sensory, motor, and emotional fragments." Second, once they were struck by the consistency of this observation, clinician-scientists looked for theoretical constructs to make sense of the data.

Initially, the constructs of repression and dissociation were the best they could find. It is not that pioneering students of traumatic memory ignored laboratory evidence, or that they did not search among laboratory scientists' constructs for ones that could help them explain the data they were encountering. It is just that when it came to delayed recall and the *fragmentary* nature of many traumatic memories, clinician-scientists encountered a conceptual void in the laboratory memory research literature. Laboratory scientists had studied memories for events they had created under controlled conditions, and thus had never encountered fragmentary traumatic memories. In short, laboratory scientists never had a reason to create constructs explicitly addressing fragmentary traumatic memories.

After first encountering inescapable empirical evidence of how traumatic memories can differ from non-traumatic ones, and second, searching for constructs to describe and explain their observations, more recent students of traumatic memory then set out to conduct systematic research on the characteristics of traumatic memory. Early studies focused on the controversial phenomena of amnesia and delayed recall (e.g., Briere & Conte, 1993; Elliott, 1997; Feldman-Summers & Pope, 1994; Williams, 1994, 1995). Laboratory memory scientists like Kihlstrom (1995) and Loftus (1993) have vigorously attacked this line of research. However, others including Freyd (1991, 1994, 1996), Morton (1994) and Schooler (1994) have taken seriously the observations of clinicians and clinician-scientists' research on traumatic memory. These researchers have led the way in applying cognitive science constructs to the full complexity of traumatic memories, including phenomena like delayed recall and fragmentation.

Despite or perhaps because of the traumatic memory debate's polarized nature and the associated dismissals of existing studies, the central questions remain: (1) Can sensory imprints in the form of vivid fragments or flashbacks of images, sounds, smells, bodily sensations and affects properly be classified as "memories"? (2) In what ways are memories of traumatic experiences qualitatively different from those of ordinary events? (3) Do traumatic memory fragments change in character over time, as narratives are known to do? (4) Could there be sensory imprints that disappear and are later retrieved as pristine representations of what actually happened?

How can we begin to approach these questions? Answers will only come from integrative studies that combine the most appropriate ideas and methods of both clinicians and laboratory researchers. Our laboratory has made an attempt by developing an instrument called the Traumatic Memory Inventory (TMI; van der Kolk & Fisler, 1995) to enable detailed examination of the nature of traumatic and non-traumatic memories. The original TMI was designed to capture the richness and complexity of traumatic memories as experienced by traumatized people and observed by clinicians on a daily basis. It provided a structured way of recording whether and how memories of traumatic experiences are retrieved differently from memories of personally significant but non-traumatic events. In order to examine the retrieval of traumatic memories in a systematic way, the TMI specifically inquires about sensory, affective and narrative ways of remembering, about triggers for unbidden recollections of traumatic memories, and about ways of dealing with them.

The TMI gathers data on several characteristics of traumatic memories that distinguish them from non-traumatic memories. It begins by probing for background and contextual information, including (1) the nature and (2) duration of the trauma(s); (3) whether the subject had always remembered ("Have you always known that this trauma happened to you in all of its details?"), and if not, when and where the subject became conscious of the trauma; (4) the circumstances under which subject first experienced intrusive memories, and circumstances under which they occur presently. It then inquires in detail about (5) the sensory modalities in which memories were and are currently experienced, that is, (a) as images ("What did you see?"), (b) as sounds ("What did you hear?"), (c) as smells ("What did you smell?"), (d) as tactile or bodily sensations ("What did you feel in your body?"), and (e) as emotions ("What did you feel emotionally?"). Next subjects are asked whether they experienced all of the components present together ("Did you see, feel, smell and hear at the same time?"), and if they remembered it as a coherent narrative ("Were you capable of telling other people what had happened?"). The sensory, affective, fragmentation and narrative data are collected for how subjects remembered the trauma (a) initially, (b) while most bothered by the memory or at "peak" intensity, and (c) currently. The original TMI gathered data as well on related clinical information, including (1) the nature of nightmares, (2) the precipitants of flashbacks and nightmares, and (3) ways the subject attempts to gain mastery over intrusive recollections (e.g., by eating, working, taking drugs or alcohol, cleaning, etc.). Finally, the original TMI inquires about confirmation, including court or hospital records, direct witnesses, a relative who went through the same trauma, or other forms of definite or probable confirmation.

The strengths and weaknesses of the original TMI both stem from its origins in clinical observation of fragmentary traumatic memories. With its detailed exploration of memory characteristics, like each sensory and affective component, and its linking of these phenomena to specific and quite different remembering contexts (initial, most distressing, and current), the TMI respected the richness and complexity of fragmentary traumatic memories. On the other hand, like data available in the clinical setting, those gathered with the original TMI are retrospective, with all the potential for distortion that entails. Still greater threats to validity and reliability come from the fact that the TMI is not only retrospective, but relies on subjects' *memories of how they remembered,* sometimes years or even decades in the past.

PREVIOUS STUDIES AT THE TRAUMA CENTER:
THE TMI AND SCRIPT-DRIVEN IMAGERY

Our research group has been interested in describing how memories of traumatic events are similar to and different from memories of ordinary experiences. We have published two previous articles (van der Kolk & Fisler, 1995; van der Kolk, Burbridge, & Suzuki, 1997) describing how memories of traumatic events, but not ordinary ones, are initially primarily retrieved as isolated sensations–as visual images, smells, sounds, affective states, and bodily sensations– and how, only with time, are many traumatized individuals able to construct a narrative that verbally describes their traumatic experience in communicable language.

In our previous studies utilizing the TMI, as described above, we asked our subjects the same questions about a personally highly significant experience, such as a wedding or graduation ceremony, and collected the same information about those memories. We have consistently found that subjects tend to consider these questions about the non-traumatic memory nonsensical: none has olfactory, visual, auditory, kinesthetic re-living experiences related to such events. Subjects also deny having vivid dreams or flashbacks about them. They never claim to have periods in their lives when they have amnesia for any of those events; nor do any claim to have photographic recollections of them. Environmental triggers do not suddenly bring back vivid and detailed memories of these events, and none of the subjects ever reports feeling a need to make special efforts to suppress memories of these events.

In both of our previous studies, the first mainly of subjects with histories of severe childhood trauma, and the second of subjects with adult trauma, such as rapes, motor vehicle accidents, and physical assaults, many subjects reported that they initially had no narrative memory at all for the event: they could not tell a story about what had happened, regardless of whether they always knew that the trauma had happened, or whether they retrieved memories of the trauma at a later date. All these subjects, regardless of the age at which the trauma occurred, claimed that they initially "remembered" the trauma in the form of somatosensory and affective flashback experiences. These flashbacks occurred in a variety of modalities: visual, olfactory, affective, auditory and kinesthetic, but often these modalities did not initially occur together. As the traumatic memories came into consciousness with greater intensity, more sensory modalities were activated along with the affective component, and over time there emerged a capacity to tell themselves and others about what had happened.

Other investigators have reported similar findings. Roe and Schwartz (1996) found that 60% of their abused inpatients reported that their first recovered memory of abuse occurred in the form of a somatosensory flashback, and that only over time were they able to articulate a narrative memory. Cameron (1996) similarly found that initially amnestic sexual abuse survivors, compared to those with continuous memories, were significantly more likely to have memories manifest as "sensory memories," and to have narrative memories initially return in "bits and pieces." Christianson (1992b) also reported that the recovered memories of their subjects initially returned in the form of flashbacks, body-sensory experiences, dreams, sudden intense emotions, or avoidance behaviors, and with respect to narrative memory, as fragments. Koss et al. (1996) found that the severity of the rape experience per se, as well as the victim's appraisal of the event, independently contributed to the lack of clarity of detail and disorganization of the narrative rape memory. Foa and colleagues (Foa, Molnar, & Cashman, 1995) developed a coding system to assess changes in rape narratives associated with exposure treatment for PTSD, and found that significant improvement in PTSD symptoms was associated with significant decreases in the fragmentation of narratives.

In an attempt to elucidate neurobiological underpinnings of these phenomena, we asked some subjects with PTSD from our prior studies to undergo a procedure in which we made Positron Emission Tomography (PET) images of their brains while we evoked memories of traumatic and neutral events (Rauch et al., 1996). We then compared levels of region-specific brain activation in each condition, and found that, compared to the neutral memory, during the traumatic memory subjects with PTSD had decreased activation of Broca's area and increased activation in the right medio-temporal region. Consistent with this and other neuroimaging studies (Shin et al., 1997; Shin et al., 1999), and neurobiological models of emotional memory (e.g., LeDoux, 1996; Squire & Zola-Morgan, 1991), we have proposed (van der Kolk, 1994, 1996) the following model. Under conditions of extreme stress there is failure of hippocampal memory processing, which results in an inability to integrate incoming sensory input into a coherent autobiographical narrative, leaving the sensory elements of experience unintegrated and unattached. These sensory elements then are prone to return during flashbacks, which occur when a sufficient number of sensory elements of the trauma are activated by current reminders.

Our PET study incorporated an important methodological innovation, script-driven imagery, to evoke both traumatic and control neutral memories in an individualized yet standardized way. Script-driven imagery is a laboratory method pioneered by Lang and colleagues (e.g., Lang, Levin, Miller, & Kozac, 1983) and applied to the psychophysiology of PTSD by Pitman, Orr and colleagues (e.g., Pitman, Orr, Forgue, de Jong, & Claiborn, 1987), who were co-investigators on this study. This study demonstrated that although researchers cannot control the events that create traumatic memories, using this approach they *can* exert considerable control over the conditions under which those memories are evoked and phenomenological data about them are gathered (see Hopper & van der Kolk, 2001, this volume).

THE CURRENT STUDY:
MEMORIES FOR "AWARENESS"
DURING ANESTHESIA

In this study we used the original TMI with a homogeneous group of subjects who were not victims of interpersonal abuse, as were most of our previous subjects, but who regained consciousness in the middle of surgical procedures (known euphemistically in the anesthesia literature as "awareness").

The aim of this study was to replicate the findings of our prior research (van der Kolk & Fisler, 1995; van der Kolk et al., 1997) on the characteristics of traumatic memories, but in a sample of homogenous, non-interpersonal abuse memories that, if they involved delayed recall, were not recovered in therapy. The subjects of this study had woken up from general anesthesia while still in surgery. Research has shown that even those who do not suffer physical pain during their aware experience report experiences of extreme fear and helplessness (Ranta et al., 1998; Schwender et al., 1998). In this study we used the original TMI to gather retrospective data on memories of awareness at three points in time: when they initially remembered awakening from anesthesia, when they were most disturbed by their memory, and at the time of the study.

Method

Design. Retrospective self-report data on memories of awareness under anesthesia were compared for subjects with and without current PTSD secondary to their awareness experiences. Six characteristics of memories of awareness under anesthesia were compared in subjects with and without PTSD, at three points in time. Two hypotheses were made about all subjects' memories: First, that compared to initial and peak intensity memories, current memories would include a coherent verbal narrative. Second, that sensory and affective components of memory would be more prevalent initially and at peak intensity than currently. Two related predictions were made about differences between the memories of subjects with and without current PTSD for their experiences of awareness under anesthesia across all stages of remembering (initial, peak and current). First, subjects with PTSD would be less likely than those without to report having a coherent narrative. Second, subjects with PTSD would be more likely than those without to remember their awareness experience as sensory and affective components.

Participants. Sixteen subjects reporting awareness under anesthesia were recruited via advertisements in newspapers and fliers posted in hospitals, self-referral following exposure to print and television news stories, or referral by anesthesiologists. The subjects were men and women 18 years of age or older who had experienced awareness under general anesthesia. Three subjects were younger than 18 at the time of surgery (two eight and one 16 years old). Subjects were interviewed between 3 months and 35 years postoperatively (mean of 17.9 years). The subjects with awareness were subsequently divided into two groups, those with ($N = 9$) and without ($N = 7$) current PTSD diagnosis. IRB approval was obtained from both institutions where the study was performed, and written informed consent was obtained from all subjects. Interviews were conducted at a public university teaching hospital and a private outpatient psychiatric clinic specializing in the treatment of traumatized populations, and in community settings.

Materials. Subjects were assessed by trained interviewers for PTSD diagnosis and severity of PTSD symptoms with the Clinician Administered PTSD Scale (CAPS; Blake et al., 1995), a structured interview which has been shown to yield reliable data and has been validated for the purpose of assessing PTSD symptoms and their severity. The target PTSD "Criterion A" event for the CAPS was the subject's experience of awareness under anesthesia. CAPS items concerning reexperiencing (criterion B), avoidant and numbing (C), and hyperarousal (D) symptoms were focused on the effects of experiencing awareness. Characteristics of subjects' memories of the awareness experience were assessed with the original TMI (described above). The TMI was used to gather data on the presence or absence of six experienced characteristics of the memories, including four sensory components (visual images, sounds, bodily sensations, smells), an affective component, and access to a verbal narrative.

Results

This study's small sample size and the categorical nature of its variables of interest precluded statistical analyses of the hypotheses. That is, chi square statistics are only valid when all cell sizes are greater than five, a condition not met because, as we discovered, people who have experienced awareness during surgery with general anesthesia tend to avoid contact with health professionals. Indeed, this was the most difficult trauma population from which we have ever attempted to recruit subjects.

Participant characteristics. There was a trend for subjects with current PTSD to be younger than subjects without current PTSD (means of 44 and 53.4 years, respectively, $t(14) = 2.06, p = .059$), but no significant difference was found for years since the surgery (means of 15.8 and 20.6 years, respectively). Subjects with PTSD had a mean total CAPS score of 75.9 (range = 57-96, *SD* = 12.52), compared to the mean of 21.7 (range = 9-41, *SD* = 11.32) for subjects without current PTSD, *t*(14) = 8.94, *p* < .001. The range of CAPS scores in the subjects with PTSD indicate a moderate to severe range of symptomatology, based on normative data from a large-scale psychometric study (Blake et al., 1995).

Amnesia and delayed recall. Six of 16 or 37.5% of the subjects reported a period of amnesia, during which they "had no memories" and did not even "know that something had happened." Four of those six subjects had PTSD at the time of the study. One subject reported that she had always known that it happened, but didn't remember some of the details. The remaining nine (56.3%) said they had always known that it happened in all of its details.

Changes in memory characteristics over time. Three subjects reported that their "initial" and "peak" memory was the same; that is, they remembered their earliest memory as most disturbing. For those cases, the same values were entered for both initial and peak periods. Figure 1 depicts the sensory, affective and narrative modalities for all subjects over the three time periods assessed with the TMI. Of 16 subjects, 18.8% (3 of 16) reported having no narrative for the experience of awareness when they first remembered it (were not "able to tell another person a story about what had happened"). Two subjects were not sure and 68.8% (11 of 16) reported initially having a narrative memory. As predicted, over time subjects acquired the ability to communicate their memory as a narrative, with 87% having a narrative at peak intensity and 100% at the time of the study. In contrast to our prediction, on the whole subjects reported surprisingly little change in other modalities of memory over time. The one

FIGURE 1. Modalities of Memory in Subjects with Awareness Under Anesthesia

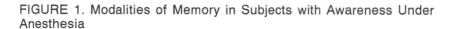

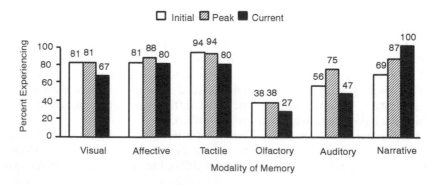

exception appeared to be the auditory component, which was experienced by more subjects when the memory was most disturbing than initially or currently.

Comparisons of memory characteristics in subjects with and without PTSD. Though the numbers in each group were small (9 with PTSD and 7 without), changes in memory characteristics over time were compared between them. As predicted and shown in Figure 2, subjects with PTSD were more likely than those without to report that initially they did not have a narrative memory. All but one of the seven non-PTSD subjects initially had a narrative memory (one was unsure), compared to five of nine subjects with current PTSD (again, one was unsure). At peak intensity, all non-PTSD subjects but only three-quarters of the current PTSD subjects reported having a narrative memory. At the time of the study, as noted above, all subjects in both groups had narratives. In this small sample, differences were not found between groups for the prevalence of sensory and affective modalities. However, we did find that most subjects with PTSD relived the surgery in the form of sensations and affects–when they initially remembered, when the memory was most disturbing to them, and at the time of the study. By definition, subjects with current PTSD had traumatic memories at the time of the study. Subjects without PTSD, in contrast, currently had distressing but not traumatic memories, and there was a trend for fewer of them to report reliving of sensations and affects from the surgery in their current memories (i.e., somewhat lower percentages for tactile, olfactory and affective modalities; data not shown).

FIGURE 2. Narrative Memory in Subjects with Awareness Under Anesthesia

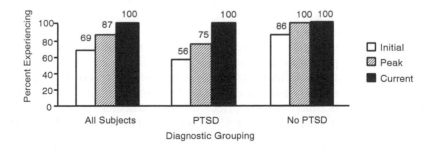

DISCUSSION

This study confirms that traumatic memories associated with Post-Traumatic Stress Disorder may initially lack narrative elements, even as the trauma is intrusively relived as sounds, smells, bodily sensations and visual images. The most unexpected finding was that all memories for traumatic experiences–whether subjects met criteria for PTSD or not–tended to have sensory and affective components. We consider the possible reasons for these findings and their implications for future research.

Narrative memory. Consistent with our prediction, six out of seven subjects without PTSD had an initial verbal narrative of the trauma, compared with five out of nine of those with current PTSD. In our first study using the original TMI (van der Kolk & Fisler, 1995), all subjects met criteria for current PTSD, and none reported having an initial narrative memory. This discrepancy may be accounted for by two differences in the nature of the subjects' traumatic experiences. All but one of the subjects in this study experienced the trauma of awareness in adulthood, while over 75% of the subjects in the first study were traumatized as children. In addition, the nature of the traumas were different, with most subjects in the first study having experienced assault by a caregiver or family member, as opposed to the accidental and undetected trauma of awareness under anesthesia. In both studies, however, there was a clear pattern of narrative formation over time, even though sensory and affective intrusions continued in subjects with PTSD.

The results of our second study using the TMI (van der Kolk et al., 1997) appear to fall somewhere in the middle. The sample consisted of adults with PTSD secondary to childhood trauma with a period of amnesia, childhood trauma without amnesia, or adult trauma. Every subject in both child trauma groups initially lacked a narrative, compared to 78% of subjects with adult traumas. At the time of the study, every subject with adult trauma or continuous memories for childhood trauma had a narrative, versus 83% of those who had experienced amnesia for childhood traumas. In addition, all subjects with childhood trauma had experienced sexual or physical abuse, while some of the adult trauma group had experienced accidents rather than assaults. Still, the majority of subjects in all three groups of this second study reported that they initially experienced their memories as sensations and affects.

Taken together, these findings from the first three TMI studies suggest that future research should determine whether the absence of narrative in a traumatic memory is independently affected by (a) whether or not the trauma involved interpersonal violence, and (b) whether it occurred in childhood or adulthood.

Sensory and affective modalities of traumatic memory. In contrast to our prior TMI research, in the present study we found no changes in sensory and affective memory modalities over time. Interestingly, we did not find differences in these memory components between subjects with PTSD and non-PTSD at any stage of remembering. These results are inconsistent with over 100 years of clinical observation and the findings of our two previous TMI studies. One possible explanation is the small sample size and the fact that half of the sample did not have PTSD. Most likely, this discrepancy is a function of a limitation of the original TMI: it assesses whether sensory and affective memory components were present or absent, but not how intensely these intrusions were experienced. For example, a subject who initially remembered, "hearing the surgeon's voice as if he were in the room with me," might currently report having "a sense of hearing his voice again." However, both were scored as a "yes" on auditory re-living.

Clearly there is a need to develop laboratory methods that can capture the potential complexity of the changes in traumatic memories over time. We believe that a standardized method of evoking memories, when combined with an instrument that rates the relative intensity of memory components, allows more precise assessment of the nature of traumatic intrusions. We discuss the development of such a method in a companion paper (Hopper & van der Kolk, 2001, this volume). The approach detailed there allows us to capture, both qualitatively and quantitatively, changes in traumatic remembrance due to effective treatment or the passage of time, and to correlate these changes with alterations in brain activation and physiological activity.

GENERAL DISCUSSION

The nature of traumatic memories has preoccupied psychiatrists since the very beginnings of their discipline. Over a hundred years ago the French psychiatrist Pierre Janet (1889) proposed that when people experience "vehement emotions" their minds may become incapable of matching their frightening experiences with their existing cognitive schemes. As a result, he proposed, the memories of the experience cannot be integrated into personal awareness. Instead, they were split off (dissociated) from conscious awareness and from voluntary control. Thus, the first comprehensive formulation of the effects of trauma on the mind was based on the notion that failure to integrate traumatic memories due to extreme emotional arousal results in the symptoms of what we call PTSD today. Janet stated, "they are unable to make the recital which we call narrative memory, and yet they remain confronted by [the] difficult situation" (1919/1925, p. 661). This results in "a phobia of memory" (1919/1925, p. 661) that prevents the integration ("synthesis") of traumatic events and splits these traumatic memories off from ordinary consciousness (1898, p. 145). As a result, Janet claimed, the memory traces of the trauma linger as terrifying perceptions, obsessional preoccupations and somatic reexperiences such as anxiety reactions, and cannot be "liquidated" as long as they have not been translated into a personal narrative (Janet, 1889, 1930).

Around this time as well, Breuer and Freud wrote their 1893 monograph, "On the nature of hysterical phenomena," worth quoting at length:

Hysterics suffer mainly from reminiscences.

At first sight it seems extraordinary that events experienced so long ago should continue to operate so intensely–that their recollection should not be liable to the wearing away process to which, after all, we see all our memories succumb. The following considerations may perhaps make this a little more intelligible.

The fading of a memory or the losing of its affect depends on various factors. The most important of these is *whether there has been an energetic reaction to the event that provokes an affect.* By "reaction" we understand the whole class of voluntary and involuntary reflexes . . . in which . . . the affects are discharged. If this reaction takes place to a sufficient amount a large part of the affect disappears as a result. . . .

"Abreaction," however, is not the only method of dealing with the situation that is open to a normal person who has experienced a psychical trauma. A memory of such a trauma, even if it has not been abreacted, enters the great complex of associations, it comes alongside other experiences, which may contradict it, and is subjected to rectification by other ideas. . . . In this way a normal person is able to bring about the disappearance of the accompanying affect through the process of association.

We must, however, mention another remarkable fact,. . . namely, that these memories, unlike the memories of their lives, are not at the patients' disposal. On the contrary, *these experiences are completely absent from the patient's memory when they are in a normal psychical state, or are only present in a highly summary form.* . . .

It may therefore be said that the ideas which have become pathological have persisted with such freshness and affective strength because they have been denied the normal wearing-away processes by means of abreaction and reproduction in states of uninhibited association (1893, pp. 7-11, italics in original).

Every contemporary study of traumatic memories has essentially corroborated Janet's and Freud's initial observations that traumatic memories persist primarily as implicit, behavioral and somatic memories, and only secondarily as vague, overgeneral, fragmented, incomplete, and disorganized narratives. Previous work by Foa (1995) and our case studies (Hopper & van der Kolk,

2001, this volume) suggest that these memories change as people recover from their PTSD.

The critical issue in studying traumatic memories, then, is to harmonize clinicians' observations and clinician-scientists' investigations with the exploding knowledge about the psychology and psychobiology of post-traumatic stress. For some time, the investigation of traumatic memory seems to have taken a detour by focusing on the issue of the "repression" or "dissociation" of traumatic memories. However, methods for assessing past amnesia for traumatic events are easier to develop than those for measuring the complexity of traumatic memory–what happens to the encoding and retrieval of memories related to overwhelming emotional experiences.

There is a need to develop new methodologies, which cannot consist of exposure to laboratory-generated stressful stimuli, but must be grounded in subjects' actual traumatic experiences. The field of PTSD has already developed standardized methods of memory evocation (e.g., individualized scripts) and structured interviews designed to assess traumatic memory characteristics (e.g., the TMI). Two other design features hold the key to valid and reliable research on the nature of traumatic memories. The first is prospective assessment of memories and changes in them over time. The second is to conduct such assessments in controlled outcome studies of treatments capable of transforming traumatic memories into relatively normal memories. Our laboratory has begun to conduct research incorporating all four of these methods (Hopper & van der Kolk, 2001, this volume).

It is also necessary to correlate the nature of retrieved memories with reliable and valid measures of PTSD and dissociative symptomatology. Finally, researchers need to correlate the mental phenomena of traumatic remembrances with biological parameters. The latter include measures of regional brain activation (e.g., functional Magnetic Resonance Imaging [fMRI], electroencephalogram [EEG], and magnetoencephalogram [MEG]), and peripheral physiological responses (e.g., heart rate, heart rate variability, skin conductance, blood pressure, and muscular activity).

Memories of traumatic experiences may not be primarily retrieved as narratives. Our own and others' research has suggested that PTSD traumatized people's difficulties with putting memories into words are reflected in actual changes in brain activity. In our PET neuroimaging study (Rauch et al., 1996), during exposure to traumatic reminders we found marked lateralization with increased activation in the right hemisphere (thought to be dominant for evaluating the emotional significance of incoming information and regulating the autonomic and hormonal responses to that information). In contrast, Broca's area (in the left inferior frontal cortex) had a simultaneous significant decrease in oxygen utilization, a finding replicated in two subsequent PET studies (Shin et al., 1997; Shin et al., 1999). This could signify that, during activation of a traumatic memory, the brain is "having" its experience: the person may feel, see, or hear the sensory elements of the traumatic experience, but he or she may be physiologically impaired from being able to translate this experience into communicable language. When they are "having" their traumatic recall, victims may suffer from "speechless terror" in which they may be literally "out of touch with their feelings." Their bodies may respond as if they are being traumatized again, with the secretions of the various neurohormones that are mobilized on those occasions, but the retrieval of the memory is dissociated, and the victim does not seem to be able to "own" what is happening.

How can we understand these findings? We previously have proposed the following understanding of these phenomena from a neurobiological information processing point of view (van der Kolk et al., 1996). When the brain processes incoming information, sensory input enters the CNS via the sensory organs. After initial processing by the thalamus, sensory information is evaluated for its existential relevance both by the amygdala and the prefrontal cortex. It has been well established that the amygdala attaches emotional significance to sensory input. The information evaluated by the amygdala is then passed on to areas in the brainstem that control behavioral autonomic and neurohormonal response systems. By way of these connections, the amygdala transforms sensory stimuli into emotional and hormonal signals, thereby initiating emotional responses (LeDoux, 1992).

LeDoux (1992) proposes that, since input from the thalamus arrives at the amygdala before information from the neocortex, this earlier arrived sensory input from the thalamus "prepares" the amygdala to process the later arriving information from the cortex. Thus, the emotional evaluation of sensory input precedes conscious emotional experience: people may become autonomically and hormonally activated before having been able to make a conscious appraisal of what they are reacting to. Thus, a high degree of activation of the amygdala and related structures can generate emotional responses and sensory impressions that are based on fragments of information, rather than full-blown perceptions of objects and events.

After the amygdala assigns emotional significance to sensory input, other brain structures further evaluate the meaning of this information. This includes the hippocampus, whose task it is to begin organizing and categorizing this information with previously existing information about similar sensory input. The strength of the hippocampal activation is affected by the intensity of input from the amygdala: the more significance assigned by the amygdala, the stronger the input will be attended to, and the better the memory will be retained. However, this interaction has an inverted U-shaped function: in animals, high levels of stimulation of the amygdala interfere with hippocampal functioning (Adamec, 1991; Squire & Zola-Morgan, 1991). This means that very high levels of emotional arousal may significantly disrupt the proper evaluation and categorization of experience by interfering with hippocampal function. We have hypothesized (van der Kolk, 1994) that, when this occurs, sensory imprints of experience are stored in memory, but because the hippocampus is impaired in its integrative function, these various imprints are incompletely unified into a whole. The experience may be laid down, and later retrieved, largely or primarily as isolated images, bodily sensations, smells and sounds that feel alien, and separate from other life experiences. Because the hippocampus was impaired in its usual role in helping to localize the incoming information in time and space, these fragments continue to lead an isolated existence. This would render traumatic memories timeless, and ego-alien.

CONCLUSIONS

Incoming sensory input ordinarily is analyzed and automatically synthesized into the large store of pre-existing information. When sensory input is personally significant these sensations may be transcribed into a personal narrative, without the subject having conscious awareness of the processes that translate sensory impressions into a personal story. Our research as shown that, in contrast with the way people seem to process ordinary information, traumatic experiences are often initially imprinted as sensations or feeling states, and are not collated and transcribed into personal narratives. Both our interviews with traumatized people, and brain imaging studies of them, seem to confirm that traumatic memories come back as emotional and sensory states, with limited capacity for verbal representation. We have proposed that this failure to process information on a symbolic level, which is essential for proper categorization and integration with other experiences, is at the very core of the pathology of PTSD.

The irony is that, while the sensory perceptions reported in PTSD may well reflect the actual imprints of sensations that were recorded at the time of the trauma, all narratives that weave sensory imprints into a socially communicable story are subject to condensation, embellishment and contamination. While trauma may leave an indelible imprint, once people start talking about these sensations, and try to make meaning of them, it is transcribed into ordinary memory, and, like all ordinary memory, it is prone to become distorted. People seem to be unable to accept experiences that have no meaning: they will try to make sense of what they are feeling. Once people become conscious of intrusive elements of the trauma, they are liable to try to fill in the blanks, and complete the picture.

Like all stories that people construct, our autobiographies contain elements of truth, of things that we wish did happen, but that did not, and elements that are meant to please the audience. The stories that people tell about their traumas are as vulnerable to distortion as people's stories about anything else. However, the question of whether the brain is able to take pictures, and whether some smells, images, sounds, or physical sensations may be etched onto the mind, and remain unaltered by subsequent experience and by the passage of time, still remains to be answered.

REFERENCES

Adamec, R. E. (1991). Partial kindling of the ventral hippocampus: Identification of changes in limbic physiology which accompany changes in feline aggression and defense. *Physiology and Behavior, 49*, 443-453.

American Psychiatric Association. (1994). *Diagnostic and statistical manual of mental disorders* (4th ed.). Washington, DC: Author.

Blake, D. D., Weathers, F. W., Nagy, L. M., Kaloupek, D. G., Gusman, F. D., Charney D. S., & Keane, T. M. (1995). The development of a Clinician-Administered PTSD Scale. *Journal of Traumatic Stress, 8*, 75-90.

Breuer, J., & Freud, S. (1893). On the psychical mechanism of hysterical phenomena: Preliminary communication. In J. Strachy (Ed. and Trans.) *The standard edition of the complete psychological works of Sigmund Freud* (Vol. 2.) (pp. 3-17). London: Hogarth Press.

Briere, J., & Conte, J. (1993). Self-reported amnesia for abuse in adults molested as children. *Journal of Traumatic Stress, 6*, 21-31.

Brown, R., & Kulik, J. (1977). Flashbulb memories. *Cognition, 5*, 73-99.

Brown, D., Scheflin, A. W., & Hammond, C. (1998). *Memory, trauma treatment, and the law.* New York: Norton.

Burgess, A. W., Hartman, C. R. & Baker, T. (1995). Memory presentations of childhood sexual abuse. *Journal of Psychosocial Nursing, 33*, 9-16.

Cameron, A. (1996). Comparing amnesic and nonamnesic survivors of childhood sexual abuse: A longitudinal study. In. K. Pezdek & W. P. Banks (Eds.), *The Recovered Memory/False Memory Debate*, pp. 41-68. New York: Academic Press.

Christianson, S. A. (1992a). Emotional stress and eyewitness memory: A critical review. *Psychological Bulletin, 112*, 284-309.

Christianson, S. A. (1992b). Remembering emotional events: Potential mechanisms. In S. A. Christianson (Ed.), *Handbook of emotion and memory: Research and theory* (pp.307-340). Hillsdale, NJ: Erlbaum.

Elliott, D. M. (1997). Traumatic events: Prevalence and delayed recall in the general population. *Journal of Consulting and Clinical Psychology, 65*, 811-820.

Feldman-Summers, S., & Pope, K. S. (1994). The experience of "forgetting" childhood abuse: A national survey of psychologists. *Journal of Consulting and Clinical Psychology, 62*, 636-639.

Foa, E. B., Molnar, C., & Cashman, L. (1995). Change in rape narratives during exposure therapy for posttraumatic stress disorder. *Journal of Traumatic Stress, 8*, 675-690.

Freyd, J. J. (1991, August 21-22). Memory repression, dissociative states, and other cognitive control processes involved in adult sequelae of childhood trauma. Invited paper given at the Second Annual Conference on A Psychodynamics-Cognitive Science Interface, Langley Porter Psychiatric Institute, University of California, San Francisco.

Freyd, J. J. (1994). Betrayal trauma: Traumatic amnesia as an adaptive response to childhood abuse. *Ethics & Behavior, 4*, 307-329.

Freyd, J. J. (1996). *Betrayal trauma: The logic of forgetting childhood abuse.* Cambridge: Harvard University Press.

Harvey, A. G., Bryant R. A., & Dang, S. T. (1998). Autobiographical memory in acute stress disorder. *Journal of Consulting and Clinical Psychology, 66*, 500-506.

Hopper, J. W., & van der Kolk, B. A. (2000). Retrieving, assessing, and classifying traumatic memories: A preliminary report on three case studies of a new standardized method. *Journal of Aggression, Maltreatment & Trauma.*

Janet, P. (1889). *L'Automatisme psychologique* [Psychological automatisms]. Paris: Félix Alcan.

Janet, P. (1898). *Névroses et idées fixes* [Neuroses and fixed ideas] (Vols. 1 & 2). Paris: Félix Alcan.

Janet, P. (1911). *L'état mental des hysteriques* [The mental state of hysterics] (2nd ed.). Paris: Félix Alcan.

Janet, P. (1919/1925). *Psychological healing* (Vols. 1 & 2). New York: MacMillan. (Original book, *Les médications psychologiques,* published in 1919).

Janet, P. (1930). Autobiography. In C.A. Murchinson (Ed.), *A history of psychology in autobiography, vol 1.* Worcester, MA: Clark University.

Kihlstrom, J. F. (1995). The trauma-memory argument. *Consciousness & Cognition, 4*, 63-7.

Koss, M. P., Figueredo, A. J., Bell, I., Tharan, M., & Tromp, S. (1996). Traumatic memory characteristics: A cross-validated mediational model of response to rape among employed women. *Journal of Abnormal Psychology, 105*, 421-432.

Koss, M. P., Tromp, S., Figueredo, A. J., Bell, I., & Tharan, M. (1995). Are rape memories different? A comparison of rape, other unpleasant, and pleasant memories among employed women. *Journal of Traumatic Stress, 8*, 607-627.

Lang, P. J., Levin, D. N., Miller, G. A., & Kozac, M. J. (1983). Fear behavior, fear imagery, and the psychophysiology of emotion: The problem of affective-response integration. *Journal of Abnormal Psychology, 92*, 275-306.

LeDoux, J. E. (1992). Brain mechanisms of emotion and emotional learning. *Current Opinion in Neurobiology, 2*, 191-197.

LeDoux, J. (1996). *The Emotional Brain.* New York: Simon and Schuster.

Loftus, E. F. (1975). Leading questions and the eyewitness report. *Cognitive Psychology, 7*, 560-572.

Loftus, E. F. (1979). *Eyewitness testimony.* Cambridge, MA: Harvard University Press.

Loftus, E. F. (1993). The reality of repressed memories. *American Psychologist, 48*, 518-537.

Loftus, E. F., & Ketcham, K. (1994). *The myth of repressed memory: False memories and allegations of sexual abuse.* New York: St. Martin's Press.

Loftus, E. F., Loftus, G. R., & Messo, J. (1987). Some facts about "weapon focus." *Law and Human Behavior, 11*, 55-62.

McFarlane, A.C., Weber, D. L., & Clark, C. R. (1993). Abnormal stimulus processing in posttraumatic stress disorder. *Biological Psychiatry, 34,* 311-320.

Mechanic, M. B., Resick, P. A., & Griffin, M. G. (1998). A comparison of normal forgetting, psychopathology, and information-processing models of reported amnesia for recent sexual trauma. *Journal of Consulting and Clinical Psychology, 66,* 948-957.

Morton, J. (1994). Cognitive perspectives on memory recovery. *Applied Cognitive Psychology, 8,* 389-398.

Myers, C. S. (1915). A contribution to the study of shell-shock. *Lancet, 185,* 316-320.

Pitman, R. K., Orr, S. P., Forgue, D. F., de Jong, J., & Claiborn, J. M. (1987). Psychophysiologic assessment of posttraumatic stress disorder imagery in Vietnam combat veterans. *Archives of General Psychiatry, 44,* 970- 975.

Ranta, S. O., Laurila R., Saario J., Ali-Melkkilä, T., & Hynynen, M. (1998). Awareness with recall during general anesthesia: Incidence and risk factors. *Anesthesia and Analgesia, 86,* 1084-1089.

Rauch, S., van der Kolk, B. A., Fisler, R., Alpert, N., Orr, S., Savage, C., Jenike, M., & Pitman, R. (1996). A symptom provocation study of posttraumatic stress disorder using positron emission tomography and script-driven imagery. *Archives of General Psychiatry, 53,* 380-387.

Roe, C. M., & Schwartz, M. (1996). Characteristics of previously forgotten memories of sexual abuse: A descriptive study. *Journal of Psychiatry and Law, 24,* 189-206.

Sargant, W., & Slater, E. (1941). Amnesic syndromes in war. *Proceedings of the Royal Society of Medicine,* 34, 757-764.

Schooler, J. W. (1994). Seeking the core: The issues and evidence surrounding recovered accounts of sexual trauma. *Consciousness and Cognition, 3,* 452-469.

Schwender D., Kunze-Kronawitter H., Dietrich P., Klasing S., Frost H., & Madler C. (1998). Conscious awareness during general anaesthesia: Patients' perceptions, emotions, cognition and reactions. *British Journal of Anaesthesia, 80,* 133-139.

Shin, L. M., Kosslyn S. M., McNally, R. J., Alpert N. M., Thompson, W. L., Rauch S. L., Macklin, M. L., & Pitman, R. K. (1997). Visual imagery and perception in posttraumatic stress disorder. A positron emission tomographic investigation. *Archives of General Psychiatry, 54,* 233-241.

Shin, L. M., McNally, R. J., Kosslyn, S. M., Thompson, W. L., Rauch, S. L., Alpert, N. M., Metzger, L. J., Lasko, N. B., Orr, S. P., & Pitman, R. K. (1999). Regional cerebral blood flow during script-driven imagery in childhood sexual abuse-related PTSD: A PET investigation. *American Journal of Psychiatry, 156,* 575-584.

Shobe, K. K., & Kihlstrom, J. (1997). Is traumatic memory special? *Current Directions in Psychological Science, 6,* 70-74.

Southard, E. E. (1919). *Shell-shock and other neuropsychiatric problems.* Boston: W.W. Leonard.

Spitzer, R. L., Williams, J. B. W., & Gibbon, M. (1987). *Structured Clinical Interview for DSM-III-R.* New York: New York State Psychiatric Institute, Biometrics Research Department.

Squire, L. R., & Zola-Morgan, S. (1991). The medial temporal lobe memory system. *Science, 153,* 2380-2386.

van der Kolk, B. A. (1987). *Psychological trauma*. Washington, DC: American Psychiatric Press.

van der Kolk, B. A. (1994). The body keeps the score: Memory and the emerging psychobiology of posttraumatic stress. *Harvard Review of Psychiatry, 1*, 253-265.

van der Kolk, B. A., McFarlane, A. C., & Weisaeth, L. (1996). *Traumatic Stress: The effects of overwhelming experience on mind, body and society*. New York: Guilford Press.

van der Kolk, B. A., Burbridge, J. A., & Suzuki, J. (1997). The psychobiology of traumatic memory: Clinical implications of neuroimaging studies. In R. Yehuda & A. C. McFarlane (Eds.), *Annals of the New York Academy of Sciences (Vol. 821): Psychobiology of Posttraumatic Stress Disorder* (pp. 99-113). New York: New York Academy of Sciences.

van der Kolk, B. A., & Fisler, R. (1995). Dissociation and the fragmentary nature of traumatic memories: Overview and exploratory study. *Journal of Traumatic Stress, 8*, 505-536.

Williams, L. M. (1994). Recall of childhood trauma: A prospective study of women's memories of child sexual abuse. *Journal of Consulting and Clinical Psychology, 62*, 1167-1176.

Williams, L. M. (1995). Recovered memories of abuse in women with documented child sexual victimization histories. *Journal of Traumatic Stress, 8*, 649-673.

Yuille, J. C., & Cutshall, J. L. (1986). A case study of eyewitness memory of a crime. *Journal of Applied Psychology, 71*, 291-301.

Retrieving, Assessing, and Classifying Traumatic Memories: A Preliminary Report on Three Case Studies of a New Standardized Method

James W. Hopper
Bessel A. van der Kolk

SUMMARY. The study of traumatic memories is still an emerging field, both methodologically and theoretically. Previous questionnaire and interview methods for studying traumatic memories have been limited in their ability to evoke and assess remembrances with the characteristics long observed by clinicians. In this article, we introduce a new standardized method that incorporates a laboratory procedure for retrieving memories of traumatic events and a clinically informed measure for assessing these memories' characteristics. We present three case studies to demonstrate the data yielded by script-driven remembering and the Traumatic Memory Inventory–Post-Script Version (TMI-PS). We then discuss subjects' script-driven remembrances in terms of methodology, theoretical classification of traumatic memories, and the inter-

---

The authors would like to thank Joseph Spinazzola and Toni Luxenberg for their helpful comments on drafts of this manuscript, and Martine Hueting for her valuable contribution to the design of the TMI-PS.

Address correspondence to: James W. Hopper, PhD, Research Associate, The Trauma Center, 227 Babcock Street, Brookline, MA 02446 (E-mail: jhopper@trauma center.org).

[Haworth co-indexing entry note]: "Retrieving, Assessing, and Classifying Traumatic Memories: A Preliminary Report on Three Case Studies of a New Standardized Method." Hopper, James W., and Bessel A. van der Kolk. Co-published simultaneously in *Journal of Aggression, Maltreatment & Trauma* (The Haworth Maltreatment & Trauma Press, an imprint of The Haworth Press, Inc.) Vol. 4, No. 2 (#8) 2001, pp. 33-71; and: *Trauma and Cognitive Science: A Meeting of Minds, Science, and Human Experience* (ed: Jennifer J. Freyd, and Anne P. DePrince) The Haworth Maltreatment & Trauma Press, an imprint of The Haworth Press, Inc., 2001, pp. 33-71. Single or multiple copies of this article are available for a fee from The Haworth Document Delivery Service [1-800-342-9678, 9:00 a.m. - 5:00 p.m. (EST). E-mail address: getinfo@haworthpressinc.com].

33

play between the two. Finally, we critique our method in detail and offer suggestions for future research. If validated as a method for evoking and assessing traumatic memories, and shown to yield reliable data, this integrative method shows great promise for advancing both clinical and cognitive research on traumatic memories. *[Article copies available for a fee from The Haworth Document Delivery Service: 1-800-342-9678. E-mail address: <getinfo@haworthpressinc.com> Website: <http://www.HaworthPress. com>   © 2001 by The Haworth Press, Inc. All rights reserved.]*

KEYWORDS. Traumatic memories, autobiographical memory, post-traumatic stress disorder, research methodology

In recent years, much of the research on traumatic memories has focused on recovered memories, true or false, and much of the theory on speculations about encoding and storage processes responsible for amnesia and delayed recall. This state of affairs has largely been a function of social and cultural factors. Scientifically speaking, however, the cart may have been put before the horse. That is, even though research on episodic traumatic memories is dependent on subjects' reports of memories they have just retrieved, research has shed little light on the processes and contents of memory retrieval in traumatized individuals. In this article, we present a new method for evoking traumatic memories and assessing some of their basic characteristics. Our method brings together a laboratory procedure for standardized retrieval of memories, and a semi-structured interview for assessing memory characteristics based on well-established observations by clinicians dealing with traumatized patients. We offer this easily adapted approach to promote controlled research on the characteristics of traumatic memories, particularly prospective studies of their transformations over time.

Endel Tulving's (1972) classic chapter on episodic and semantic memory begins, "One of the unmistakable signs of an immature science is the looseness of definition and use of its major concepts" (p. 381). This certainly appears to be the case today for the scientific study of traumatic memories. Use of the unitary construct of "traumatic memory" is common, though clinical experience and recent empirical and theoretical work suggest that memories for traumatic experiences are complex and heterogeneous phenomena, which change over time in a variety of ways. At this early stage, it might be more helpful to use the super-ordinate and plural construct of "traumatic memories" and methodically build a definitional taxonomy–just as traditional memory researchers have done since Tulving's incisive statement nearly 30 years ago.

A primary goal of this article is to demonstrate that progress toward an empirically derived taxonomy of traumatic memories will be advanced by more attention to the following: (1) memory retrieval or evocation methods, and (2) instruments for assessing memory characteristics. We also aim to show that the former must draw more from laboratory research, and the latter from clinical experience and understanding–otherwise a shift in emphasis from encoding and storage to the processes and contents of retrieval cannot realize its potential. We believe such changes in shared theoretical and methodological frameworks can foster the understanding, communication and collaboration needed to advance the field.[1]

Pierre Janet (1889, 1919/1925) was the first clinician to clearly articulate differences between ordinary and traumatic memories. He described memories that were inaccessible to retrieval under ordinary conditions and beyond conscious control. The memories of his patients, he noted, consisted of sensory experiences, emotional states, intrusive recollections, and behavioral reenactments (Janet, 1889, 1919/1925; van der Kolk & van der Hart, 1989, 1991). Janet wrote of memory fragments that were remembered with particular vividness, yet resisted integration into existing mental structures, leaving the person "incapable of making the necessary narrative which we call memory regarding the event. . ." (1919/1925, p. 663). It is important to note, however, that Janet's lucid descriptions were limited to the kinds of traumatic memories he could observe in his severely traumatized patients.

In the literature review that follows, we begin by examining the work of three research groups that have investigated the characteristics of traumatic memories in some depth. Next we outline a recent theory of posttraumatic stress disorder which offers a framework for classifying traumatic memories and points to a critical limitation of current methods for assessing those memories' characteristics. We then recount our discovery of a procedure that overcomes this limitation through standardized evocation and assessment of traumatic memories, particularly their somatosensory and affective characteristics.

PRIOR METHODS FOR RETRIEVING
AND ASSESSING CHARACTERISTICS
OF TRAUMATIC MEMORIES

To date, few researchers have studied in depth the characteristics that, according to clinicians, distinguish many traumatic memories from non-traumatic memories. Fewer still have investigated the characteristics of memories for traumatic events in non-clinical samples. During the last decade three research groups have attempted to capture the nature of traumatic memories by investigating qualities such as intensity and vividness of somatosensory and affective components, fragmentation and disorganization, and the ability to share memories as coherent narratives. Table 1 provides an overview of their studies, and Table 2 details how they have assessed traumatic memory characteristics. The following brief review is not focused on study results, but on some strengths and limitations of these investigators' methods for retrieving traumatic memories and assessing their characteristics.

Two studies by Koss, Tromp and colleagues (Koss et al., 1996; Tromp et al., 1995) compared characteristics of rape memories and memories for other unpleasant events. Both studies were conducted on the same two samples of respondents to surveys mailed to all female employees of a medical center (N = 1,047) and all female employees of a university (N = 2,142). Such large non-clinical samples offered these researchers the possibility of discovering characteristics of traumatic memories that have not been observed in clinical populations. The other major strength of this work was the use of a detailed measure for assessing memory characteristics (see Table 2). It consisted of 23 items, most taken from a measure proven useful for differentiating real from imagined memories (Suengas & Johnson, 1988), and six items relating to flashbulb memory qualities. Each item was rated on a 1 to 7 scale, which makes for greater sensitivity (than dichotomous or categorical scoring) to gradations of difference between types of memories. Continuous scoring also permitted factor analyses, and four distinct but correlated factors were confirmed: Clarity, Affect, Reexperiencing, and Nonvisual Sensory.

The major limitation of these studies concerns the conditions for retrieval of memories. Subjects first read a series of detailed behavioral descriptions of

TABLE 1. Overview of In-Depth Studies of Traumatic Memory Characteristics

Research Group and Study	Type of Event	Method of Cueing	Memories Assessed
Tromp, Koss et al. (1995)	rape	questionnaire	current memory of event
Koss, Tromp et al. (1996)	rape	questionnaire	current memory of event
Reynolds & Brewin (1998)	various stressful and traumatic	interview	current most disturbing intrusion
			initial most disturbing intrusion (cognitions as well as memories)
Reynolds & Brewin (1999)	various stressful and traumatic	interview	current two most disturbing intrusive memories
van der Kolk & Fisler (1995)	various adult and childhood traumas	interview	current memory of event most distressing memory of event initial memory of the event
van der Kolk et al. (1997)	same as above	interview	same as above
van der Kolk et al. (2000)	awareness under general anesthesia	interview	same as above

TABLE 2. Memory Characteristics Assessed and Types of Variables Used in In-Depth Studies

Characteristics	Research group, measure used, and coding of variables		
	van der Kolk et al. Traumatic Memory Inventory Memories Interview	Tromp, Koss et al. Memory Characteristics	Reynolds & Brewin Life Events and Questionnaire (adapted)
Visual memory	dichotomous		
Affective/emotional memory		dichotomous	
Auditory/sound memory	dichotomous	continuous	
Bodily memory	[incl. in "tactile"]		
Tactile/touch memory	dichotomous	continuous	
Taste memory		continuous	
Olfactory/smell memory	dichotomous	continuous	
Components together	dichotomous		
Able to tell coherent story	dichotomous		
Order of events		continuous	
Feelings at time		continuous	free recall
Feelings now		continuous	free recall
Affect intensity then		continuous	
Reexperiencing physical	[incl. in "tactile"]	continuous	
Reexperiencing feelings	[incl. in "affective"]	continuous	
Memory clarity		continuous	
Visual detail		continuous	
Color/BW memory		continuous	
Vividness of memory		continuous	
Affect intensity now		continuous	
Unexpectedness		continuous	
Consequences, valence		continuous	
Thoughts about since		continuous	
Overall memory		continuous	
Talked about since		continuous	
How long memory lasted			graded categorical (5 levels)
Frequency of memory			graded categorical (2 levels)
Clarity and vividness			graded categorical (3 levels)
Strong physical sensations			dichotomous
Feeling of reliving			dichotomous
How distressing			continuous
Specific associated emotions			free recall
Accompanied by out-of-body experience			dichotomous

possible experiences of attempted and completed rape, and indicated if they had experienced any of them. For subjects victimized in this way, that section of the survey constituted a cued recall intervention. In contrast, respondents who did not report sexual victimization were simply asked to pick another significant memory–i.e., to engage in free recall–then to rate its emotional valence as pleasant or unpleasant, and to respond to the same memory items as the victimized subjects. These different recall strategies may have fostered better retrieval of rape memories than other pleasant or unpleasant ones (Tulving, 1976), and in turn may have biased their comparative data on memory characteristics. Researchers using questionnaire or interview measures to assess and compare traumatic memories and non-traumatic memories need to be alert to this potential problem, and whenever possible to control for recall strategy across types of memories. The other limitation related to conditions of retrieval is that subjects were asked to rate characteristics of their memory as called up and experienced while filling out the questionnaire. A remembrance cued via survey questions is not likely to be representative of some traumatic memories, i.e., flashbacks and other reexperiencing phenomena associated with posttraumatic stress disorder. To summarize, behaviorally descriptive recall cues for the rape memories would be expected to enhance their retrieval relative to unpleasant memories; and traumatic remembrances evoked by survey items should yield less retrieval of somatosensory and affective components than, for example, a method capable of evoking a flashback. Both features are likely to shape these researchers' findings.

The most important finding of the Tromp et al. (1995) study, that the Clarity factor best discriminated between rape and other unpleasant memories, was both against their prediction and in the opposite direction of the divergent recall biases for the two types of memories. That is, they reported that rape memories "were *less* clear and vivid, *less* likely to occur in a meaningful order, *less* well-remembered, *less* thought about and *less* talked about" (Tromp et al., 1995, p. 622, italics in original). These findings were unexpected. In the clinical literature, from Janet (1889, 1919/1925) to the present (e.g., van der Kolk & van der Hart, 1989, 1991), *more* clarity and vividness have tended to be associated with less meaningful ordering and incompleteness. However, this discrepancy could be partly an artifact of methodology and semantics. First, the items of the Clarity factor associated with these researchers' terms "clear" and "vivid" were phrased in terms of the memory *as a whole*, while the clinical literature has focused on the clarity and vividness of memory *fragments* in the *absence* of an overall clear and vivid memory. Second, questionnaire cueing would not be expected to evoke the types of remembrances described by clinicians. Tromp and colleagues (1995) interpreted their findings primarily in terms of avoidance coping. However, from a methodological perspective attentive to factors influencing memory retrieval, it may be that surveys in general, even when they involve numerous cues to recall, tend to *reveal, but not challenge* avoidant coping strategies that constrain the accessibility of traumatic memories–particularly distressing somatosensory and affective aspects. Indeed, this could be true of many interview measures as well.

Taking a different approach, Reynolds and Brewin developed (1998) and revised (1999) a structured interview to assess relationships among several phenomena: the type of event recalled, diagnosis of posttraumatic stress disorder (PTSD) versus major depression, and the contents and characteristics of intrusive memories (Table 2). In their second study, in contrast to the approach of Koss and colleagues (Koss et al., 1996; Tromp et al., 1995), Reynolds and Brewin (1999) had subjects identify actual intrusive memories they had experienced over the past week, then answer questions about each of the two most prominent ones. The memories retrieved with this method are more likely than survey-evoked ones to be flashbacks or other memories characterized by intense somatosensory and affective representations. In addition, their revised interview included a simple yet powerful feature: a free recall item that asked subjects to "name any emotions they associated with" their intrusive memory (Reynolds & Brewin, 1999, p. 206). Responses to this item revealed that memories associated with fear were not associated with sadness and vice versa. This finding suggests that assessing a memory's general "emotional intensity," without *also* assessing the presence and intensity of certain key emotions, may obscure important characteristics of traumatic memories and their transformations over time.

Our research group has always assumed that to document the characteristics that distinguish traumatic memories from non-traumatic memories, it would be necessary to show changes in memory characteristics over time. To that end, we developed a retrospective interview measure, the Traumatic Memory Inventory (TMI) (van der Kolk & Fisler, 1995; see Table 2). Subjects were asked about how they had remembered the trauma at three times: initially, peak (i.e., when it was most distressing), and at the time of the study. The idea was to investigate the characteristics of particular remembrances over the entire "life of the memory." The TMI's focus on assessing changes in the characteristics of traumatic memories over time is its greatest strength *and* weakness. In terms of the heterogeneity of traumatic memories, this constitutes a strength because, as clinicians know, traumatic memories may change over time, and they can be transformed into relatively normal memories, sometimes very slowly and at others quite rapidly (e.g., with effective treatment). Yet the biggest weakness of the TMI is the *extent* to which it asks subjects to look back over time. It requires subjects to *remember how they remembered up to years or decades in the past.* This sort of retrieval task increases the threats to validity and reliability already associated with retro-spective reports and their potentials for inaccuracy and distortion.

In the first two studies using the TMI (van der Kolk & Fisler, 1995; van der Kolk, Burbridge, & Suzuki, 1997), both conducted with subjects current-ly suffering from PTSD, the findings corresponded to classical clinical knowledge about the characteristics of traumatic memories. Many subjects reported that they initially had no narrative memory at all for the event. They could not tell a story about what had happened, regardless of whether they always knew that the trauma had happened, or whether they retrieved memo-ries of the trauma at a later date. Further, the TMI data suggested that all of these subjects initially "remembered" the trauma in the form of flashback experiences in a variety of modalities: visual, affective, auditory, olfactory and kinesthetic. At the same time, subjects reported that these modalities initially tended not to occur together. Finally, the TMI data suggested that as the traumatic memories came into consciousness with greater intensity, more sensory modalities were activated along with the affective component, and over time there emerged a capacity to tell others about what had happened in narrative form.

However, the most recent TMI study (van der Kolk, Hopper, & Osterman, this volume) failed to replicate some key findings of the earlier studies. In a sample of subjects who had experienced the trauma of awareness of surgery under general anesthesia, some with PTSD and some without, no differences were found between groups in the prevalence of sensory and affective memory modalities for reports over time, i.e., initial, peak, and current mem-ories. Nor were significant differences found between the memory character-istics of subjects with and without PTSD at any of the stages of remembering. We concluded that these negative findings stemmed, in part, from a limitation of the TMI: constrained by a dichotomous scoring system, it assessed only whether sensory and affective memory components were present or absent, not the *intensity* with which these components were experienced.

From this brief review, it is clear that these three research groups have already revealed–in their methods, their findings, and evidence of interplay between the two–several of the complexities of traumatic memories and attempts to study them. To make sense of such complexities, and to think clearly about the challenges to research methodology that they pose, we must draw on theory. Given this paper's primary concern with methods for retriev-ing and assessing characteristics of traumatic memories, the theoretical focus will be limited to the work of Brewin and his colleagues (Brewin, Dalgleish, & Joseph, 1996). Their theory is accessible to cognitive scientists, clinical re-searchers and clinicians; relevant to memory retrieval and assessment meth-odology; and contributes to the development of more refined definitions and classifications of traumatic memories.

DUAL REPRESENTATION THEORY:
MEMORY REPRESENTATION SYSTEMS
AND PROCESSING OUTCOMES

Brewin and colleagues (Brewin et al., 1996), in line with earlier descriptions (van der Kolk & van der Hart, 1991), formulated a "dual representation theory" of PTSD. They cite lines of well-established research in several areas of cognitive psychology, social psychology, clinical psychology, and neuropsychology which support the view that sensory input is subject to both conscious and nonconscious processing. They propose that two types of memory representations are the "minimum cognitive architecture" within which the complex memory and other phenomena of PTSD can be understood: verbally accessible memories and situationally accessible memories. By verbally accessible memories of trauma, Brewin and colleagues mean a set of representations of a person's conscious experience of the trauma, which consists of "a series of autobiographical memories that can be deliberately and progressively edited" (Brewin et al., 1996, p. 677). Situationally accessible memories, in contrast, are defined as a different set of representations that cannot be accessed deliberately, but may be accessed automatically when sufficient retrieval cues are present.[2]

The other major feature of Brewin and colleagues' (1996) theory consists of three proposed outcomes of the emotional processing of traumatic events: completed processing, chronic emotional processing, and premature inhibition of processing. They characterize completed processing or integration, well-described in clinical literature from Janet to the present, as "the ideal stage in which the memories of trauma have been fully processed, or worked through, and integrated with the person's other memories and sense of self in the world" (Brewin et al., 1996, p. 679). At this stage, a person may still experience situationally accessible somatosensory memories that are unexpected and distressing, but these will not be overwhelming or strongly avoided; rather, they can be placed within a network of organized and personally meaningful verbally accessible memories, and processed further if needed or desired. As Janet noted, "It is not enough to be aware of a memory that occurs automatically in response to particular current events; it is also necessary that the personal perception 'knows' this image and attaches it to other memories" (translation from Janet, 1898, p. 135).

The second outcome described by Brewin and colleagues (1996), chronic emotional processing, is when both verbally and situationally accessible memories of the trauma are chronically processed, and the person is preoccupied with the trauma and its consequences. Whether ruminating about a past trauma, flooded with intrusive memories, or consciously and deliberately restricting one's life to avoid such memories being triggered, one is preoccupied with the trauma. People in this stage have classic PTSD reexperiencing symptoms and/or avoidance symptoms, and are more likely to seek therapy or volunteer for researcher on PTSD.

The notion of prematurely inhibited processing of traumatic memories, that is, the *sustained and automatic* suppression of situationally accessible or intrusive fragmentary memories, is an uncommon one in the literature on psychological trauma. An exception is the work of Creamer and colleagues (Creamer, Burgess, & Pattison, 1990, 1992), who, like Brewin et al. (1996), describe this outcome as the result of long-sustained efforts to avoid both verbally and situationally accessible memories. But while Creamer et al. (1992) propose a general theory of posttraumatic outcomes based on this concept, Brewin and colleagues (1996) view prematurely inhibited processing as a particular outcome that can result from combinations of psychological and social factors. Creamer and colleagues' (1992) theory is largely based on their longitudinal study of office-shooting victims, a sample less likely than clinical ones to include subjects who chronically or completely process the trauma. Similarly, many of the rape victims whose memories were studied by Koss, Tromp and colleagues (Koss et al., 1996; Tromp et al., 1995) may have fit into this category. Indeed, Tromp et al. (1995) cited Creamer and colleagues' (1992) work in their discussion of avoidance coping as an explanation of their findings.

Brewin and colleagues' (1996) theory, with its two types of traumatic memory representations (situationally and verbally accessible) and three processing outcomes (premature inhibition, chronic and completed), can provide a preliminary framework for classifying traumatic memories. However, dual representation theory focuses on the two memory systems as corresponding to distinct types of remembrance (Brewin et al., 1996; Reynolds & Brewin, 1999, p. 204). In contrast, we focus on how these different types of representations can also be mixed together within particular remembrances, and this perspective informs our framework for describing traumatic memories and investigating their characteristics. That is, each processing outcome can be described in the following terms: (1) the nature of the relationship between the memory systems, and (2) how situationally and verbally accessible traumatic memories are experienced. The chronic processing outcome is characterized by (1) dominance of situationally accessible memory, or fluctuating dominance of situationally accessible memories and verbally accessible memories marked by intense secondary emotions like sadness, shame or anger, and (2) both forms of memory being experienced as distressing, and situationally accessible as very dangerous. In the case of premature inhibited processing, (1) verbally accessible memory is dominant and situationally accessible memory is suppressed, but more as one would control a violent prisoner who could some day attack with terrible consequences, and (2) neither form of traumatic memory is consciously experienced as dangerous. Finally, with completion/

integration, (1) verbally accessible memories are dominant, and situationally accessible memories arise seldom, only with strong cueing, and are easily coded into narrative memory, while (2) neither form of memory is experienced as dangerous, and verbally accessible memory is experienced as a vehicle for mastery. Not only processing *outcomes*, however, but every stage of memory processing should be the focus of research on characteristics of traumatic memories and their transformations over time. There is a great need for prospective research of this kind.

Many critical methodological issues stem from potential interactions among key factors: *sample type* (e.g., clinical vs. non-clinical), *traumatic event type* (e.g., single incident vs. chronic exposure, accident vs. interpersonal violence), *memory representation type* (verbally vs. situationally accessible), *memory retrieval method* (e.g., questionnaire vs. interview) and *instrument for assessing memory characteristics* (e.g., questionnaire vs. interview, probing primarily for verbally accessible vs. situationally accessible representations). For example, because "existing scales do not capture" the distinction between situationally and verbally accessible traumatic memories, Brewin and colleagues suggested "it may be profitable to examine the phenomenology of intrusive memories in more detail, with a view to developing more comprehensive data" (Brewin et al., 1996, p. 683).

HOW MEMORIES ARE RETRIEVED DETERMINES THE MEMORY CHARACTERISTICS AVAILABLE FOR ASSESSMENT

While we agree that new measures are needed to assess the characteristics of traumatic memories, the creation of better *scales*–whether questionnaires or interviews, however strong the psychometric properties–is insufficient. Our position is best summed up in two questions:

1. What kind of instruments enable valid and reliable assessment of the characteristics of both (a) verbally accessible and (b) situationally accessible somatosensory and affective traumatic memory representations?
2. Which retrieval-facilitation methods enable valid and reliable *evocation* of these two types of memory systems, particularly situationally accessible somatosensory and affective representations, so that they *can* be assessed with appropriate instruments?

One possible answer to the second question emerged from our Positron Emission Tomography (PET) study of PTSD (Rauch, van der Kolk et al., 1996), which we conducted in an attempt to elucidate neurobiological substrates of the traumatic memory characteristics we had previously investigated with the TMI (van der Kolk & Fisler, 1995). This neuroimaging study incorporated "script-driven imagery," a laboratory research method, to retrieve both traumatic and control neutral memories in an individualized yet standardized way. Script-driven imagery is a method pioneered in the field of psychophysiology by Lang and colleagues (e.g., Lang, Levin, Miller, & Kozac, 1983) and later applied to the psychophysiology of PTSD by Pitman, Orr and colleagues (e.g., Pitman, Orr, Forgue, de Jong, & Claiborn, 1987), who were co-investigators on the PET study. This study taught us that researchers can exert considerable control over the retrieval of traumatic memories, and that a standardized retrieval-facilitation method can provide an excellent opportunity to gather phenomenological data on the characteristics of memories. We realized that, when linked to such a method, the TMI or a similar instrument could be used to assess how subjects remembered their trauma *immediately after a controlled retrieval process*, which we saw as an advance over prior methods.

THREE CASE STUDIES USING A NEW METHOD FOR STANDARDIZED RETRIEVAL AND ASSESSMENT

We present three cases of subjects whose script-driven traumatic memories were assessed with an adapted version of the TMI, before and after treatment with Eye Movement Desensitization and Reprocessing (EMDR) (Shapiro, 1995), an intervention that fosters processing of traumatic memories. Our aim is to provide sufficient preliminary data for readers to evaluate whether this new method warrants further study.

Method

Design. Characteristics of traumatic memories were prospectively assessed by script-driven remembering and a brief structured interview, and compared for differences between pre- and post-treatment. Data on three cases were qualitatively analyzed. There were comparisons of responses to free-recall questions, and continuous indices of the intensity of somatosensory and affective memory components.

Participants. Three of 12 participants in a functional neuroimaging study of treatment outcome of PTSD were given the Traumatic Memory Inventory–Post-Script Version (TMI-PS) immediately after script-driven remembering, both before and after a course of three 90-minute sessions of EMDR treatment. Subjects were recruited via advertisements in newspapers and fliers posted in public spaces. As in previous research with the TMI (van der

Kolk & Fisler, 1995), the advertisements and fliers prominently featured descriptions of intrusive PTSD reexperiencing symptoms, and all subjects were men and women 18 years of age or older who met DSM-IV criteria for PTSD. All had continuously remembered the traumatic experiences for which memories were retrieved and assessed. Procedures were conducted at an outpatient psychiatric clinic specializing in the treatment of traumatized populations and at the nuclear medicine department of an academic hospital. Human subjects approval was obtained from both institutions where the study was performed, and written informed consent was obtained from all subjects. Exclusion criteria included scores over 35 on the Dissociative Experiences Scale, suicidal or self-mutilating behaviors in the past six months, and active substance abuse in the past six months (DSM-IV criteria).

Materials. Subjects were assessed by trained interviewers for PTSD diagnosis and severity of PTSD symptoms with the Clinician Administer PTSD Scale (CAPS; Blake et al., 1995), a structured interview which has been shown to yield reliable data and has been validated for the purpose of assessing PTSD symptoms and their severity. The CAPS was administered at the initial assessment, and immediately before and after treatment. Comorbidity of DSM-III-R Axis I disorders was assessed with the SCID-I for DSM-III-R (Spitzer, Williams, & Gibbon, 1987).

Procedure. Subjects completed all eight visits of the neuroimaging study. These visits included (1) initial assessment, (2) laboratory psychophysiology assessment, (3) pre-treatment SPECT scan of neutral memory, (4) pre-treatment assessment, including SPECT scan of script-driven remembering, (5-7) three EMDR sessions, and (8) post-treatment assessment, including a SPECT scan of script-driven remembering. Data reported below were gathered in the fourth and eighth visits, when SPECT scans were conducted to assess CNS correlates of script-driven remembrance of the trauma addressed in treatment.

Script-Driven Remembering. At visit 1 the subject and a research assistant composed an individualized script portraying the most traumatic experience the subject could recall, after the method of Lang's group (e.g., Lang et al., 1983), as adapted for PTSD psychophysiology research by Pitman, Orr, and colleagues (for details of the methodology, see Pitman et al., 1987, and Orr, Pitman, Lasko, & Herz, 1993). Subjects were asked to describe their target traumatic experience in writing on script preparation forms (for current version, see Appendix A). Each form has two pages. The first page has directions for writing a description that includes contextual information, sensations, bodily experiences, emotions, and cognitions. The second page consists of a "menu" of subjective visceral and muscular reactions (associated with physiological arousal), from which subjects select those they remembered having accompanied the experiences. The research assistant reviewed subjects' forms and asked them to clarify or expand on the details where necessary for script construction.

The research assistant then composed a written script of the traumatic experience, which portrayed the experiences in the second person and present tense. Scripts were written to maximize accessibility of episodic, situationally accessible memory representations. Each script began with information that set the context of time, place and situation. Then it narrated the event by incorporating, in the sequence specified by the subject, sensory, affective, cognitive and physiological details from the subject's description (including five visceral and muscular reactions, or as many as the subject selected, whichever was less). Each script, approximately 30 seconds in length when read aloud, was then narrated onto an audiotape for later playback.

The subject was seated in a comfortable chair in an examination room that did not include scanning equipment. After a baseline rest period, the subject listened to the taped script with eyes closed. The subject was instructed to "remember the experience as vividly as you can, in all of its details–all the sensations, feelings, etc.," while the tape played, and to continue remembering in this way until signaled to "relax" by a research assistant. In this study subjects received an intravenously administered injection of a radioactively labeled tracer immediately before the tape started, and had a script-driven remembering period of 3 minutes, including 2 1/2 minutes after the tape. (This long post-tape period may not be optimal, but was necessary because it takes nearly 3 minutes for 80% of the tracer to absorb into brain tissue.)

Administration of the Traumatic Memory Inventory–Post-Script Version. Immediately after a memory was evoked by the standardized script method, the TMI-PS was administered (for current version, see Appendix B). First, subjects were asked a free-recall question, "When you remembered the traumatic experience today, listening to the tape and/or during the imaging phase, how did you remember it?" Next, they were asked to report whether or not their experience included content in various modalities (visual, etc.), and if so, what they had experienced. At the level of the whole memory, these modality-specific inquiries constitute cued recall prompts; at the level of the memory modalities, they are free recall questions. In contrast to the original TMI, which only has subjects report the absence or specific content of each memory component, the TMI-PS followed up on these responses by having subjects go back and provide intensity/vividness ratings for each component. The interviewer said, "Now I'd like you to go back and rate the intensity of each aspect of the memory, with 0 being not at all present and 10 being as intense or vivid as the original event." This rating is intended to allow more valid and reliable determination of the extent to which contents of a particular memory modality were experienced as relived sensory or affective fragments versus less intense and vivid recollections (perhaps partly derived from a semantic memory schema). Subjects were next asked three questions related to fragmentation and narrative incoherence (see Appendix B). As a validity check on subjects' compliance with the task, and to probe for additional important but unexpected data, subjects were then asked, "Were you thinking about or remembering anything else while listening to the tape and/or during the imagining phase?" (Please note: The TMI-PS in Appendix B is a revision of this earlier version, with changes in the wording and ordering of some items; as discussed below, ethical considerations may also dictate modifications, e.g., removing free-recall questions if the data will not be analyzed).

Eye Movement Desensitization and Reprocessing. EMDR is a comprehensive treatment approach to PTSD (Shapiro, 1995) that involves exposing people to memories of their trauma (Chemtob, Tolin, van der Kolk, & Pitman, 2000). Patients rapidly move their eyes back and forth during exposure to their traumatic memories, including visual, affective and physiological components. "Desensitization and reprocessing" refers to reducing the distress associated with a traumatic memory and integrating it into autobiographical memory. A memory previously experienced as a traumatizing intrusion to be assiduously avoided should become, after successful EMDR, a less painful or even painless memory that one can remember without being overwhelmed, or choose to stop remembering without engaging in debilitating avoidance. Successful treatment should render a memory less intense and fragmented in its somatosensory and affective aspects, and more dominated by verbal narrative constructions. In short, successful and completed treatment is indicated by transformation of a traumatic memory into a more normal memory. Subjects received three EMDR sessions, which were expected to transform their memories to varying degrees partly dependent on the severity of their trauma histories and PTSD.

Results

Three cases are presented, each beginning with identifying information and CAPS scores indicating severity of PTSD symptoms before and after treatment (measured the same day memory characteristics were assessed). Then TMI-PS data are presented, in the following order: first, quotations from responses to the first, open-ended TMI-PS question about how the subject remembered; second, verbatim descriptions of the reported contents of memory components (no subject reported an olfactory memory component); third, a bar graph depicting intensity ratings for somatosensory and affective modalities. And finally, one subject's particularly illuminating responses to TMI-PS questions about whether (a) she experienced the components of the memory separately or together, and (b) she could "tell it to someone as a coherent story."

Subject 1 was a 50-year-old married man who worked as a computer programmer. He had experienced repeated sexual abuse by a 19 year old male babysitter over a period of 2 years. His script narrated an incident that occurred when he was 5 years old, the incident he found most upsetting and remembered most vividly. Subject 1 had a history of alcohol abuse from adolescence to age 38, and he continued to struggle with compulsive sexual behaviors, a source of intense shame. He had been in psychotherapy for 1 1/2 years before entering the study, and though he had discussed his traumatic experiences and their effects often in therapy, he had no prior experience with any exposure therapies, including EMDR. He had been on 60mg of fluoxetine (Prozac) since 3 1/2 months prior to entering the study. When entering the study he met criteria for Dysthymia and Obsessive Compulsive Disorder, though neither condition was severe. On the day of his pre-treatment memory assessment, his CAPS score was 54, indicating PTSD of mild to moderate severity, and at post-treatment it was 16, a sub-clinical level of symptomatology.

In his responses to the initial, open-ended TMI-PS question about his experience of the memory, this subject focused on his reactions to the memory.

> *Pre-treatment*: "Pretty much the way I always do, as far as the pictures. I didn't feel as intense or as involved as I normally do. . . . I think there was an undercurrent of knowledge where I was. But, I'm not sure. It was a very strange feeling for me to hear it being narrated. . . . In one respect I think it was almost lifting some burden, hearing it, but on the other hand I wanted to run away from hearing it. I felt like I wanted to escape. . . ."
>
> *Post-treatment*: "I remembered it as though it was a real memory, but it was a little distant, and more manageable. There wasn't the vividness I am used to having. And there wasn't the bright light–remember the bright light?. . . . I guess a clear way of putting that very simply is, I typically drown in it, and this time I was floating on top."
>
> ". . . .There's another thing that was very foreign to me in terms of this particular memory. I'm reluctant to say it: There was a certain *power* in calling up the memory. I didn't feel as helpless. Right now I'm feeling angry" (spoken emphasis).
>
> "I felt difficulty in connecting to it. I was remembering the emotions as opposed to experiencing the emotions. I didn't feel like it was happening all over again. That's probably where the power came from."

In response to specific probes about each potential sensory and affective modality, he only reported experiences of visual and affective components (intensity ratings are in parentheses):

Pre-treatment visual (8): "I swear there was a multi-colored comforter. I saw my baby-sitter next to me–same thing as I always see. I think what strikes me is that the room is incredibly bright."

Post-treatment visual (3): "No bright light. I saw the same snapshot I always see. It was subdued, darker. It was harder to connect with it in terms of getting emotionally involved with it. And it didn't feel as real as it used to."

Pre-treatment affective (8): "Embarrassed, frightened, helpless. Maybe disgust. Upset."

Post-treatment affective (1): "I felt sad. If I had to say there was one consistent emotion, it was sadness. I really didn't seem to get involved. It was pretty difficult for me to connect with it. But some anger. I am still feeling that. Intensifies and subsides."

Bar graph A of Figure 1 visually depicts differences between the subject's pre- and post-treatment remembrances, i.e., greater intensity ratings in the visual and affective modalities for the pre-treatment than the post-treatment remembrance.

Subject 2 was a 55-year-old single woman who worked as a childcare provider and had been collecting disability since 1994. She used the EMDR sessions to address the effects of a brutal rape by her ex-husband at age 33. She had experienced significant emotional abuse by both parents in childhood, and had a history of substance abuse (alcohol, amphetamines and marijuana) which began immediately after the rape and ended at age 39. Subject 2 had been in supportive therapy several times, and had seen her current therapist bi-weekly for 5 years. That therapy had focused sporadically on how the rape continued to affect her and how to manage related symptoms, but little progress had been made in terms of her intrusive symptoms and intense shame and self-hate. When entering the study she met criteria for Dysthymia and Past Major Depressive Episode, for which she had been taking 300 mg of bupropion (Wellbutrin) daily for 2 years. At pre-treatment her CAPS score was 64, and at post-treatment it had dropped to 30.

For this case, we include her traumatic script, which ends moments before her ex-husband initiates the rape, to illustrate this method:

It is October of 1976, and after coming home late you are taking a shower in the bathroom off the master bedroom. You have locked the door, but suddenly hear your husband smashing through it. You are seized with terror and your heart pounds as he breaks through the door, piece by piece. You are unable to escape and can only freeze. He pulls you from the shower, throws you on the floor, kicks you and drags you into the bedroom. Your body is shaking and he's got you up against the wall. You're naked though he's clothed, and he's punching you.

FIGURE 1. Transformations of Traumatic Memories as Measured by TMI-PS Intensity Ratings

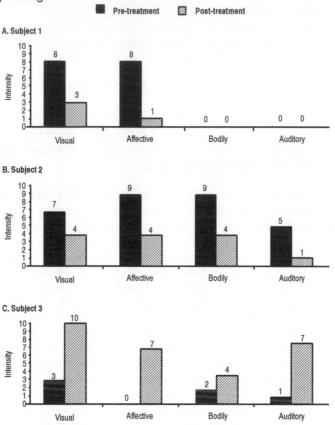

Both before and after treatment, this subject's response to the initial open-ended TMI-PS question focused on affective aspects of the memory. Her post-treatment response to this question also addressed the issue of fragmentation versus cohesion over time.

> *Pre-treatment*: "As soon as I heard it, just the date, I got really anxious and sad. I got all choked up. I think that's masked anger. Powerless. Real powerless. Part of it was kind-of a reenactment. I was definitely there.
>
> "There aren't too many incidents where I haven't been able to take control. You know what, I just flashed back to a drunk experience. Woke up with someone, there were these attack dogs growling at me, he

had me in a headlock. I was around 35. . . . I think I was so traumatized and freaked out that I've chosen not to remember that."
Post-treatment: "Vividly, pretty vividly. And I was surprised that it stirred me to the degree it did. But my body didn't tremble and shake like it did the first time . . . Less traumatic. I don't think I've cried–it's the first time I've cried about it. . . ."

"More sadness than horror. It was unsettling, mostly because I thought I was gonna sail through, which was unrealistic."

"This time it was like a cohesive unit. You know what I mean? Before, I felt each and every step of it. Now it's like an event. It's like a whole instead of fragments, so it's more manageable. In the past, five years ago, I would *think* of it as an event, but wouldn't allow myself to go there" (spoken emphasis).

Asked specifically about each sensory and affective modality, she reported experiences in each modality except olfactory:

Pre-treatment visual (7): "I saw myself really skinny and naked in the shower. What I saw was trouble coming. I just see me with my skin kind of glistening. He was dressed and I wasn't. He was dressed and waiting for me."
Post-treatment visual (4): "It wasn't as vivid. I didn't see myself on the floor, skinny and wet and frightened. I just kind of listened to it and didn't see anything, until he slammed me against the wall. I saw him clothed on top of me, which the tape brought back. So the beating part was blurrier, but the rape was clear."
Pre-treatment affective (9): "I was only conscious of how I was feeling today. Just this horrible overwhelming sadness."
Post-treatment affective (4): "I said there wasn't any horror. I think it's more sadness. I didn't feel disgust. I didn't feel anger. . . . I think the other part of the sadness is that I waited 22 years to go through this. . . ."
Pre-treatment bodily (9): "I was trying not to just burst out crying. My whole body was pulsing!" [Interviewer asks, "Did you remember how your body felt then?"] "No. I think I try to block that out. I sort-of won't go there."
Post-treatment bodily (4): "I felt myself kind of shaking, but nothing like the first time."
Pre-treatment auditory (5): "Not many, not real vivid. I did hear the wood breaking and cracking."
Post-treatment auditory (1): "I didn't hear him crashing the door. I didn't hear much. I guess I did hear him say, 'You're just like my mother.' I heard less, and it was less significant. No grunting, no animal sounds."

Bar graph B of Figure 1 conveys significant differences between pre- and post-treatment intensity ratings for the sensory, bodily and affective representations in subject 2's remembrances.

Subject 3 was a 25-year-old woman severely physically and emotionally abused by both parents throughout childhood and adolescence. She had no prior psychotherapy experience and entered the study hoping to reduce post-traumatic symptoms, particularly intrusive memories of an incident of sadistic emotional abuse by her mother. Thus, the event she focused on was not a "Criterion A event," that is, not traumatic according to the DSM-IV definition, but experienced by her as traumatic because of its *meaning* to her and its thematic linkage to many other traumatic experiences involving her mother. Subject 3 was employed as a temporary office worker at the time of the study, and was struggling to finish a senior thesis, her final requirement at a prestigious college. She met criteria for current major depressive disorder (recurrent), past simple phobia, and agoraphobia without panic, but had never taken psychiatric medications. She entered the study with an extremely high CAPS score of 122 (maximum score is 136), which after three EMDR sessions had dropped to 75, still in the moderate to severe range of PTSD symptomatology.

This subject had a very different pre-treatment script-driven memory experience than the other two subjects. Theirs were primarily characterized by reexperiencing phenomena (i.e., PTSD Criterion B). Her response to the opening TMI-PS question indicates that her pre-treatment response to the script was a numbing one (i.e., PTSD Criterion C). However, on the same day as the pre-treatment memory assessment, she reported frequent and severe reexperiencing symptoms for the past week on the CAPS, including flashbacks with extremely intense visual and affective components. Thus the comparisons she draws below in her post-treatment comments refer to her more typical intrusive memories.

> *Pre-treatment*: "It was hard to get into it this time. It can be hardest to psych into it if I'm feeling safe. . . ."
>
> "Either I'm really worked up, or I'm really calm. But there's nothing else. I felt more numb."
>
> "When I'm calm about it, I don't feel anything and I can function. But I don't *feel* anything. Like in high school. . . . I really had a grip on things, but in gym class I couldn't function. . . . "(spoken emphasis).
>
> "The decision I made [only recently]: I'd rather be fucked up but feel something. . . . I didn't react to anything in the past."
>
> *Post-treatment*: "Just calmer. That's the biggest thing. I can think of it and it's not gripping me. Be able to think about it, and not be controlled when it's happening. It's like, I feel fine now, like, I feel safer about it is

probably the biggest thing. Like if I walk outside it's not going to happen again. But it's still there. It's going to be there a long time."

In terms of specific sensory and affective components, the contrast between the pre- and post-treatment remembrances is quite striking, though again a reversal of the pattern for the other two subjects.

Pre-treatment visual (3): "I tried to hold an image of her in front of me of her looking at me. It was silence, looking at her through a glass wall, so it couldn't affect me, couldn't touch me."

Post-treatment visual (10): "Her, looking at me, not from the outside, more her in front of me. I think I saw her body more so, not just her face. I can remember her body now–it didn't remain as part of the memory. It's not realistic, a lot of darks and lights."

Pre-treatment affective (0): "It was like an anti-emotional effect, total calmness like wanting really badly to sleep. Feeling of emptiness."

Post-treatment affective (7): "I feel like I'm in the memory now, instead of her totally taking over the situation. I felt sorry for myself. I usually don't feel bad for myself. I felt kind-of a little bit sad, sad for myself."

Pre-treatment bodily (2): "Just stiff, and sometimes really calm. There's part of me that feels it will totally psychologically destroy me."

Post-treatment bodily (4): "I could feel myself breathing. I felt a lot more stable physically. Usually I don't feel there, but this time I felt physically calm, like I was there, calm in a settled way. Sometimes I feel calm in a numb way."

Pre-treatment auditory (1): "Silence. Nothingness. Instead of hearing her talking to me, it was coming from me."

Post-treatment auditory (7): "Her voice. More background noise. Her voice was dimmed. It's like it used to be like in movies, that overvoice, thundcrous, but now it's less like that."

Bar graph C of Figure 1 depicts the intensity ratings of subject 3, which are quite different from those of subjects 1 and 2, both in terms of magnitudes at pre- and post-treatment and which of the two remembrances had higher ratings.

Finally, this subject, who still had a relatively high CAPS score of 75 at post-treatment, gave the following answers to TMI-PS questions about whether she had experienced the memory components together and whether she could tell someone the experience as a "coherent story":

Post-treatment, components together? (No): "It's not cohesive. It's definitely pretty fragmented. I just don't see it being any other way for a while, because personally I just want to deal with a little at a time. Like I don't want to get overwhelmed by it again. Only recently have I felt like I can choose not to get into it. There's actual distance now. It's so little, but very significant. I feel like I have a little layer of skin on me now."

Post-treatment, tell coherent narrative? (No): "I think I'd start crying. But I'd much rather cry than laugh about it. No. Too much. I'd have to stop."

DISCUSSION

What are the characteristics of traumatic memories? Are there different subtypes? How are traumatic memories different from normal memories? How do we know when traumatic memories have *become* normal memories, or have changed in less dramatic but clinically significant ways? Traumatized individuals and the clinicians who treat them continually attempt to answer such questions, and the clinical literature addressing these issues is over a century old (e.g., Breuer & Freud, 1893; Janet, 1889, 1898). Yet valid and reliable methods for answering these questions with empirical research are just beginning to be developed. The cases presented here demonstrate that a clinically informed memory assessment instrument, when combined with a laboratory science method for retrieving memories, can yield phenomenological data that are complex, true to the experiences of traumatized people, yet quantifiable. Such integrative methods–if shown to yield reliable data and validated as assessments of traumatic memories–could provide a sound basis for more systematic and comprehensive classification traumatic memories, for distinguishing them from non-traumatic ones, and for discerning stages and outcomes of processing.

Retrieving Traumatic Memories

Distressing memories are the hallmark of posttraumatic stress disorder. "Reexperiencing" symptoms are listed first in the DSM-IV (APA, 1994), and all of them involve distress associated with remembering or being reminded of the traumatic event. Just as people with panic disorder suffer mainly from panic attacks, people with PTSD, as Breuer and Freud commented over a century ago, when the disorder had a different name, "suffer mainly from reminiscences" (1893, p. 7). Though not every remembrance of a traumatic event is a *traumatic remembrance,* such remembrances are important types of traumatic memories–and the characteristics of such memories (not only recovered ones) have been a topic of heated debate between psychological trauma researchers and cognitive scientists (e.g., Shobe & Kihlstrom, 1997).

To investigate *these* sorts of traumatic memories the procedures for memory retrieval are crucial. In research on panic disorder, researchers have developed methods to provoke panic attacks so they can assess their phenomenology and biological correlates (e.g., Lindsay, Saqi, & Bass, 1991; Reiman et al., 1989; Verburg, Pols, de Leeuw, & Griez, 1998). In contrast, for the study of traumatic memories, *how to evoke the memories to be assessed* is neither obvious nor straightforward. A questionnaire or interview can be used to assess characteristics of a memory evoked by the questionnaire or interview itself (e.g., Koss et al., 1996; Tromp et al., 1995), or a remembrance the subject experienced in the past week (e.g., Reynolds & Brewin, 1999). An interview might have subjects "call the memory to mind," and then pose questions about its characteristics, or it might direct and redirect subjects to narrate the trauma out loud, in the present tense, as if it were happening again (e.g., Foa et al., 1995). Clearly each method utilizes very different strategies to evoke remembrances of traumatic events, and we should not be surprised if assessment of identical characteristics yields data that are different or apparently contradictory.

Several features of script-driven remembering appear to make this a uniquely effective method for evoking traumatic memories in the laboratory. The method is both individualized and standardized, thus capable of evoking memories for unique events using highly structured procedures. Three features of script-driven remembering are designed to channel the retrieval process rapidly from contextual information directly into situationally accessible event-specific knowledge: (1) the directions given to the subject, (2) the present-tense narration of the script, and (3) the sequential specification of somatosensory and affective details. When subjects listen to the tape, they experience a memory evocation procedure that is directive rather than interrogative, and that employs detailed and sequentially unfolding cues to retrieve an episodic memory that is "script-driven." The fundamental goal of script-driven remembering is not perfect matching between cue and memory store, but as full as possible activation of the episodic memory system under well-controlled conditions. That is a task for which questionnaire and interview measures alone are not well suited. The superficial cueing of questionnaires is likely to undermine their validity, and interviews are likely to lack reliability because an interactive conversation of several minutes cannot approach the standardization of listening to a brief and formulaic script. This individualized, standardized and adaptable method warrants further research to determine its validity as a method for evoking traumatic memories, and the reliability of the data it yields.

The greatest strength of the TMI-PS, the "assessment side" of our evocation-assessment methodology, is its "delegation" of memory retrieval to the preliminary procedure of script-driven remembering. In prior research, the procedure for evoking a remembrance has been embedded in the instrument used to assess the same remembrance's characteristics. The TMI-PS acquires data on particular remembrances *already* evoked under very controlled conditions, and is minimally retrospective–minutes at most. Further, its intensity ratings of somatosensory and affective modalities are meant to provide data on characteristics of traumatic memories long observed by clinicians. Thus we also believe that the TMI-PS warrants further research on its validity as a measure of these memory characteristics and the reliability of the data it yields.

Script-Driven Remembrances and the Classification of Traumatic Memories

In the absence of empirical research demonstrating the validity and reliability of our method, we cannot draw definitive conclusions from the case data presented here. We do not know whether these subjects' pre- or post-treatment responses to script-driven remembering would have demonstrated stability over time. And even if we did, we would have no way of knowing, for example, whether a simple habituation effect accounted for any differences between observed pre- and post-treatment remembrances. Indeed, strictly speaking, we cannot even say that we measured characteristics of memories, only that *we evoked remembrances with certain characteristics, some of which we attempted to measure.* Therefore, in discussing our case data, we only *describe* these subjects' remembrances, sparingly using theoretical constructs in order to suggest how researchers might approach the interpretation of such findings. Only the unexpected pre-treatment numb remembrance of subject 3 is used for tentative theoretical speculation, and in that case, mainly because of the possible implications of such remembrances for the research required to establish the reliability of script-driven remembering.

Though designed to assess script-driven remembrances, the TMI-PS itself is necessarily a collection of memory retrieval methods. These methods include an opening free recall question, several items concerning the contents of somatosensory and affective modalities, and cues that elicit intensity ratings for the contents of each modality. Besides its delegation of memory evocation to script-driven remembering and its minimally retrospective nature, the major advance of the TMI-PS (over the original TMI) is the elicitation of somatosensory and affective intensity ratings in addition to modality contents reports. Therefore, we focus our discussion on the data yielded by this section of the instrument.

Figure 1's bar graphs warrant two observations: First, for all subjects, the pre-treatment traumatic memory does not resemble the post-treatment memory on somatosensory and affective intensity ratings. Second, subject 3's pre-treatment memory is strikingly different from those of subjects 1 and 2. As the validity of the method and the reliability of these data are not established, causality cannot be established either. However, we believe it is worthwhile to describe differences between each subject's pre- and post-treatment remembrances. Thus we will not discuss "changes in memories" from pre- to post-treatment, but "differences in remembrances" assessed at two times.

Subject 1's reports of modality contents and intensities suggest two differences between the remembrances, in terms of relative dominance of verbally versus situationally accessible memories. First, the intensity ratings for visual and affective modalities were less in the post- than the pre-treatment remembrance; second, different affective experiences were reported for each memory. At pre-treatment, subject 1 referred to a "bright light" and at post-treatment to its absence, and he gave visual intensity ratings of 8 and 3, respectively. His affective intensity rating at pre-treatment was 8, compared to 1 at post-treatment. However, the *types* of affects he experienced were different as well: "frightened" and "upset" at pre-treatment versus "sadness" and "some anger" at post-treatment–that is, feelings experienced *during* the original event versus feelings *about* the event based on what it means to him now. This distinction fits with that of Brewin and colleagues' between "conditioned emotional reactions corresponding to the activation of specific emotional states. . . experienced during the trauma," and "secondary emotions," which "follow from the consequences and implications of the trauma," and are part of verbally accessible memories (Brewin et al., p. 677). The different types of affects experienced by subject 1 at pre- and post-treatment also fit with an empirical finding (Reynolds & Brewin, 1999), that memories associated with fear were not associated with sadness, and vice versa. Any future research with this method should probably evaluate the utility of the *combination* of the affective intensity rating and content report, particularly for categorizing traumatic memories into different types.

Subject 2 described her pre-treatment auditory memory of "wood breaking and cracking" as "not real vivid," but gave an intensity rating of 5, much higher than the rating of 1 at post-treatment, when she "didn't hear him crashing the door." It is notable that those sounds were missing from the memory evoked at post-treatment, even though the script *suggested* that she hear them. For the bodily modality, at pre-treatment subject 2 reported "trying not to burst out crying," and exclaimed, "My whole body was pulsing!" Interestingly, she did *not* report that fear accompanied these intense somatosensory representations, but that she was "only conscious of what I was feeling today . . . horrible overwhelming sadness." Recall that for subject 1, a pre- versus post-treatment difference in the affective intensity rating (8 versus 1) corresponded to a difference in affective content, of primarily fear in the first remembrance and sadness and anger in the second. In contrast, subject 2 reported different intensities of 9 at pre-treatment versus 4 at post-treatment in both affective and bodily modalities, but with *consistency* of content: "horrible overwhelming sadness" versus "sadness" but not "horror"; and "whole body . . . pulsing" versus "kind of shaking." It appears, then, that the relationships of sadness and fear to somatosensory and affective contents may be quite complex within and across remembrances. The finding of sadness co-occurring with intense somatosensory representations also suggests that situationally and verbally accessible memory representations may be simultaneously activated and blended together within the same remembrance.

Before discussing subject 3's data, two tentative conclusions are warranted concerning methodology. First, script-driven remembering appears capable of *eliciting* remembrances that are characterized by (a) intensely experienced somatosensory and affective contents, and (b) the presence of affects associated either with the traumatic event or subsequent interpretations of its meaning. Second, the TMI-PS appears capable of *detecting*, in particular script-driven remembrances, gradations in the intensities of sensations, bodily experiences and emotions.

Subject 3's pre-treatment remembrance can be interpreted in two ways: (1) as evidence that our method lacks validity and/or reliability; (2) as an example of a type of traumatic memory not adequately addressed by current theories of PTSD or traumatic memory. It is worth considering each interpretation to shed light on methodological and theoretical issues related to our method. How does her pre-treatment remembrance cast doubt on script-driven remembering as a method for evoking traumatic memories? Subject 3 was found to have extremely severe PTSD, including *frequent and intense intrusive memories*, on a validated and reliable measure for assessing PTSD diagnostic status and symptom severity (i.e., a CAPS score of 122). If someone with such extreme reexperiencing symptoms does not respond or does not consistently respond to script-driven remembering with an intrusive memory characterized by intense somatosensory and affective experiences, then there may be something wrong with the method.

On the other hand, subject 3 herself said spontaneously that her pre-treatment remembrance was familiar to her, indeed, as familiar as having an intense intrusive memory. That is, responding to the opening free-recall question of the TMI-PS, she said, "Either I'm really worked up, or I'm really calm. But there's nothing else. I felt more numb." Subject 3 presents a clear picture of extreme numbing. Of the visual images she said, "It was silence, looking at her through a glass wall," and rated their intensity at 3. Asked what she felt emotionally, she began, "It was like an anti-emotional effect," and gave *zero* as the intensity. For the auditory modality, she rated it a 1 and began, "Silence. Nothingness." If this sort of remembrance is fairly typical for this subject, then at least two possible explanations arise: (1) script-driven remembering may be an effective method for evoking such a remembrance; (2) her numbing may only be *incidentally* related to the procedure, i.e., she was numb before, during and afterward. Only controlled studies with sufficient power to detect such possible effects are adequate to investigate these sorts of remembrances in people who have experienced traumatic events.

However, *it may not be possible* to separate the issue of numb remembrances from the studies required to establish the validity and reliability of script-driven remembering and the TMI-PS. If numb remembrances *are* a type of traumatic remembrance, then their occurrence *despite* the script-driven remembering procedure–a method designed to evoke intense somatosensory and affective representations–might constitute a robust phenomenon measurable by the TMI-PS (or other measures). In that case, subjects who exhibit such remembrances *and* classic intrusive remembrances would not be expected to provide data supporting the test-retest reliability of script-driven remembering–but neither should their data be considered evidence of the *un*reliability of script-driven remembering. Clinicians have long noted the tendency of some traumatized people to alternate between intrusive remembrances characterized by intense somatosensory and affective fragments, on the one hand, and highly schematized memories that, when spoken, are superficial narratives devoid of feeling, on the other. Two passages from Breuer and Freud's classic 1893 paper capture this paradoxical situation:

> At first sight it seems extraordinary that events experienced so long ago should continue to operate so intensely–that their recollection should not be liable to the wearing away process to which, after all, we see all our memories succumb. . . .
> We must, however, mention another remarkable fact . . . *these experiences are completely absent from the patient's memory when they are in a normal psychical state, or are only present in a highly summary form.* (1893, pp. 7 & 10, italics in original)

The dual representation theory (Brewin et al., 1996) offers a clear framework with its two types of memory representations and three processing outcomes. However, it does not clearly articulate a place for numb remembrances among people in the *chronic emotional processing outcome*, the outcome that includes people with PTSD. Thus "trauma-related scripts" (Brewin et al., 1996, p. 679) are described as effectively and *continually* preventing the activation of situationally accessible intrusive memories, and only associated with the prematurely inhibited processing outcome. Their theory does not address numbing or dissociative symptoms in detail, and they only propose in passing that numbing or dissociative responses to a specific trauma may be "coded within" situationally accessible memories and reinstated when triggered by an appropriate cue (Brewin et al., 1996, p. 680). In our prior work (e.g., van der Kolk & van der Hart, 1991; van der Kolk & Fisler, 1995), we have focused on relationships between peritraumatic dissociation and later retrieval of intense and intrusive fragmentary memories, but not posttraumatic remembrances characterized by numbing and *lack* of intensity in somatosensory and affective modalities. Therefore, the *possibility* needs to be kept in mind that numb remembrances are a distinct type of traumatic remembrance. Failure to consider this possibility could result in misinterpreting data from such remembrances as indicating the unreliability of script-driven remembering.

A Preliminary Taxonomy of Traumatic Memories

To guard against this potential threat to valid interpretation of data generated by script-driven remembering and the TMI-PS, and to clarify relationships between methodology and theory in the study of traumatic memories, we offer in Table 3 a preliminary taxonomy of traumatic memories. This classification scheme has four major features. First, the framework is organized around the three processing outcomes and the two types of memory systems described in dual representation theory. Second, each processing outcome has different types of remembrances associated with it. Third, the relationship between situationally and verbally accessible memories, and how these are experienced in particular forms of remembrance, delineate the basic phenomenological parameters of the model. Finally, based on our experience with subject 3 (as well as clinical experience and data from other subjects not presented), we conceptualize the chronic processing outcome as encompassing two basic types of remembrance: "over-aroused remembrance" and "under-aroused remembrance." While the typical reexperiencing symptoms of PTSD are associated with the "over-aroused remembrance" category, subject 3's pre-treatment remembrance belongs to the category of "under-aroused remembrance."

At the heart of this preliminary classification system is our conviction that distinguishing the constructs of memories and remembrances is essential for sound research and theory in the study of traumatic memories. *Researchers can only infer the nature of encoded and stored memories for particular traumatic events by evoking and assessing particular remembrances under particular conditions.* Our taxonomy of traumatic memories is admittedly speculative and incomplete, but our main purpose here is to stimulate new empirical and theoretical work. Our goal is to help advance the study of

TABLE 3. A Preliminary Taxonomy of Traumatic Memories

Processing Outcomes and Remembrance Categories	Characteristics of Memories Evoked with Script-Driven Remembering			
	Situationally Accessible	Verbally Accessible	Relationship of SA to VA	Subject Descriptions
1. Prematurely inhibited processing				
Superficial remembrance	suppressed	schematized "script" with no emotions	VAMs dominant	"I would <u>think</u> of it as an event, but wouldn't allow myself to go there."
2. Chronic emotional processing				
A. Over-aroused remembrance (i.e., typical reexperiencing symptoms of PTSD)	intense and easily accessed	suppressed <u>or</u> preoccupation with secondary emotions and attributions	SAMs dominant or alternating dominance of SAMs and VAMs	"A reenactment. I was definitely there." "wood breaking and cracking"
B. Under-aroused remembrance				
(i.e., numbing and/or dissociation as chronic symptoms, responses to triggers or memories, or reexperiencing phenomenon)	relatively muted, suppressed, or inaccessible	relatively suppressed, schematized script, or inaccessible	both relatively "shut down" in context of numbing or dissociation	"anti-emotional effect "numb" "through a glass wall"
3. Successful completed processing				
Integrated remembrance	seldom emerges; no longer overwhelming	narrative that integrates event into life story; not preoccupied	VAMs dominant without suppressing SAMs or secondary emotions	[no data from current sample]

traumatic memories, so that it might progress beyond the current "looseness of definition and use of its major concepts," just as the study of non-traumatic memory has since Tulving (1972) made his observation and introduced the distinction between episodic and semantic memory.

Methodological Issues and Limitations

In this section, we critically evaluate script-driven remembering and the TMI-PS as research methods, particularly ways that specific components of each may enhance or threaten validity and reliability in a variety of research contexts.

Script-Driven Remembering. A few features of the script-driven remembering method, besides those discussed as strengths above, could have significant effects on characteristics of the evoked memories subsequently assessed with the TMI-PS. These call out for critical appraisal and component analyses, which could help others who adopt this approach to avert unnecessary problems.

The first potential limitation of the method is that the data for making scripts were collected *in writing*, which could reduce subjects' access to non-verbal situationally accessible memory representations. The script construction form does employ a recognition format for selection and inclusion of physiological responses in the written account, increasing the likelihood that these nonverbal representations will be retrieved. (The current version [see Appendix A] explicitly directs subjects to review and circle physiological response items on the second page *before* writing their description.) Still, an interview procedure in which subjects are directed to talk about the traumatic event as if it were happening (Foa, Molnar, & Cashman, 1995; Harvey & Bryant, 1999) could yield more somatosensory and affective representations for incorporation into scripts. However, subjects may not feel comfortable saying key details out loud, and the cases presented here suggest that form-derived scripts can effectively retrieve intense sensory, bodily and emotional representations.

Because the 30-second scripts are designed to end right at the worst part of the memory, researchers must choose between inquiring about (a) the entire remembering experience across both the "script listening" and the "post-script remembering" periods, (b) only one period, or (c) each period separately. Certainly these two periods are different conditions. Some subjects report experiencing the most intense and vivid sensations and emotions during the script-listening period, while others say things like, "I had to wait for the tape to end before I could really get into the memory." We chose to inquire about the whole experience for two reasons. First, we did not want to overburden subjects by inquiring about both separately. Second, we were not confident in the reliability of recall for the two periods separately (given the longer interview and potential for contamination effects). Finally, shorter tapes with fewer cues provide fewer opportunities for distraction and distortion of memory content or sequencing, and we believed this consideration trumped the two-period problem.

Indeed, the potential for script-driven remembering to introduce suggestion and distortion into memories should be considered very thoughtfully. In some ways, the method is inherently suggestive, from the second-person present-tense language (i.e., "You are . . .") to the fact that the script only selectively incorporates somatosensory and affective contents written on the form. Subjects having difficulty accessing situationally accessible memories may write sensations and emotions that they believe they "probably," "must have" or "should have" experienced during the event. To prevent this, the directions on the script construction form should include instructions not to guess, and researchers can inquire about this after its completion (included in current version; see Appendix A). If a subject's memory is already distorted, the problem could be reinforced or worsened by a script incorporating the errors. Such uncertainties about accuracy are endemic to research on traumatic and many other memories, but this method's potential for reinforcing distortions should be kept in mind and guarded against. Strictly speaking, the scripts provided a "narrative," but only of an unfolding temporal sequence. They did *not* suggest that the subject experience a "narrative memory"–that is, memories organized by meaning propositions that thematically integrate the event with other autobiographical memories. Finally, subsequent playings of the script may suggest sensory, bodily or emotional representations that have been neutralized by desensitization or memory processing. In that sense, a suggestive aspect of script-driven remembering could make it a conservative test of treatment outcome.

Probably a greater threat to validity than suggestion is *habituation to the script*. In general each subsequent playing should be less effective at retrieving situationally accessible memory representations. This could threaten both validity and test-retest reliability. In treatment outcome studies, researchers should use two pre-treatment and two post-treatment assessments, and a matched non-treatment group. Control non-traumatic memories can indicate whether habituation effects differ for traumatic and non-traumatic memories of different kinds (stressful, non-stressful, etc.). However, as demonstrated by subject 3, other factors may mask or counter the habituation effect, including symptomatic responses such as numbing, avoidance or dissociation. Clearly the issue is not simple, and appropriate reliability studies are needed.

Other components of the method might be systematically manipulated to understand better its mechanisms for shaping the characteristics of evoked memories. How might remembrances differ if somatosensory and affective representations were played to subjects *without* initial contextual information (i.e., time and place), *without* a particular order, or both? How might remembrances differ if the script were to suggest an emotion that was *not* named on the script form, but which follows from the event? Indeed, experiments with these dimensions of memory scripts may reveal the extent to which traumatized individuals are vulnerable to suggestion, and their remembrances to distortion.

Traumatic Memory Inventory-Post-Script Version. We selected subsets of original TMI items for the TMI-PS, and added three new features. The opening free-recall question was new, and allowed subjects to make unexpected and valuable observations about their memories and how they changed over time. Items focused on the *contents* of somatosensory and affective representations were retained from the original TMI; the modality *intensity* ratings were new. Together these features of the interview provided rich qualitative data and continuous variables that show promise for quantitative analyses.

A closer and more critical look, however, suggests that the language for eliciting intensity ratings should be refined and that a dichotomous "reliving" item should be added. We have revised the TMI-PS in light of these issues. We replaced the phrase "intense or vivid" with "intense," because the contents of a modality might be experienced quite intensely but given a lower rating if lacking in clarity of detail. These ratings are now followed by inquiries about remembering versus reliving contents of particular modalities, to better assess a characteristic of some traumatic memories cited in the clinical literature (e.g., van der Kolk & van der Hart, 1991) and assessed by Reynolds and Brewin (1999). (See Appendix B for the revised TMI-PS.)

Three conceptually related TMI-PS items that we retained from the original TMI share limitations that undermine their validity as measures of their respective constructs. These were the questions concerning fragmentation of memory components and capacity to tell the experience as a coherent story and without interruption. The meaning of "all at the same time" is not clear in the question, "Of the components present, did you remember them all at the same time?" Any memory lasting more than a few moments will necessarily include different sensations and emotions being experienced at different times. Similar lack of clarity characterizes the other two questions, meant to assess for "narrative memory." Thus more valid measures are necessary for investigation of memory fragmentation and narrative incoherence. Fortunately, two studies have been published that used systems for coding the "utterance units" of narrated traumatic memories on indices of fragmentation and disorganization, both with positive results. Foa and colleagues' (Foa, Molnar, & Cashman, 1995) study of rape victims with PTSD, the first prospective study of treatment-induced transformations of traumatic memories, found that decreases on indices of narrative memory fragmentation were highly associated with improvement in PTSD symptoms. Harvey and Bryant (1999), in a study of motor vehicle accident survivors, found greater disorganization in the narratives of subjects with acute stress disorder (ASD) than those without, and significant relationships between disorganized memory structure, severity of ASD, and meeting criteria for the dissociative symptom cluster of ASD. Perhaps before dropping the related TMI-PS questions, subjects who give "yes" and "no" responses could be compared on fragmentation and disorganization indices derived from their *actual* spoken narratives.

We believe it is important to retain the last two TMI-PS questions. One question asked subjects if their "response to the memory" was "typical" or "different than" how they usually "respond to a strong reminder." The final question inquired about whether they were "thinking about or remembering anything else while listening to the tape and/or during the post-tape remembering phase?" These questions can provide a validity check on the previously collected data, and are potential sources of unexpected information that could spur refinements of methodology or theory. Objective rules should be developed for deciding when to discard TMI-PS data based on answers to these questions.

Ethical Issues. For subjects with PTSD and those with prematurely inhibited processing, it is possible that reexperiencing and other PTSD symptoms will be triggered or exacerbated by script-driven remembering. Subjects can find TMI-PS questions about details of their traumatic remembrances quite intrusive and distressing. If researchers are not confident they will be using data on the *contents* of somatosensory modalities (i.e., particular images, sounds, etc.) this information should not be gathered. Fortunately, with its intensity ratings and reliving/remembering items, the TMI-PS can gather valuable data *without* asking about particular sensations and bodily experiences. However, inquiring about particular emotions is less intrusive, and the distinction between primary and secondary emotions, for example fear and sadness, may provide important information about the memory.

Future Directions

A top priority for future research on this method is to determine the validity of script-driven remembering and the TMI-PS as methods for evoking and measuring characteristics of traumatic memories long observed by clinicians. To establish the divergent and convergent validity of script-driven remembering, the TMI-PS and other assessment measures might be used to compare characteristics of remembrances evoked by script-driven remembrance with those evoked by (1) completing a memory assessment questionnaire and (2) narrating the trauma out loud in an interview. Convergent validity could also be assessed by whether changes in pre- and post-treatment script-driven remembrances are paralleled by similar changes in PTSD symptoms. Reliability studies should be informed by an appreciation of individuals' potentially complex and variable responses to traumatic reminders. Indeed, for some subjects with PTSD, a reexperiencing response to the first script might be *expected* to lead to an avoidant, numb or dissociative response the second time. To assess for distinct types of traumatic remembrances shaped by such symptoms, we are developing the Responses to Script-Driven Remembering Scale (RSDR) (Hopper, unpublished), a brief structured interview which assesses PTSD reexperiencing, avoidant and numbing symptoms, and dissociative symptoms. Finally, if validity and appropriate indications of reliability are established, the use of this method in prospective studies could significantly advance the study of traumatic memories. Naturalistic longitudinal studies could reveal how experiences of traumatic events lead to the creation of traumatic memories, and treatment outcome studies how traumatic memories can be transformed into more normal memories.

CONCLUSION

In order for the study of traumatic memories to become a mature field, capable of fostering more systematic classification and comprehensive understanding of the varieties of traumatic memories and remembrances, more researchers must draw on clinical *and* scientific experience and knowledge, and employ more integrative methods of retrieval and assessment. We offer this new method as a step in that direction.

NOTES

1. For the purposes of this introduction, "traumatic memories" refers to autobiographical memories of events originally encoded under conditions meeting the definition of "extreme trauma," specified under Criterion A for acute and posttraumatic stress disorders (ASD & PTSD), in the *Diagnostic and Statistical Manual of Mental Disorders, Fourth Edition* (DSM-IV; APA, 1994). Case data below will address some limitations of this definition.

2. See also Brewin and Andrews' (1998) more recent paper, in which they make the case, in effect, that the barrier between verbally and situationally accessible representations is maintained in part by processes familiar to cognitive psychologists, including not only the commonly cited implicit memory, but also retrieval inhibition and post-retrieval decisional processes.

REFERENCES

American Psychiatric Association. (1994). *Diagnostic and statistical manual of mental disorders* (4th ed.). Washington, DC: Author.

Blake, D. D., Weathers, F. W., Nagy, L. M., Kaloupek, D. G., Gusman, F. D., Charney, D. S., & Keane, T. M. (1995). The development of a Clinician-Administered PTSD Scale. *Journal of Traumatic Stress, 8,* 75-90.

Breuer, J., & Freud, S. (1893). On the psychical mechanism of hysterical phenomena: Preliminary communication. In J. Strachy (Ed. and Trans.) *The standard edition of the complete psychological works of Sigmund Freud* (Vol. 2., pp. 3-17). London: Hogarth Press.

Brewin, C. R., & Andrews, B. (1998). Recovered memories of trauma: Phenomenology and cognitive mechanisms. *Clinical Psychology Review, 4,* 949-970.

Brewin, C. R., Dalgleish, T., & Joseph, S. (1996). A dual representation theory of posttraumatic stress disorder. *Psychological Review, 103,* 670-686.

Chemtob, C. M., Tolin, D. F., van der Kolk, B. A., & Pitman, R. K. (2000). Eye Movement Desensitization and Reprocessing. In E. B. Foa, T. M. Keane, & M. J. Friedman (Eds.), *Effective treatments for PTSD: Practice guidelines from the International Society for Traumatic Stress Studies* (pp. 139-154). New York: Guilford Press.

Creamer, M., Burgess, P., & Pattison, P. (1990). Cognitive processing in post-trauma reactions: Some preliminary findings. *Psychological Medicine, 20,* 597-604.

Creamer, M., Burgess, P., & Pattison, P. (1992). Reaction to trauma: A cognitive processing model. *Journal of Abnormal Psychology, 101,* 452-459.

Foa, E. B., Molnar, C., & Cashman, L. (1995). Change in rape narratives during exposure therapy for posttraumatic stress disorder. *Journal of Traumatic Stress, 8,* 675-690.

Harvey, A. G., & Bryant, R. A. (1999). A qualitative investigation of the organization of traumatic memories. *British Journal of Psychiatry, 38,* 401-405.

Hopper, J. W. (2000). Responses to Script-Driven Remembering Scale. Unpublished Manuscript.

Janet, P. (1889). *L'Automatisme psychologique* [Psychological automatisms]. Paris: Félix Alcan.

Janet, P. (1898). *Névroses et idées fixes* [Neuroses and fixed ideas] (Vols. 1 & 2). Paris: Félix Alcan.

Janet, P. (1919/1925). *Psychological healing* (Vols. 1& 2). New York: MacMillan. (Original book, *Les médications psychologiques,* published in 1919).

Koss, M. P., Figueredo, A. J., Bell, I., Tharan, M., & Tromp, S. (1996). Traumatic memory characteristics: A cross-validated mediational model of response to rape among employed women. *Journal of Abnormal Psychology, 105,* 421-432.

Lang, P. J., Levin, D. N., Miller, G. A., & Kozac, M. J. (1983). Fear behavior, fear imagery, and the psychophysiology of emotion: The problem of affective-response integration. *Journal of Abnormal Psychology, 92,* 275-306.

Lindsay, S., Saqi, S., & Bass, C. (1991). The test-retest reliability of the hyperventilation provocation test. *Journal of Psychosomatic Research, 35,* 155-162.

Orr, S. P., Pitman, R. K., Lasko, N. B., & Herz, L. R. (1993). Psychophysiological assessment of posttraumatic stress disorder imagery in World War II and Korean combat veterans. *Journal of Abnormal Psychology, 102*, 152-159.

Pitman, R. K., Orr, S. P., Forgue, D. F., de Jong, J., & Claiborn, J. M. (1987). Psychophysiologic assessment of posttraumatic stress disorder imagery in Vietnam combat veterans. *Archives of General Psychiatry, 44*, 970-975.

Rauch, S., van der Kolk, B. A., Fisler, R., Alpert, N., Orr, S., Savage, C., Jenike, M., & Pitman, R. (1996). A symptom provocation study of posttraumatic stress disorder using positron emission tomography and script-driven imagery. *Archives of General Psychiatry, 53*, 380-387.

Reiman, E. M., Raichle, M. E, Robins, E., Mintun, M. A., Fusselman, M. J., Fox, P. T., Price, J. L., & Hackman, K. A. (1989). Neuroanatomical correlates of a lactate-induced anxiety attack. *Archives of General Psychiatry, 46*, 493-500.

Reynolds, M., & Brewin, C. R. (1998). Intrusive cognitions, coping strategies and emotional responses in depression, post-traumatic stress disorder and a non-clinical population. *Behaviour Research and Therapy, 36*, 135-147.

Reynolds, M., & Brewin, C. R. (1999). Intrusive memories in depression and post-traumatic stress disorder. *Behaviour Research and Therapy, 37*, 201-215.

Shapiro, F. (1995). *Eye movement desensitization and reprocessing.* New York: Guilford Press.

Shobe, K. K., & Kihlstrom, J. (1997). Is traumatic memory special? *Current Directions in Psychological Science, 6*, 70-74.

Spitzer, R. L., Williams, J. B. W., & Gibbon, M. (1987). *Structured Clinical Interview for DSM-III-R.* New York: New York State Psychiatric Institute, Biometrics Research Department.

Suengas, A. G., & Johnson, M. K. (1988). Qualitative effects of rehearsal on memories for perceived and imagined complex events. *Journal of Experimental Psychology*: *General, 117*, 377-389.

Tromp, S., Koss, M. P., Figueredo, A. J., Bell, I., & Tharan, M. (1995). Are rape memories different? A comparison of rape, other unpleasant, and pleasant memories among employed women. *Journal of Traumatic Stress, 8*, 607-627.

Tulving, E. (1972). Episodic and semantic memory. In E. Tulving & W. Donaldson (Eds.), *Organization of memory* (pp. 381-403). New York: Academic Press.

Tulving, E. (1976). Ecphoric processes in recall and recognition. In J. Brown (Ed.), *Recall and recognition* (pp. 37-73). London: Wiley.

van der Kolk, B. A., Burbridge, J. A., & Suzuki, J. (1997). The psychobiology of traumatic memory: Clinical implications of neuroimaging studies. In R. Yehuda & A. C. McFarlane (Eds.), *Annals of the New York Academy of Sciences (Vol. 821): Psychobiology of posttraumatic stress disorder* (pp. 99-113). New York: New York Academy of Sciences.

van der Kolk, B. A., & Fisler, R. (1995). Dissociation and the fragmentary nature of traumatic memories: Overview and exploratory study. *Journal of Traumatic Stress, 8*, 505-536.

van der Kolk, B. A., Hopper, J. W., & Osterman, J. E. (2001). Exploring the nature of traumatic memory: Combining clinical knowledge and laboratory methods. *Journal of Aggression, Maltreatment & Trauma 4(8)*, 9-31.

van der Kolk, B. A., & van der Hart, O. (1989). Pierre Janet and the breakdown of psychological adaptation in psychological trauma. *American Journal of Psychiatry, 146,* 1530-1540.

van der Kolk, B. A., & van der Hart, O. (1991). The intrusive past: The flexibility of memory and the engraving of trauma. *American Imago, 48,* 425-454.

Verburg, K., Pols, H., de Leeuw, M., & Griez, E. (1998). Reliability of the 35% carbon dioxide panic provocation challenge. *Psychiatry Research, 78,* 207-214.

APPENDIX A

Traumatic Scene Form

We would like you to write a description of the most traumatic event you have experienced in your life. We may ask you more detail about this experience later.

If you find it difficult to think of something to write, it may help to close your eyes and imagine yourself back in the situation. Try to generate the same sensations and feelings that you experienced at the time. While the image is vivid in your memory, jot down the details of the scene and the sensations you experienced at the time. Also, on the next page are bodily experiences you may have had; please circle any that apply.

Describe the traumatic situation. Include such details as *when* it happened (age and date), *where* you were, *who* was there (names), *what* you were doing, how things looked, what you heard, what you were feeling, etc. Please *do not guess* or include anything about which you are not *positive.*

Please write things in the order they happened, and include bodily sensations from the next page at the appropriate times (turn to that page first). Continue your description on the reverse side of this page if necessary.

Listed below are a number of bodily sensations that people may experience in various situations. Please circle all of the responses that you experienced in the situation you described, <u>and include</u> several in your description.

APPENDIX A (continued)

heart stops	breath faster	whole body shakes
heart pounds	breath slower	eye twitches
heart beats slower	pant	eyes burn
heart skips a beat	shallow breathing	eyes wide open
heart races	labored breathing	eyes water
heart quickens	gasping for air	body feels heavy
feel sweaty	feel tense all over	feel hot all over
palms are clammy	feel relaxed all over	blood rushing to head
beads of perspiration	tension in forehead	arms and legs warm and relaxed
sweat pours out	clenched fist	flushed face
feel warm	tension in back	head pounds
nauseous	grit my teeth	feel restless
stomach is in a knot	clenched jaw	jittery
butterflies in stomach	tension in the arms	calm
cramps in stomach	tightness in face	
constriction in chest	hands trembling	

APPENDIX B

Traumatic Memory Inventory – Post-Script Version

Hopper and van der Kolk, 2000

Subject ID:_____Interviewer:_____Date of assessment:___/___/___

When you remembered the traumatic experience today, how did you remember it? (Listen for subject's report, and write below. Ask follow-up clarifying questions sparingly, and record them as well.)

Memories can have a variety of components. They may include visual images, physical sensations, sounds, etc. The next questions are about these possible components of your memory.

<u>Int</u>   <u>Re</u>

___ ___ Were there visual images? Y N (Visual) What did you see?
_____

___ ___ Were there physical sensations? Y N (Bodily) What did you feel in your body?_____

___ ___ Were there smells? Y N (Olfactory) What did you smell?
_____

___ ___ Were there sounds? Y N (Auditory) What did you hear?____

___ ___ Were there emotions? Y N (Affective) How did you feel emotionally?_____

Y   N   Were there thoughts about the situation? (Cognitive) What did you remember thinking?_____

Y   N   Components together? Of those components present, did you remember all of them at the same time?

Y   N   As a story? (Narrative) Could you tell it to someone as a coherent story?

Y   N   Would you be able to talk about what happened today, without being interrupted by associated feelings or perceptions?

Explain

I'm going to ask you two questions about some components of the memory. First, I will ask you to rate their intensity, with 0 being not at all present, and 10 being the most intense possible.

Now, I'm going to ask you whether you *re-lived* any images, sensations, etc., as opposed to just remembering them. For example, you may have felt like you were hearing the *same* sound *all over again*, or just *remembering* hearing that sound. Do you understand the difference?

Summary: **Intensity**   **Reliving**   **Coherence**

_____Visual   Y N   Components together

_____Tactile   Y N   Narrative

_____Olfactory   Y N   Without interruptions

_____Auditory   _____

_____Affective   _____

Y N   Cognitive

Was your response to the memory today a typical response for you, or was it different than how you usually respond to a strong reminder?   **Typical   Not typical   How?** (Listen for subject's report, and write below. Ask follow-up clarifying questions sparingly, and record them as well.)

Were you thinking about or remembering anything else while listening to the tape and/or during post-tape remembering phase? (Listen for subject's report first. . .)

A Cognitive Analysis
of the Role of Suggestibility
in Explaining Memories for Abuse

Kathy Pezdek

SUMMARY. In this article, the phenomenon of delayed recall for traumatic memories is considered, and the recovered memory interpretation and the false memory interpretation for this phenomenon are articulated. A major tenet in the false memory interpretation is the claim that delayed recall of traumatic memories results from the suggestive planting of memories for events that did not actually occur. However, this view assumes a very powerful construct of suggestibility. In this chapter, recent research from our laboratory on the suggestibility of memory is reviewed to assess if the construct of suggestibility is sufficiently robust to account for this effect. In particular, four constraints on the suggestibility of memory are discussed and related to memory for traumatic events. These constraints are (a) the familiarity of the original event, (b) whether the original event is consistent or inconsistent with expectations, (c) whether the suggestion is to change or to plant a memory for the original event, and (d) the plausibility of the suggested false event. Research on each of these constraints is presented. Based on this cognitive analysis of the recovered memory/ false memory debate, it is concluded that suggestibility does not appear to be a sufficiently strong cognitive construct to explain the delayed recall phenomenon. *[Article copies available for a fee from The Haworth*

Address correspondence to: Kathy Pezdek, Department of Psychology, Claremont Graduate University, Claremont, CA 91711-3955 (E-mail: kathy.pezdek@cgu.edu).

The author thanks the Fletcher Jones Foundation for their support during this project.

[Haworth co-indexing entry note]: "A Cognitive Analysis of the Role of Suggestibility in Explaining Memories for Abuse." Pezdek, Kathy. Co-published simultaneously in *Journal of Aggression, Maltreatment & Trauma* (The Haworth Maltreatment & Trauma Press, an imprint of The Haworth Press, Inc.) Vol. 4, No. 2, (#8), 2001, pp. 73-85; and: *Trauma and Cognitive Science: A Meeting of Minds, Science, and Human Experience* (ed: Jennifer J. Freyd, and Anne P. DePrince) The Haworth Maltreatment & Trauma Press, an imprint of The Haworth Press, Inc., 2001, pp. 73-85. Single or multiple copies of this article are available for a fee from The Haworth Document Delivery Service [1-800-342-9678, 9:00 a.m. - 5:00 p.m. (EST). E-mail address: getinfo@haworthpressinc.com].

Document Delivery Service: 1-800-342-9678. E-mail address: <getinfo@ haworthpressinc.com> Website: <http://www.HaworthPress.com> © 2001 by The Haworth Press, Inc. All rights reserved.]

KEYWORDS. Recovered memory, false memory, sexual abuse, amnesia, delayed recall, trauma

A number of critical questions have been raised over the past decade regarding the credibility of adults' memory for their childhood experiences. These questions have been raised by members of the False Memory Syndrome Foundation (see for example, Loftus, 1993) and others, who have claimed that childhood memories are simply not reliable, and in particular, that it is relatively easy to suggestively plant memories for events that did not occur. The context for this claim is the increase in the past ten years in the number of cases of people, who in their adulthood, have recovered access to previously inaccessible memories of having been sexually abused as children. In response to these claims, parents of some of the alleged victims have asserted that they did not sexually molest their children, but that these ideas were suggested to their children by overzealous therapists, the media, or by self-help books on the topic of sexual abuse. The ensuing debate has been termed "the recovered memory/false memory debate" (Pezdek & Banks, 1996).

One step toward solving this debate would be to develop a Pinocchio test for determining whether each account relates a true or a false event, and some steps have been taken in this direction. However, although accounts of memories for true and false events tend to differ in predictable and statistically significant ways, the tools available for determining the veracity of memory accounts are far less than perfect (see Pezdek & Taylor, 2000, for a discussion of this work).

In this debate we have a classic case of two interpretations of the same effect, and the task is to discern which interpretation can best account for the available data. This is the type of problem that scientists approach on a daily basis; such problems are the driving force behind the scientific method. In this article each side of the recovered memory/false memory debate will be summarized and then some of the recent research that addresses the constraints on suggestibility in accounting for memories for abuse will be examined.

Although the type of traumatic events cited herein are primarily those related to childhood sexual abuse, it is important to remember that a range of other sources of psychogenic amnesia have also been identified (see Arrigo & Pezdek, 1997, for a recent review of this research). Psychogenic amnesia refers to a deficit in memory that is precipitated by psychological stressors rather than by organic insult, and has as its major symptom the loss of memory for information acquired normally prior to the onset of the stressors. The models, processes, and mechanisms developed to account for amnesia and recovery of memory for sexual abuse should account for psychogenic amnesia from other traumatic events as well.

At the outset, three disclaimers are warranted. First, I want to clarify that the research upon which this chapter is based is not research that involves memories for real traumatic events. It is research that has focused on isolating specific cognitive factors that affect the suggestibility of memory. This work has been conducted using controlled studies so that the underlying cognitive processes can be identified and assessed. Research on memory for real traumatic events has an important role in the field, however it does not inform the specific issue at hand. Second, although allegations of false memories have, by and large, been raised against adults, the work reported here includes research conducted with both adults and children. Third, an important factor in relating suggestibility to memory for abuse involves the time interval between the alleged event and the suggestion. Unfortunately, this factor has not received sufficient attention in the research literature.

THE RECOVERED MEMORY INTERPRETATION

According to the recovered memory interpretation, a traumatic event did actually occur, but due to the traumatic nature of the event, the event was made inaccessible for some period of time. Often some years later, often in adulthood, a triggering event stimulates memory for the event and the memory becomes accessible. There have been numerous interpretations of why traumatic events are sometimes rendered inaccessible in memory and subject to psychogenic amnesia. One interpretation is that the traumatic memory is repressed or dissociated from consciousness to defend against awareness (see, for examples, Freud, 1896 and Janet, 1904, for discussions of this position) or to maintain attachment with an individual that the victim's survival depends upon (Freyd, 1996). Another interpretation is based on the finding that active attempts to inhibit retrieval of information from memory can reduce access to that information (see Michael Anderson's article in this volume for a discussion of this notion of retrieval induced forgetting). Several neurobiological models are available as well to account for the inaccessibility of memories for traumatic events (Bremner, Krystal, Charney, & Southwick, 1996; van der Kolk, 1993).

The False Memory Interpretation

According to the false memory interpretation, a traumatic event did not actually occur. Rather, memory for the event was suggestively planted. Ordinarily the traumatic event is suggestively planted in relative close temporal proximity to when the event is actually reported. This would explain why for many years, often from childhood to adulthood, there was no memory for the event; the event simply never occurred. This interpretation is most clearly articulated by Loftus (1993). Loftus has suggested that the two major sources of false memories are popular writings, such as *The Courage to Heal* (Bass & Davis, 1988), and suggestive therapeutic techniques. According to the recovered memory interpretation, traumatic memories may occur during therapy or after exposure to self-help books on sexual abuse, because something in this material serves as an effective retrieval cue to trigger a previously inaccessible memory. On the other hand, Loftus, and those who hold the false memory interpretation, posit that traumatic memories are not triggered by this material, rather, they are suggestively planted by it.

The false memory interpretation assumes a very powerful construct of suggestibility. Given the large number of people who have reported that they recovered in adulthood traumatic memories for events such as sexual abuse that occurred in their childhood, suggestibility would have to be an extremely robust cognitive construct. Before we can adopt the false memory interpretation we need to test if the construct of suggestibility is sufficiently robust to account for this effect.

The Cognitive Construct of Suggestibility

The large majority of the cognitive research conducted on the suggestibility of memory has employed a three phase procedure modeled after methods used by, for example, Loftus (1975), Loftus, Miller, and Burns (1978), and Pezdek (1977). Using this procedure, participants first view a sequence of slides, a videotape, or a film of an event. After viewing this event, they read a narrative or are asked some questions that intentionally mislead them about the identity of a small set of target items viewed in the original event (the misled condition), or they do not receive the misleading information (the control condition). The major dependent variable in this research is the signal detection measure of d'. This measure, d', is an index of the extent to which participants can discriminate between memory for old and new information. The principal result is that participants are more accurate (i.e., higher d' values) recognizing the original target item in the control condition than in the misled condition; that is, they are misled by the postevent information presented in the narrative or questions. But, even in these laboratory experiments, typical differences in the rate of false assents to the suggested item of only 20%-30% have been reported between the misled and control conditions. And in these experiments, subjects were simply misled, for example, to believe that a stop sign was really a yield sign (Loftus et al., 1978) or that a peripheral male bystander was a female bystander (Pezdek, 1977). In reviewing this work, Lindsay (1993) reported:

> At present, we can conclude that under some conditions MPI (misleading postevent information) can impair people's ability to remember what they witness and can lead them to believe that they witnessed things they did not, but that neither of these effects is as large or robust as earlier research suggested. (p. 89)

Further, there are numerous constraints on the suggestibility of memory, constraints that in fact are related to the occurrence of childhood sexual abuse. Four of these constraints will be discussed here: (a) the familiarity of the original event, (b) whether the original event is consistent or inconsistent with expectations, (c) whether the suggestion is to change a memory or to plant a memory for the initial event, and (d) the plausibility of the suggested false event.

Suggestively Changing Memory for Familiar versus Unfamiliar Events

Pezdek and Roe (1995) recently conducted a study to test how vulnerable events are to suggestibility as a function of their familiarity. This issuc is relevant to memory for traumatic events such as sexual abuse because perpetrators of sexual abuse often repeatedly abuse a child; sexual abuse is rarely an isolated event. In this study, the typical suggestibility paradigm was used with the modification that in the presentation phase target items were presented either one or two times each. It has been demonstrated in previous studies (cf. Ebbinghaus, 1964, originally published 1885) that the strength of memory increases with the familiarity or frequency of presentation. If stronger memories are more likely to resist suggestibility than weaker memories, then the difference in recognition memory between misled and control test items would be predicted to be greater under less memorable conditions (with frequency one) than under more memorable conditions (with frequency two).

Four- and ten-year-old children viewed a slide sequence in which four target slides were presented one or two times each. The slide sequence presented an individual moving about a house performing a sequence of activities. In a postevent narrative, participants were misled about two target items, and two target items served as controls. In a subsequent recognition memory test, the hypothesis was confirmed. The d' difference between control and misled items was greater for frequency one ($d' = 3.8$ versus -2.8) than for frequency two ($d' = 5.2$ versus 1.6); stronger memories were more resistant to suggestibility than weaker memories. This pattern was consistent for both four- and ten-year-old children, indicating that similar cognitive processes underlie suggestibility at each age.

These results suggest that children are significantly more likely to be misled about unfamiliar events than about events that are more familiar to them. Generalizing to the situation of memory for childhood abuse, an event would be familiar if a child had experienced the event or a similar event multiple times. An event would be unfamiliar if it was experienced less often, or perhaps only a single time. Accordingly, if a child reports memory for multiple alleged incidents of having been abused, these memories are less likely to have been suggestively planted than if the child is reporting memory for a single such alleged incident. Of course it would also be important to evaluate the strength of the suggested information in memory relative to the strength of the original information. Zaragoza and Mitchell (1996) for example, reported that repeated exposure to suggestive questions increased adult subjects' recollection that a suggested event occurred. Accordingly, when a suggestive interview has been repeated numerous times, the strength of the suggested item may exceed that of the original item.

Suggestively Changing Memory for Events That Are Consistent or Inconsistent with Expectations

In a number of studies, it has been reported that inconsistent items are more accurately recognized than consistent items. For example, Pezdek, Whetstone, Reynolds, Askari, and Dougherty (1989) introduced adult participants to two real world environments, a graduate student's office or a preschool classroom. In each setting some of the items were consistent with expectations and some were inconsistent with expectations. Later they were given a recognition memory test in which the distractor items were different exemplars of the original items viewed. This type of recognition memory test assesses whether participants remember the physical appearance of the items viewed. Inconsistent items were recognized significantly more accurately than consistent items. This phenomenon is referred to as the consistency effect. Inconsistent information appears to be encoded into memory with more of the physical details preserved. Consistent information, on the other hand, appears to be encoded more generically with less of the physical details preserved.

If stronger memories are more likely to resist suggestibility than weaker memories, and the physical details of inconsistent events are remembered better than those of consistent events, then memory for inconsistent events should be more resistant to suggestibility than memory for consistent events. This issue is relevant to memory for traumatic events such as sexual abuse because in most home environments, sexual contact between an adult and a child would be inconsistent with children's expectations. This hypothesis was tested in a Masters Thesis by Taylor (1998).

In this study, participants were shown a slide series depicting a woman returning home and performing several specific chores. The series included two schema-consistent target items and two schema-inconsistent target items. Participants later read a post event narrative containing two misleading statements and two control statements. Each misleading statement suggested that a different item had been presented in one of the target slides. In each control statement no suggestion was made. A recognition memory test followed in which each distractor picture was identical to the matched target picture presented except that the target item in the picture (e.g., tennis shoe) was replaced by a different exemplar of that items (e.g., running shoe). It was predicted that participants would more likely be misled regarding schema-consistent than schema-inconsistent items.

The results confirmed this hypothesis. The d' data were analyzed using a 2 (consistent versus inconsistent items) $\times$ 2 (misled versus control condition) analysis of variance. Both main effects were significant in the predicted direction. In addition, the interaction of consistency with the misled versus control condition was also significant. The d' difference between the control and the misled conditions was greater in the consistent condition ($d' = 2.39$ versus .73) than in the inconsistent condition ($d' = 2.83$ versus 2.39). These findings suggest that participants were indeed more likely to be suggestively misled about schema-consistent information than about schema-inconsistent information. Our interpretation of these results is that inconsistent information is encoded in memory with more of the physical details preserved thus producing a stronger memory trace. Consequently, inconsistent information is less vulnerable to the suggestive influence of misleading information.

These findings have implications for memory for childhood abuse. For a child with no history of inappropriate and abusive contact with an alleged perpetrator, the occurrence of an abusive incident would be inconsistent with expectations. Accordingly, the child's memory for this inconsistent event would be expected to be more reliable than would be their memory for an event that is more consistent with their expectations of this person.

Suggestively Changing versus Suggestively Planting Memories

There is an important difference between the research on the suggestibility of memory using the typical suggestibility paradigm discussed above, and the situation of suggestively planting memories for events that did not occur. In the typical suggestibility paradigm, an item that was observed (e.g., a stop sign) is suggested to be a different and related item (e.g., a yield sign). However, suggestively planting memories involves the situation in which (a) an event never occurred; (b) it is later suggested that the event did occur; and then (c) memory is tested for whether the event occurred or not. There is a significant difference between the structure of these two situations that would restrict the generalization of the results regarding suggestibility obtained from the first situation (i.e., something happened and it is suggested that a different thing happened) to the second situation (i.e., nothing happened and it is suggested that something did happen).

In a recent study (Pezdek & Roe, 1997), we examined the probability of suggestibility under three conditions:

1. Event A occurred, event B was suggested (the *changed* memory condition).
2. Event A did not occur, event A was suggested (the *planted* memory condition).
3. Event A occurred, it was suggested that event A did not occur (the *erased* memory condition).

These were compared with two control conditions:

4. Event A occurred, nothing was suggested (control condition for experimental conditions 1 and 2).
5. Event A did not occur, nothing was suggested (control condition for experimental condition 3).

The two events, A and B were specific types of physical touches by the experimenter administered while each participant was read directions, a touch on the hand versus the shoulder.

The participants in each experiment were 80 4-year-old children and 80 10-year-old children. The suggestibility effect occurred only in the changed memory condition; the difference between the experimental changed condition ($d' = -.85$) and the corresponding control condition ($d' = .88$) was significant. In the erased memory condition, no suggestibility effect occurred; the d' difference between the experimental group ($d' = .19$) and the corresponding control conditions ($d' = .88$) did not approach significance. Similarly, in the planted memory condition, no suggestibility effect occurred; the d' difference between the experimental group ($d' = .44$) and the corresponding control conditions ($d' = 1.68$) did not approach significance. Thus, although it is relatively easy to suggest to a child a change in an event that was experienced, it is less likely that an event can be planted in or erased from memory. It is thus inappropriate to generalize regarding the probability of suggestively planting false memories based on the typical suggestibility research that has largely been restricted to the study of suggestively changing memories.

So, what evidence is there that events can be suggestively planted in memory? One of the most highly cited study in the psychological literature this decade is the "lost-in-a-shopping-mall study" by Loftus and Pickrell

(1995). In this study, 24 volunteers suggested to offspring or younger siblings that they had been lost in a shopping mall when they were about 5 years old. Six of the 24 subjects reported either full or partial memory for the false event. The results of this study are frequently cited to support the claim that false memories can be planted with ease. Similarly, Hyman, Husband, and Billings (1995) asked college students about their memory for numerous true events and two false events. The percentage of subjects who recalled the false events as real was 20% in Experiment 1 and 25% in Experiment 2. Ceci, Huffman, Smith, and Loftus (1996) read preschool children a list of true and false events and asked them to "think real hard about each" event and "try to remember if it really happened." In the initial session, 44% of the children age 3 to 4 years old and 25% of the children age 5 to 6 years old remembered at least one of the false events, however, with repeated suggestions over seven sessions, there was a significant 7% increase in false assents for older children but an 8% decrease in the incidence of false assents for the younger children. Nonetheless, these studies demonstrate that it is possible to suggestively plant false events in memory.

Suggestively Planting Plausible versus Implausible Events

Although it is clear that some events can be suggestively planted in memory, it is not clear what factors affect the probability of suggestively planting false memories. In a study that we recently conducted (Pezdek, Finger, & Hodge, 1997), we investigated a specific factor that affects the probability of suggestively planting a false event in memory, the plausibility of the event attempting to be suggestively planted. Plausibility is relevant to memory for traumatic events such as sexual abuse because for most children, sexual contact with an adult is undoubtedly an implausible event.

This study tested the hypothesis that events will be suggestively planted to the degree that they are plausible and script-relevant knowledge exists in memory. This hypothesis is derived from the notion that an asserted event must first be evaluated as true before it can be incorporated into autobiographical memory, and if an event is implausible, it is not likely to be evaluated as true. Further, it should be easier to form a memory trace for an event that is plausible and about which one has a well-developed generic script than to form a memory trace for an event that is implausible and about which one does not have a generic script.

In Experiment 1, 22 Jewish and 29 Catholic high school students were read descriptions of three true events and two false events reported to have occurred when they were eight years old. One false event described a Jewish ritual, and one described a Catholic ritual. Results for the false event showed the predicted asymmetry: Whereas seven Catholics but zero Jews remembered only the Catholic false event, three Jews but only one Catholic remembered only the Jewish false event. Two subjects recalled both events.

Experiment 2 provided an additional test of the hypothesis that events will be suggestively planted in memory to the degree that they are plausible and script-relevant knowledge exists in memory, and specifically tested the generalizability of the results of Loftus and Pickrell (1995). The false event suggested by Loftus and Pickrell was being lost in a shopping mall at about the age of 5. We contend that this event is familiar to most people, and therefore should be relatively easy to plant in memory. Children are often warned about the dangers of getting lost, have fears about getting lost, read classic tales about children who get lost (e.g., Hansel and Gretel, Snow White and the Seven Dwarfs, Pinocchio, Goldilocks and the Three Bears), and often do get lost, if only for a few frightening minutes.

In Experiment 2, each of 20 confederates tested the memory of a younger sibling or close relative (the subject). The mean age of the subjects at the time of this study was 28.5 years. Confederates read descriptions of three events that they reported had happened when the subjects were 5 to 6 years old. Subjects were asked to recall everything they could remember about each event. One event was true; two events were false. One false event, an incident very similar to that used by Loftus and Pickrell (1995), described the subject being lost in a mall while shopping with a parent (the relatively plausible event). The other false event described the subject receiving a rectal enema for constipation (the relatively implausible event). Because much of the research on planting false memories is used to evaluate the probability of planting false memories for childhood sexual abuse, we selected a false event that approaches this experience. This particular false event was suggested because, like sexual abuse, being given a rectal enema is shameful and embarrassing and involves discomfort to a private part of the body. The results are simple: Only three events were falsely remembered; all were the more plausible event regarding being lost in a mall while shopping.

Pezdek and Hodge (1999) replicated the above study with children in two age groups, five to seven years of age and nine to twelve years of age, to see if plausible events were more likely to be suggestively planted with children as well as with adults. The children were read descriptions of two true events and two false events, reported to have occurred when they were four years old. The plausible false event described the child lost in a mall while shopping; the implausible false event described the child receiving a rectal enema. The majority of the 39 children tested (54%) did not remember either false event. However, whereas 14 children recalled the plausible but not the implausible false event, only one child recalled the implausible but not the plausible false event; this difference was statistically significant. Three additional children (all in the younger age group) recalled both false events.

Together, these two studies indicate that with children as well as adults, false memories are more likely to be planted if they involve events that are relatively plausible. As demonstrated by Pezdek and Hodge (1999) and Pezdek et al. (1997) in Experiment 2, although it may be relatively less effortful to plant a false memory that someone had been lost in a mall when he or she was a child, it is more difficult to plant a false memory in someone that he or she had received a rectal enema as a child. Because the findings of Loftus and Pickrell (1995) are frequently applied to cases involving adults' memory for childhood sexual abuse (Loftus, 1993), it is especially important to empirically consider the appropriateness of this generalization.

CONCLUSIONS

Several conclusions follow from the experiments presented here. First, surely there have been some false memories for sexual abuse and other traumatic events that have been suggestively planted, whatever their cause. And surely some therapeutic techniques are more likely to support false memories than others. Also, it is surely possible to find some individuals who are so suggestible that it is possible to get them to believe almost anything. But the claim of those who promote the false memory interpretation, that is, that it is relatively easy to plant memories for childhood sexual abuse and other traumatic events that did not occur, assumes an extremely strong construct of suggestibility, one that is just not supported by the data.

The results presented here demonstrate that suggestibility is not an especially robust phenomenon. Yes, researchers have obtained 20-30% reductions in the likelihood that someone thought they saw a yield sign when they had in fact seen a stop sign, but even this probability is substantially reduced with events that are experienced more frequently, with events that are inconsistent with expectations, and with implausible events. Also, although it is relatively easy to suggest that a stop sign was really a yield sign, it is relatively more difficult to plant a memory for an event that did not occur at all, especially if the event is an implausible one. In conclusion, suggestibility does not appear to be a sufficiently strong cognitive construct to explain the delayed recall phenomenon considered here.

REFERENCES

Arrigo, J. M., & Pezdek, K. (1997). Lessons from the study of psychogenic amnesia. *Current Directions in Psychological Science, 6,* 148-152.

Bass, E., & Davis, L. (1988). *The courage to heal.* New York: Harper & Row.

Bremner, J. D., Krystal, J. H., Charney, D. S., & Southwick, S. M. (1996). Neural mechanisms in dissociative amnesia for childhood abuse: Relevance to the current controversy surrounding the "false memory syndrome." *American Journal of Psychiatry, 153,* 71-82.

Ceci, S. J., Huffman, M. L. C., Smith, E., & Loftus, E. F. (1996). Repeatedly thinking about a non-event: Source of misattributions among preschoolers. In K. Pezdek, & W. P. Banks (Eds.). *The recovered memory/false memory debate* (pp. 225-244). San Diego: Academic Press.

Ebbinghaus, H. F. (1964). *Memory: A contribution to experimental psychology.* New York: Dover. (Original work published 1885).

Freud, S. (1896). The aetiology of hysteria. In J. Strachey (Ed. & Trans.). *The standard edition of the complete psychological works of Sigmund Freud* (Vol. 3, pp. 191-221). New York: Norton.

Freyd, J. J. (1996). *Betrayal trauma: The logic of forgetting childhood abuse.* Cambridge, MA: Harvard University Press.

Hyman, I. E., Jr., Husband, T. H., & Billings, F. J. (1995). False memories of childhood experiences. *Applied Cognitive Psychology, 9,* 181-197.

Janet, P. (1904). Amnesia and the dissociation of memories by emotion. *Journal de Pschologie, 1,* 417-453.

Lindsay, D. S. (1993). Eyewitness suggestibility. *Current Directions in Psychological Science, 2,* 86-89.

Loftus, E. F. (1975). Leading questions and the eyewitness report. *Cognitive Psychology, 7,* 560-572.

Loftus, E. F. (1993). The reality of repressed memories. *American Psychologist, 48,* 518-537.

Loftus, E. F., Miller, D., & Burns, H. (1978). Semantic integration of verbal information into a visual memory. *Journal of Experimental Psychology: Human Learning and Memory, 4,* 19-31.

Loftus, E. F., & Pickrell, J. E. (1995). The formation of false memories. *Psychiatric Annals, 25,* 720-725.

Pezdek, K. (1977). Cross-modality semantic integration of sentence and picture memory. *Journal of Experimental Psychology: Human Learning and Memory, 3,* 515-524.

Pezdek, K., & Banks, W. P. (1996). *The recovered memory/false memory debate.* San Diego: Academic Press.

Pezdek, K., Finger, K., & Hodge, D. (1997). Planting false childhood memories: The role of event plausibility. *Psychological Science, 8,* 437-441.

Pezdek, K., & Hodge, D. (1999). Planting false childhood memories in children: The role of event plausibility. *Child Development, 70,* 887-895.

Pezdek, K., & Roe, C. (1995). The effect of memory trace strength on suggestibility. *Journal of Experimental Child Psychology, 60,* 116-128.

Pezdek, K., & Roe, C. (1997). The suggestibility of children's memory for being touched: Planting, erasing, and changing memories. *Law and Human Behavior, 21*, 95-106.

Pezdek, K., & Taylor, J. (2000). Discriminating between accounts of true and false events. In D. F. Bjorklund (Eds.), *False memory creation in children and adults: Theory, Research, and Implications,* 69-91. Mahawah, NJ: Lawrence Erlbaum and Associates.

Pezdek, K., Whetstone, A., Reynolds, K., Askari, N., & Dougherty, T. (1989). Memory for real world scenes: The role of consistency with schema expectation. *Journal of Experimental Psychology: Learning, Memory and Cognition, 15*, 587-595.

Taylor, J. K. (1998). *The suggestibility of memory for consistent versus inconsistent information.* Unpublished master's thesis, Claremont Graduate University, Claremont, CA.

van der Kolk, B. (1993). Biological considerations about emotions, trauma, memory and the brain. In S. Ablon, D. Brown, E. Khantzian, & J. Mack (Eds.), *Human feelings: Explorations in affect development and meaning* (pp. 221-240). Hillsdale, NJ: Analytic Press.

Zaragoza, M. S., & Mitchell, K. J. (1996). Repeated exposure to suggestion and the creation of false memories. *Psychological Science, 7*, 294-300.

The Role of the Self
in False Memory Creation

Mark A. Oakes
Ira E. Hyman, Jr.

SUMMARY. People will create false memories of childhood experiences. In this article, the research that demonstrates the creation of false memories is first described. Three processes that may be involved in memory creation are then outlined. First, individuals must accept a suggested event as plausible. Second, they construct an image and narrative of the false event. Third, they incorrectly attribute the source of the event to personal memory rather than external suggestion. We argue that the self plays a role in each of these processes. In addition, because memories are important components of the self, when memories change, the self changes as well. *[Article copies available for a fee from The Haworth Document Delivery Service: 1-800-342-9678. E-mail address: <getinfo@haworthpressinc.com> Website: <http://www.HaworthPress.com> © 2001 by The Haworth Press, Inc. All rights reserved.]*

KEYWORDS. Recovered memory, false memory, traumatic memory, amnesia, delayed recall

Can people create false memories of childhood experiences? Can people forget traumatic childhood experiences and many years later recover memories of the event? Often these two questions are presented as conflicting explana-

Address correspondence to: Ira E. Hyman, Jr., Psychology Department, Western Washington University, Bellingham, WA 98225 (E-mail: hyman@cc.wwu.edu).

[Haworth co-indexing entry note]: "The Role of the Self in False Memory Creation." Oakes, Mark A., and Ira E. Hyman, Jr. Co-published simultaneously in *Journal of Aggression, Maltreatment & Trauma* (The Haworth Maltreatment & Trauma Press, an imprint of The Haworth Press, Inc.) Vol. 4, No. 2, (#8), 2001, pp. 87-103; and: *Trauma and Cognitive Science: A Meeting of Minds, Science, and Human Experience* (ed: Jennifer J. Freyd, and Anne P. DePrince) The Haworth Maltreatment & Trauma Press, an imprint of The Haworth Press, Inc., 2001, pp. 87-103. Single or multiple copies of this article are available for a fee from The Haworth Document Delivery Service [1-800-342-9678, 9:00 a.m. - 5:00 p.m. (EST). E-mail address: getinfo@haworthpressinc.com].

tions of an individual discovering a childhood memory: The memory is either a false memory created in response to suggestions or a true memory recovered during adulthood (e.g., Pezdek, this issue). While the recovered memory versus false memory dichotomy may describe the quandary for any one individual, it is a false dichotomy for memory researchers. Both recovered memories and false memories occur. In this article, we will describe research investigating the creation of false childhood memories and present an overview of the processes involved in memory creation. We focus particularly on the role that the self plays in the creation of false memories.

Self is a complex set of perceptions, memories, and knowledge. James (1890) argued that the self included the physical body, the objects to which applies the term "my," the social responses made by others, one's recollections, one's thoughts and emotions, and that sense of "I" that does the thinking. Self and memory are intricately interwoven. Memory forms part of our sense of self (James, 1890; Neisser, 1988). Many clinical theorists (e.g., Adler, 1956; Spence, 1982) have argued that the memories a person chooses to recall define the individual's life. In addition, James (1890) noted that autobiographical memories provide a sense that current experience of self is continuous with the past. The self as remembered also provides for an extension of the self into the future (Neisser, 1988). Without autobiographical memories, there is no sense of where the self is going and no clear ability to plan for the future (Hirst, 1994).

Although memory contributes to our understanding of the self, the self also plays an important role in memory. Some have argued that the self is special, either because it is the central focus of autobiographical memory (Greenwald, 1980) or because we have direct access to forms of knowledge, such as thoughts and emotions, about our selves that are not directly available about others (Hyman & Neisser, 1992). At the very least, the self concept is a large set of knowledge and information that is processed in reference to the self, and is better remembered than other information (Greenwald & Banaji, 1989; Klein & Kihlstrom, 1986; Kuiper & Rogers, 1979; Rogers, Kuiper, & Kiker, 1977). Thus we will explore how various connections to the self contribute to the creation of false memories and how false memories may contribute to one's understanding of self.

We will explore the connections between the self and false memories through first describing some of the research on false childhood memories. We will then turn to a consideration of the processes involved in false memory creation. We will end with a consideration of how both recovered memories and false memories may change someone's understanding of the past, plans for the future, and thus the self. The creation of memories is a normal process. Remembering is always a constructive process, whether the content of memory is a word list, a song, a short story, or one's autobiography.

Remembering is also a social activity (Hyman, 1994) and is open to social influence (Hyman, 1999). Thus the normal activity of remembering will lead to errors. To the extent that the self is defined by memories, the self will also be a construction built through social discourse.

FALSE CHILDHOOD MEMORIES

Since remembering is a constructive process, researchers have often demonstrated errors in memory. For example, in response to suggestions, people will alter their memory for an aspect of an event, they will come to believe that they saw a stop sign rather than a yield sign in a series of slides they viewed. The events used in studying memory errors are usually unemotional and do not involve the self. Thus, there was good reason to wonder if people would create more extensive memory errors for emotional events that involve the self. Since thinking of new information in terms of the self aids memory (Greenwald & Banaji, 1989; Klein & Kihlstrom, 1986; Kuiper & Rogers, 1979; Rogers et al., 1977), self involvement in events may lead to stronger memories that are less open to suggestion. Yuille and Cutshall (1986) argued that errors will rarely be observed in memory for emotional events that involve the self. The goal of the researchers was to extend the exploration of memory errors: Will people create a complete memory, that involved the self, and that was somewhat emotional, although never traumatic?

Researchers studying the creation of false childhood memories have generally used a common methodology (Ceci, Huffman, Smith, & Loftus, 1994; Ceci, Loftus, Leichtman, & Bruck, 1994; Hyman & Billings, 1998; Hyman, Husband, & Billings, 1995; Hyman & Pentland, 1996; Loftus & Pickrell, 1995; Pezdek, Finger, & Hodge, 1997). For the most part, researchers request from family members information about events that occurred during the participant's childhood. The participant is then asked to try to recall these true events along with a false event, an event that the researchers are fairly sure did not happen to the participant. During a series of interviews the false event is presented as if it is also a true event that was obtained from the initial family solicitation. The participants are usually told that their memories will improve over time. The most meaningful result of this sort of study is how the participants respond to the false event: Do the participants come to believe that the event took place sometime during their childhood?

In order to clarify how researchers study false memories, we expand on one example of this basic approach to studying the creation of false childhood memories. In Hyman et al.'s (1995) second experiment, the researchers obtained from parent surveys descriptions of true childhood events involving introductory psychology students. When the parents returned the questionnaires, the researchers asked the students to participate in a series of interviews investigating their memory for early childhood experiences. The students were told that the goal was to see how completely and accurately they could recall childhood. In each of three interviews (separated by one day), the students were asked to remember several true events plus one false event. For all events, the interviewer provided the students with a basic description (including age, event, a few actions, other people involved, and a location) and asked the students what they remembered about the event. Three different false events were used in this study. One was called the punch bowl event: when you were 6 years old, you were at the wedding of a friend of the family, you were running around with some other kids when you bumped into the table the punch bowl was sitting on, and spilled punch on the parents of the bride. All of the false events were self-involving: the student was an active participant in the event and was asked to recall his or her own behavior. In addition, the events would have been somewhat emotional at the time of the event, although none were traumatic events. Spilling punch would have been embarrassing or funny or perhaps angering, depending on the individuals involved, but would not have been life-threatening nor involve long-term consequences.

The participants recalled a majority of the true events in the first interview and remembered even more of the true events over time. There are two ways to explain the increased recall of the true events. First, by thinking about the events over a period of time, the students provided themselves with additional memory cues that led to the recollection of previously unretrieved memories. Another possibility is that the participants created, rather than recalled, memories that matched the cues provided to them in the interviews. We cannot say whether this recovery of memory for the true experiences represents actual memories or the creation of memories.

Regarding the false events, no participants remembered the false event on its initial presentation. However, by the third interview 25% of the students remembered the event. Six students reported memories that were very clear and included the critical information (such as turning over the punch bowl) as well as consistent elaborations (such as their parents being upset). Five of the reports were less clear; the students included little of the critical suggested information although they elaborated in a consistent fashion. Two of the students created clear images, but they were not positive about whether they were remembering or simply imagining the events that had been suggested to them. Although Hyman et al. (1995) used only college students in their study, other studies using varying populations (e.g., preschool children, adults, teenagers) and different false events have found similar results (Ceci, Huffman et al., 1994; Ceci, Loftus et al., 1994; Loftus & Pickrell, 1995; Pezdek et al., 1997).

With greater pressure, the proportion of individuals who create false memories increases. Hyman and Pentland (1996) also asked college students to remember childhood experiences reported by their parents. When the students failed to remember an event, whether true or false, they were asked to imagine the event and describe their image. After three interviews, nearly 40% remembered spilling the punch bowl by the third interview.

Nonetheless, questions of generalizability still remain. Spilling a punch bowl at a wedding is not the same as being sexually abused. To this point, no researcher has attempted to have participants create memories of being sexually abused. For ethical reasons, it is unlikely that anyone ever will; if a memory impacts one's self concept and family relationships whether the memory is true or false, then experimentally inducing such memories would be atrocious. In addition, most studies of false childhood memories rely on the authority of the researchers and the parents who provided the information. We do not know how authority affects the acceptance of false memories and the willingness to construct memories. Generalizing to realistic situations will always be somewhat difficult. We believe that a general model of the processes involved in memory creation may help bridge the gap between research and practice. With a better theory of how memories are created, we can better understand the aspects of realistic situations that may increase or decrease the likelihood of false memory creation. For this reason, in the next section, we outline a theory of the processes involved in memory creation.

Three Processes Involved in Memory Creation

Hyman and Kleinknecht (1999) have described three processes that may be involved in the creation of false childhood memories: (1) plausibility judgments, (2) memory construction, and (3) source monitoring errors (i.e., identifying the constructed narrative as a personal memory). In order for a person to create a false memory, the suggested event needs to be plausible. In other words, the event needs to be something that the person believes could have happened to them. A person can believe that an event is likely, or even that the event occurred, but must still construct a memory; an image with a narrative. All autobiographical memories are constructed by combining schematic knowledge from various sources with personal experiences, suggestions, and current demands. Even if a person believes an event is plausible and constructs an image of the event, he or she still may not think that the image is a personal memory. In order to have a false memory, the participants must make a source monitoring error, they must claim the image as a personal memory. Many studies have shown that people experience difficulties remembering the source of information they have learned (see Johnson, Hastroudi, & Lindsay, 1993). The critical final error in false childhood memory cases is that the individual claims the suggestion and constructed image is a personal memory rather than just an image.

Although the processes of plausibility judgment, memory construction, and source monitoring error may occur in a linear fashion and be dependent on the preceding step, we suspect that the processes are somewhat interactive. For example, constructing a clear image may influence one's assessment of the plausibility of an event having occurred (Garry, Manning, Loftus, & Sherman, 1996). It is more correct to state that all three processes are necessary for false memory creation and that they are somewhat independent in the sense that different factors and individual differences may influence each process. In addition, we argue that making connections to the self will increase the likelihood of errors in each process. Thus, in the following pages, we describe these three processes and discuss the role of the self in each.

Plausibility Judgments. If a person is to create a false memory, then the person must first consider the suggested event plausible. For example, some of the participants in the studies in our lab did not create memories of spilling a punch bowl at a wedding because they believed that they had never attended a wedding as child (Hyman & Billings, 1998; Hyman et al., 1995; Hyman & Pentland, 1996). They refused to accept the event as a plausible personal experience. Plausibility is not, however, something that is automatically associated with an event. Instead, it is a judgment that people make based on various types of information.

Pezdek et al. (1997) demonstrated the importance of the event in plausibility judgments. In two studies they asked participants to recall true events and false events that varied in plausibility. In Experiment 1, they manipulated event plausibility based on religious background. They found that individuals were more likely to create memories for events that matched their religious background than events that did not (for a Catholic, an event involving communion as opposed to an event involving Shabbat). In Experiment 2, they manipulated plausibility by suggesting two different false events: (1) being lost, the plausible event, and (2) receiving an enema, the less plausible event. They found a tendency for people to be more likely to create a memory of being lost than a memory of receiving an enema. In both cases, Pezdek et al. argued that events that are more plausible are more likely to result in false memories.

Plausibility is not simply a matter of the event. Since plausibility is a judgment, several factors may influence whether a person sees an event as plausible. The source of the suggestion may affect plausibility assessments: The more reliable the informant the more plausible the event will seem. Whether a certain type of information is considered more plausible (e.g., scientific data vs. cultural theory) or whether the person supplying the information is critical (e.g., professor vs. undergraduate student) ultimately rests with the person's views and opinions.

In addition, group membership also may affect plausibility. If new people are introduced to a group with members similar to themselves on some dimension (common problems, experiences, world views, etc.), and if all of the other members of the group have similar childhood memories that the new members lack, then this may make the experience more plausible for the new members. This seems particularly likely if the experience is important for the group. In this case, the group's memories act as the feedback that people who share common characteristics are likely to have had a certain class of experiences. Perhaps this could provide an individual without memories of abuse, who participates in a group of survivors of sexual abuse, feedback that sexual abuse is a plausible experience for him or her.

Plausibility judgments may also depend on whether the event matches with an individual's view of the general likelihood of a class of experiences. For instance, many people do not consider abduction by extraterrestrials a likely event, while for others this may be an event that they consider relatively common. Spanos, Cross, Dickson, and DuBreuil (1993) found that belief in alien visitations was the primary variable that differentiated people who claimed memories of UFO experiences from individuals who did not claim such experiences. Thus judgments about the general frequency of an event will influence plausibility judgments. How this may impact beliefs about the plausibility of abuse is unclear. Some individuals may believe that abuse is a rare event while others may hear statistics that a surprising number of people experienced abuse in childhood.

The point we have tried to stress is that it is possible to manipulate people's plausibility judgment that a suggested event occurred. For example, consider again those students who doubted they attended a wedding and thus did not create a memory of spilling a punch bowl at a wedding. In such a case, the experimenter could manipulate the participant's judgment of the event plausibility by suggesting some reasons for their "erroneous" belief that they did not attend a wedding: perhaps the student repressed memories of weddings, or perhaps the parents were embarrassed and thus never talked about it. In addition, suggestions that the experience is not only generally likely, but also personally likely will increase willingness to believe an event may have occurred. In this fashion, studies using false feedback (e.g., Kelley, Amodio, & Lindsay, 1996) may be effective in part because the researchers provided reasons for the participants to believe that an experience occurred to them.

For this reason, one line of research in our lab has investigated how plausibility judgments can be manipulated. Our basic goal is to provide people reasons to believe that certain events are likely to have occurred to them. We do this by connecting childhood events that occur rarely to personality characteristics that we tell them they possess: tying the suggested event to the self. Thus, our investigations of plausibility judgments are based on an extension of the Barnum effect.

In a classic investigation of the Barnum effect, individuals take a personality test and are later provided feedback supposedly based on the test. The feedback is not, however, based on the personality test. Instead, all partici-pants receive identical feedback containing statements that are vague, and generally socially desirable and positive. The typical finding is that most individuals rate the resulting personality description as describing them. The effect is powerful and can be used as a teaching tool to demonstrate how people blindly accept the results of psychological tests (Forer, 1949) and horoscopes (Glick, Gottesman, & Jolton, 1989), and easily leads to a discussion of ethics in research (Beins, 1993). In addition, the effect itself has been used to under-stand a variety of situations in which people accept test results as plausible and subsequently diagnose themselves (c.f. Goodyear, 1990).

Our lab's research on plausibility judgments began as a Barnum type study (Hyman, Chesley, & Thoelke, 1997). We went into a large introductory Psychology class and administered two personality tests: The Rotter Locus of Control Scale (1966) and the Eysenck Personality Inventory (Eysenck & Eysenck, 1968) that assesses Neuroticism and Extroversion and includes a Lie scale. These scales were used because previous research has found that acceptance of a Barnum description is related to an External Locus of Control and to higher scores on Neuroticism. The students were told that we were investigating the relationships between personality and autobiographical memory. One week later all students were provided with a packet containing their "individual" feedback and a follow-up questionnaire on autobiographical memory. There were 104 students who completed the study (58 females, 46 males, mean age = 19.05, SD = 1.09). The students were asked to read their personality description and rate how well it described them on a 7-point scale from "does not describe me" (1) to "describes me very well" (7). To this point, the experiment was a standard Barnum-effect demonstration.

After the students had rated the personality description, they were asked to respond to the autobiographical memory questionnaire: this was the exten-sion we added to the standard Barnum methodology. All students were told that the autobiographical memory questionnaire included some events that we thought were likely to have happened to them, and other events that we thought were unlikely to have happened to them based on their personality type. This was the connection we made to the self. To the extent that the students accepted the personality feedback, this gave the students a reason to believe the events were personally plausible. All students were given 10 events that we told them were likely to have occurred based on their personal-ity type and 10 that we stated were unlikely based on their personality type. The events were counter-balanced across packets so that half the students received one set of ten likely and unlikely events and these were reversed for the remainder of the students. The students rated each event on a 7-point scale from "did not happen" (1) to "did happen" (7). The events we used were selected based on a pilot survey to find events that are unlikely to have occurred to students at Western Washington University. Although these students are typical middle-class college students, what counts as infrequent childhood events may vary with the background of the participants. For example, we found that Western Washington University students were unlikely to have jumped off a roof before age 10 and unlikely to have cried on the first day of kindergarten.

The first thing to note is that most of the students rated the personality feedback as a good fit. The mean rating on the 7-point scale was 5.27 (SD = 1.13), and the distribution was negatively skewed so that 84 of the 104 students rated the description as a five or higher and only two individuals gave a rating of one or two.

Although there was an overall tendency for individuals to rate the events we told them were likely as more plausible than the events we stated were unlikely, the effect was clearest for individuals who accepted the personality feedback. There was a significant correlation such that individuals who rated the personality feedback as a better description of themselves rated the events we told them were more likely as more plausible (r = .316, p = .001). Those individuals who accepted the personality feedback, also accepted the plausibility of the events that we tied to that self-description.

We also found that acceptance of the personality profile and the plausibility ratings of events were correlated with some of the actual personality measures. Acceptance of the personality profile was significantly correlated with neuroticism (r = .323, p = .001). The plausibility ratings of the events were related to the Rotter Locus of Control scale (1966), such that scores closer to the external end of the scale were related to higher plausibility ratings (r = .193, p = .049). In addition, the plausibility ratings of the likely events was also related to neuroticism (r = .317, p = .001) and negatively related to the lie index (r = −.194, p = .049).

As Pezdek and her colleagues (Pezdek, this issue; Pezdek et al., 1997) noted, event plausibility is important in the creation of false memories. Plausibility is not, however, a feature of the event, instead it is a judgment that can be manipulated. A crucial factor in plausibility judgments is the connection of the childhood event to the self. In our Barnum study, we showed that connecting events to personality feedback, whether accurate or not, led people to believe the events were more likely to have occurred.

Memory Construction

Once an individual accepts the event as plausible, she or he must construct a memory for the event. Several factors contribute to memory construction. For example, when people imagine false experiences, they are more likely to create memories (Goff & Roediger, 1998; Hyman & Pentland, 1996). In addition, social pressure may contribute to memory construction when people are told they will remember more over time or are repeatedly pressured to remember an event. Any activity that encourages people to engage in narrative creation will contribute to memory construction. Thus, when people are asked to write about an event or to describe an event in more detail, they are constructing elaborations that become part of the event description.

A disconcerting finding in the recent research on various forms of memory errors is that factors that have traditionally been found to increase memories for events seem to also increase false memories. For example, mental imagery aids memory and increases the likelihood of memory creation. Countless studies have documented that imagining the words in a list aids in remembering the items in the list (Goff & Roediger, 1988). Various imagery techniques, such as the method of loci, are staples in chapters of cognitive textbooks that focus on memory improvement strategies. When these imagery techniques are applied to false memories, they seem to aid the strength of the false memory as well (Garry et al., 1996; Goff & Roediger, 1998; Hyman & Pentland, 1996).

The self may play a similar role in memories and false memories. Generally, thinking about the connection between the self and the items in a list improves memory for the list (Greenwald & Banaji, 1989; Klein & Kihlstrom, 1986; Kuiper & Rogers, 1979; Rogers et al., 1977). In addition, information that is generated by the individual is remembered better than the same information when provided by someone else (Ross & Sicoly, 1979; Slamecka & Graf, 1978). Thus, connecting information to the self improves memory.

The self, however, also plays a critical role in the construction of memories. Greenwald (1980) argued that the ego is one of the primary biasing forces in memory. The self selects consistent information for memory and often revises the past in a favorable light (Ross & Sicoly, 1979). Ross (1989) argued that the past is constructed based on current views of the self and beliefs about whether or not things have changed during the intervening time. If one thinks of oneself in some fashion and believes that things have not changed during the last few years, then one constructs a past consistent with the present. In contrast, if a person holds a current view and believes that things have gotten worse during the last ten years, then the individual constructs a past that was much better than the present. Clearly the self is important in autobiographical memories (Hyman & Neisser, 1992).

What would be the consequence of thinking about the self when confronted with a false memory? Hyman and his colleagues (Hyman & Billings, 1998; Hyman et al., 1995) found that participants often thought and talked about the self when presented with a false childhood event. Thus they classified individuals by how the individuals responded to the false event (spilling a punchbowl at a wedding) in the first interview. They grouped people based on whether or not they connected a false event to the self. Some individuals made a connection between the false event and their life experiences; they speculated about where the wedding would have been or who would have been there, they noted that they were the type of children who would have done something like that, or they talked about weddings they remembered attending. Other individuals did not connect the false event to any aspect of their selves or their past. Participants who made such connections of the false event to the self were much more likely to create a false memory.

One explanation of this finding is to focus on the role of the self in memory construction. When individuals are asked about the false event in subsequent interviews, they construct a memory based on the false suggestion and the self-relevant knowledge they activated in the first interview. This construction is then a composite of true self-knowledge and the false event.

Source Monitoring Errors. To complete the creation of a false memory, an individual must accept the constructed memory as a personal memory. The person must fail to accurately attribute the narrative and image to the false suggestion. Johnson and her colleagues (Johnson et al., 1993; Johnson, Foley, Suengas, & Raye, 1988) have argued that the content of the memory determines the source to which individuals attribute the memory. When a memory comes to mind with clear sensory details, people assume that it is a real event that is being re-experienced. In contrast, if a memory comes to mind with information about cognitive processing, such as knowledge of imagining the event, then people are less likely to attribute the experience to memory. Various aspects of the remembering context may also affect source monitoring decisions. For example, feedback from others may lead people to accept the narrative as a personal memory.

In support of source monitoring theory, Johnson et al. (1988) asked people to rate childhood memories and false childhood experiences they imagined on a variety of measures. Johnson et al. found that people rated the sensory qualities of memories as more clear than those of imagined experiences. Based on Johnson's source monitoring theory (Johnson et al., 1993; Johnson et al., 1988), Hyman, Gilstrap, Decker, and Wilkinson (1998) investigated how people make source judgments for autobiographical knowledge. They first asked people to briefly describe a childhood event they remembered and one they knew but did not remember (the distinction is based on Tulving, 1985). The participants then rated the remember and know events on several dimensions. As predicted from source monitoring theory, the events people claimed to remember were rated as having more sensory detail and emotion.

In further work, Hyman et al. (1998) and Wilkinson and Hyman (1998) found that source judgments can be manipulated. They asked people to first describe a childhood event that they knew but did not remember. The participants were then asked to elaborate on the sensory details and their emotional response. When people imagined the experience, Hyman and his colleagues expected them to develop the sensory qualities of their knowledge of the event. At the end, the participants rated the extent to which they remembered the experience. Compared to participants who did not imagine the experience, those who imagined a "known" experience rated their re-experiencing of the event as being closer to something they remembered.

The self may also matter in source monitoring judgments. The more the self is involved in a memory, the more likely people will claim the memory as a personal recollection, as something they remember. In part, this claim follows directly from Tulving's (1985) definition of what it means to remember. Remembering is re-experiencing an event. To re-experience is to have the self's original experience re-created in the current conscious awareness. The more the self is involved in that experience, the more likely it will be judged a memory.

There is also some support for the claim that the self will influence source monitoring judgments. First, several researchers (e.g., Barclay & DeCooke, 1988; Conway, Collins, Gathercole, & Anderson, 1996) have found support in diary studies of autobiographical memory. In these studies, individuals are presented with real events from their diaries and distractors created by the researchers. The closer the distractor is to typical self events, the more likely that people will falsely claim to remember the event. Second, Conway and Dewhurst (1995) found that when people perform self-relevant processing while encoding a list of words, they not only recall more words on the list, but also are more likely to claim to remember the presentation of the word rather than report that they simply know the word was on the list. Thus the more the self is involved in the re-experiencing of an event, the more likely a person will attribute the source to memory.

CONCLUSION

People will create false memories of childhood experiences. Individual differences, the nature of the event, and the context all contribute to memory creation. Applying these findings to counseling and other interview situations is difficult. The events and the contexts differ. Recently, researchers have expanded our understanding of the contexts in which people will create false memories (Kassin & Kiechel, 1996; Mazzoni, Loftus, Seitz, & Lynn, 1999; Spanos, Burgess, Burgess, Samuels, & Blois, 1999). Nonetheless, researchers will never duplicate all clinical settings nor should they ever suggest traumatic events as potential false memories.

For this reason, we have emphasized a set of processes that may be involved in memory creation. To the extent that any situation involves conditions that increase event plausibility, encourage memory construction, and discourage careful source monitoring, that situation will increase the risk of memory creation. We suspect that the self plays an important role in each process. Connecting a false event to something about the self, real childhood memories or current self-conceptions, will make the event more plausible. The self and self-relevant autobiographical knowledge provide pieces for memory construction. When a memory contains a re-experiencing of the self, that memory will more likely be judged real.

Although the self may contribute to the creation of false memories, memories also contribute to our understanding of ourselves. Memories are important components of the self, both for defining the self in the past and projecting the self into the future (James, 1890; Neisser, 1988; Neisser & Fivush, 1994). When memories change, the self changes as well. In addition, new memories may also alter one's understanding of others and of possible futures. If a person comes to believe that he or she was abused as a child, this is a change that may have negative impacts on the self. Finding abuse memories would alter anyone's self conception, even individuals who experienced a less than ideal childhood may find child abuse a qualitative change in their understanding of their past. This is clear when considering the narratives of individuals who recover memories of abuse (e.g., Bass & Davis, 1988; Pendergrast, 1995). The abuse becomes a part of how these people define themselves, something they must integrate with their life stories.

The impact of discovered memories will be felt whether the events truly were experienced, forgotten and only recently remembered, or whether the memories have been created via memory construction. This is important to note, just as people can recover memories of traumatic childhood experiences, they can also create false memories. Pendergrast (1995) told the stories of individuals who have discovered memories that were later confirmed by external sources and of individuals who recovered memories that they eventually came to believe were false. In both cases, the self-concept was dramatically affected as people began to think of themselves as abuse survivors. In both cases, relationships with family members were affected. People can not reliably distinguish between recovered true memories and created false memories (Hyman & Pentland, 1996; Johnson et al., 1997). What people know is that the memories become their memories, thus, they act on the memories they possess. The self and family relationships are reshaped by the new memories.

These changes in self-concept and relationships with others are justified when the recovered memories are of events that actually happened. In contrast, if the individual has created false memories, then the changes are a catastrophic error. The individual develops a false sense of self based on events that never occurred. The individual interrupts relationships with important individuals for a false cause. This is the argument that has been played out in many families and in court cases across the country for the last several years. Individuals recover memories of abuse; they rewrite their personal narrative and change their relationships based on the memories.

Families often contend that the memories are false, that they are the result of suggestions and social pressure. Families argue that they have been wrongfully cut off from children, siblings, and grandchildren. In the absence of some evidence external to memory, it is difficult, if not impossible, to know which narrative corresponds to historical truth. The inability to differentiate between false memories and historically accurate memories raises the question of how to balance historical and narrative truth (Spence, 1982).

Although these cases are dramatic, they exist because they are instances of how human memory functions. Memory is always constructed. What we remember will be constructed from residual information and from general schematic knowledge structures. In addition, memory construction takes place within a social context and in response to social pressures. Thus the memories we construct reflect the suggestions and stories told by others. Many of our childhood memories may actually be stories that we heard others, such as parents or siblings, tell. Unable to remember for ourselves, we accept these stories as highly plausible. We then imagine the stories. Perhaps, we eventually adopt the image and story as our own memory and forget the source of the image. Much of the past is constructed in a social environment. This may explain how individuals fail to remember or come to mislabel abuse, perhaps they have adopted the story of the perpetrator (see Hyman & Kleinknecht, 1999). As Hyman and Pentland (1996) suggested, life is an ongoing misinformation experiment, in which the outcome is a self that is memory's illusion.

REFERENCES

Adler, A. (1956). *The individual psychology of Alfred Adler.* New York: Basic Books.

Barclay, C.R., & DeCooke, P.A. (1988). Ordinary everyday memories: Some of the things of which selves are made. In U. Neisser & E. Winograd (Eds.), *Remembering reconsidered: Ecological and traditional approaches to the study of memory* (pp. 91-125). New York: Cambridge University Press.

Bartlett, F. C. (1932). *Remembering: A study in experimental and social psychology.* Cambridge: Cambridge University Press.

Bass, E., & Davis, L. (1988). *The courage to heal: A guide for women survivors of child sexual abuse.* New York: Harper & Row.

Beins, B. C. (1993). Using the Barnum Effect to teach about ethics and deception in research. *Teaching of Psychology, 20,* 33-35.

Ceci, S. J., Huffman, M. L. C., Smith, E., & Loftus, E. F. (1994). Repeatedly thinking about non-events. *Consciousness and Cognition, 3,* 388-407.

Ceci, S. J., Loftus, E. F., Leichtman, M. D., & Bruck, M. (1994). The possible role of source misattributions in the creation of false beliefs among preschoolers. *International Journal of Clinical and Experimental Hypnosis, 42,* 304-320.

Conway, M. A., Collins, A, F., Gathercole, S. E., & Anderson, S. J. (1996). Recollections of true and false autobiographical memories. *Journal of Experimental Psychology: General, 25*, 69-95.

Conway, M. A., & Dewhurst, S. A. (1995). The self and recollective experience. *Applied Cognitive Psychology, 9*, 1-19.

Eysenck, H. J., & Eysenck, S. B. G. (1968). *Eysenck personality inventory.* San Diego, CA: Educational and Industrial Testing Service.

Forer, B. R. (1949). The fallacy of personal validation: A classroom demonstration of gullibility. *Journal of Abnormal and Social Psychology, 44*, 118-123.

Garry, M., Manning, C. G., Loftus, E. F., & Sherman, S. J. (1996). Imagination inflation: Imaging a childhood event inflates confidence that it occurred. *Psychonomic Bulletin & Review, 3*, 208-214.

Glick, P., Gottesman, D., & Jolton, J. (1989). The fault is not in the stars: Susceptibility of skeptics and believers in astrology to the Barnum Effect. *Personality and Social Psychology Bulletin, 15*, 572-583.

Goff, L. M., & Roediger, H. L., III (1998). Imagination inflation for action events: Repeated imaginings lead to illusory recognition. *Memory & Cognition, 26*, 20-33.

Goodyear, R. K. (1990). Research on the effects of test interpretation: A review. *The Counseling Psychologist, 18*, 241-257.

Greenwald, A. G. (1980). The totalitarian ego: Fabrication and revision of personal history. *American Psychologist, 35*, 603-618.

Greenwald, A. G., & Banaji, M. (1989). The self as a memory system: Powerful, but ordinary. *Journal of Personality and Social Psychology, 57*, 41-54.

Hirst, W. (1994). The remembered self in amnesiacs. In U. Neisser & R. Fivush (Eds.), *The remembering self: Construction and accuracy in the self-narrative* (pp. 252-277). New York: Cambridge University Press.

Hyman, I. E., Jr. (1994). Conversational remembering: Story recall with a peer vs. for an experimenter. *Applied Cognitive Psychology, 8*, 49-66.

Hyman, I. E., Jr. (1999). Creating false autobiographical memories: Why people believe their memory errors. To appear in E. Winograd, R. Fivush, & W. Hirst (Eds.), *Ecological approaches to cognition: Essays in honor of Ulric Neisser.* Hillsdale, NJ: Erlbaum.

Hyman, I. E., Jr., & Billings, F. J (1998). Individual differences and the creation of false childhood memories. *Memory, 6*, 1-20.

Hyman, I. E., Jr., Chesley, C. A., & Thoelke, R. S. (1997, November). *False memories: False personality feedback affects plausibility judgments.* Paper presented at the meeting of the Psychonomic Society. Philadelphia, PA.

Hyman, I. E., Jr., Gilstrap, L. L., Decker, K., & Wilkinson, C. (1998). Manipulating remember and know judgments of autobiographical memories: An investigation of false memory creation. *Applied Cognitive Psychology, 12*, 371-386.

Hyman, I. E., Jr., Husband, T. H., & Billings, F. J. (1995). False memories of childhood experiences. *Applied Cognitive Psychology, 9*, 181-197.

Hyman, I. E., Jr., & Kleinknecht, E. E. (1999). False childhood memories: Research, theory, and applications. In L. M. Williams, & V. L. Banyard (Eds.), *Trauma and memory* (pp. 175-188). Thousand Oaks: Sage.

Hyman, I. E., Jr., & Neisser, U. (1992). The role of the self in recollections of a seminar. *Journal of Narrative and Life History, 2*, 81-103.

Hyman, I. E. Jr., & Pentland, J. (1996). The role of mental imagery in the creation of false childhood memories. *Journal of Memory and Language, 35*, 101-117.

James, W. (1890). *Principles of Psychology.* New York: Holt.

Johnson, M. K., Foley, M. A., Suengas, A. G., & Raye, C. L. (1988). Phenomenal characteristics of memories for perceived and imagined autobiographical events. *Journal of Experimental Psychology: General, 117*, 371-376.

Johnson, M. K., Hastroudi, S., & Lindsay, D. S. (1993). Source monitoring. *Psychological Bulletin, 114*, 3-28.

Johnson, M. K., Nolde, S. F., Mather, M., Kounios, J., Schacter, D. L., & Curran, T. (1997). The similarity of brain activity associated with true and false recognition memory depends on test format. *Psychological Science, 8*, 250-257.

Kassin, S. M., & Kiechel, K. L. (1996). The social psychology of false confessions: Compliance, internalization, and confabulation. *Psychological Science, 7*, 125-128.

Kelley, C., Amodio, D., & Lindsay, D. S. (1996, July). *The effects of 'diagnosis' and memory work on memories of handedness shaping.* Paper presented at the International Conference on Memory, Padua, Italy.

Klein, S. B., & Kihlstrom, J. F. (1986). Elaboration, organization, and the self-reference effect in memory. *Journal of Experimental Psychology: General, 115*, 26-38.

Kuiper, N. A., & Rogers, T. D. (1979). Encoding of personal information: Self-other differences. *Journal of Personality and Social Psychology, 37*, 499-514.

Loftus, E. F., & Pickrell, J. E. (1995). The formation of false memories. *Psychiatric Annals, 25*, 720-725.

Mazzoni, G. A. L., Loftus, E. F., Seitz, A., & Lynn, S. J. (1999). Changing beliefs and memories through dream interpretation. *Applied Cognitive Psychology, 13*, 125-144.

Neisser, U. (1988). Five kinds of self-knowledge. *Philosophical Psychology, 1*, 35-59.

Neisser, U., & Fivush, R. (Eds.) (1994). *The remembering self: Construction and accuracy in the self-narrative.* New York: Cambridge University Press.

Pendergrast, M. (1995). *Victims of memory: Incest accusations and shattered lives.* Hinesburg, Vermont: Upper Access, Inc.

Pezdek, K., Finger, K., & Hodge, D. (1997). Planting false childhood memories: The role of event plausibility. *Psychological Science, 8*, 437-441.

Rogers, T. D., Kuiper, N. A., & Kiker, W. S. (1977). Self-reference and the encoding of personal information. *Journal of Personality and Social Psychology, 35*, 677-688.

Ross, M. (1989). The relation of implicit theories to the construction of personal histories. *Psychological Review, 96*, 341-357.

Ross, M., & Sicoly, F. (1979). Egocentric biases in availability and attribution. *Journal of Personality and Social Psychology, 37*, 322-336.

Rotter, J. B. (1966). Generalized expectancies for internal versus external control of reinforcement. *Psychological Monographs, 91* (1, Whole No. 609).

Slamecka, N. J., & Graf, P. (1978). The generation effect: Delineation of a phenomenon. *Journal of Experimental Psychology: Human Learning and Memory, 4*, 592-604.

Spanos, N. P., Burgess, C. A., Burgess, M. F., Samuels, C., & Blois, W. O. (1999). Creating memories of infancy with hypnotic and non-hypnotic procedures. *Applied Cognitive Psychology, 13*, 201-218.

Spanos, N. P., Cross, P. A., Dickson, K., & DuBreuil, S. C. (1993). Close encounters: An examination of UFO experiences. *Journal of Abnormal Psychology, 102*, 624-632.

Spence, D. P. (1982). *Narrative truth and historical truth: Meaning and interpretation in psychoanalysis.* New York: Norton.

Tulving, E. (1985). Memory and consciousness. *Canadian Psychology, 26*, 1-12.

Wilkinson, C., & Hyman, I. E., Jr. (1998). Individual differences related to two types of memory errors: Word lists may not generalize to autobiographical memory. *Applied Cognitive Psychology, 12*, S29-S46.

Yuille, J. C., & Cutshall, J. L. (1986). A case study of eyewitness memory of a crime. *Journal of Applied Psychology, 71*, 291-301.

Discovering Memories of Abuse in the Light of Meta-Awareness

Jonathan W. Schooler

SUMMARY. Discovered memories of abuse are often viewed with marked skepticism due to the relative dearth of well-corroborated evidence for their occurrence and the absence of a compelling theory to explain them. This article addresses these concerns by reviewing seven recovered (or, as will be explained, what I prefer to term "discovered") memory cases in which there was independent corroborative evidence for the alleged abuse. These cases are considered within the context of a theory of meta-awareness that assumes that experiential consciousness (i.e., the contents of phenomenological experience) can be distinct from meta-awareness (i.e., one's consciousness of their consciousness). In this context, discovered memories can be understood as involving changes in individuals' meta-awareness of the abuse. In some cases, discovered memories may involve *the gaining of a different meta-awareness* of the meaning of an experience. The discovery of this new meaning may become confused with the discovery of the memory itself, leading to the (sometimes erroneous) belief that the memory is just now being accessed for the first time. In other cases, the discovery may involve *the regaining of a prior meta-awareness* of the experience that either deliberately or non-deliberately may have been avoided for

The following individuals provided extremely helpful comments on earlier drafts of this article: Sonya Dougal, Christopher Brewin, Jennifer Freyd, David Halpern, Larry Jacoby, Marcel Kinsbourne, Elizabeth Loftus, J. Don Read, Daniel Wegner, and Timothy Wilson.

Address correspondence to: Jonathan W. Schooler, Learning Research and Development Center, 3939 O'Hara Street, University of Pittsburgh, Pittsburgh, PA 15260 (E-mail: Jonathan Schooler <schooler+@pitt.edu>).

[Haworth co-indexing entry note]: "Discovering Memories of Abuse in the Light of Meta-Awareness." Schooler, Jonathan W. Co-published simultaneously in *Journal of Aggression, Maltreatment & Trauma* (The Haworth Maltreatment & Trauma Press, an imprint of The Haworth Press, Inc.) Vol. 4, No. 2 (#8), 2001, pp. 105-136; and: *Trauma and Cognitive Science: A Meeting of Minds, Science, and Human Experience* (ed: Jennifer J. Freyd, and Anne P. DePrince) The Haworth Maltreatment & Trauma Press, an imprint of The Haworth Press, Inc., 2001, pp. 105-136. Single or multiple copies of this article are available for a fee from The Haworth Document Delivery Service [1-800-342-9678, 9:00 a.m. - 5:00 p.m. (EST). E-mail address: getinfo@haworthpressinc.com].

some time. In still other cases, the discovery may actually involve *the gaining of a previously non-existent meta-awareness* of the experience. A variety of factors ranging from the very straightforward (e.g., age, lack of discussion, stress) to the more esoteric (e.g., dissociation, nocturnal cognitive processing) may prevent incidents of abuse from being initially encoded with meta-awareness. Such non-reflected memories, particularly when they are aschematic and disjunctive with other experiences, may continue to elude meta-awareness until a specific (and potentially obscure) contextual retrieval cue is encountered. Once recalled in the alarming light of meta-awareness, individuals may understand what happened to them, and this discovery may fundamentally change their view of their personal histories. *[Article copies available for a fee from The Haworth Document Delivery Service: 1-800-342-9678. E-mail address: <getinfo@haworthpressinc.com> Website: <http://www.HaworthPress. com> © 2001 by The Haworth Press, Inc. All rights reserved.]*

KEYWORDS. Child abuse, sexual abuse, forgetting, amnesia, recovered memory, repressed memory

Revisiting memories from the distant past is much like rummaging through one's attic. We may be bemused by small forgotten items but we are rarely shocked by the major things we encounter. Occasionally, however, people report being truly stunned when they discover significant and disturbing recollections lurking in their memory. For example, Schooler (1994) described the case of JR who, after grappling with unpleasant feelings that followed a movie involving sexual abuse, suddenly recalled being molested by a priest as an adolescent. JR was reportedly "stunned" by this discovery noting, "If you had done a survey of people walking into the movie theater when I saw the movie . . . asking people about child and sexual abuse 'have you ever been, or do you know anybody who has ever been,' I would have absolutely, flatly, unhesitatingly said 'no.'"

What could lead to the belief that one had discovered a previously forgotten memory of something as significant as being sexually molested in one's youth? In some cases, such memories may be sincere but fallacious, the unfortunate product of therapists' overly suggestive techniques combined with patients' overly eager imaginations. (For discussions of the very real dangers of false recovered memories resulting from therapy see Lindsay & Read, 1994; Loftus & Ketcham, 1994; Schooler, Bendiksen, & Ambadar, 1997). In other cases, however (such as that of JR's for which corroborative evidence of abuse was obtained), these memories are likely to correspond to actual events. Although some have questioned whether so-called "recovered memories" are ever genuine (e.g., Ofshe & Waters, 1994; Pope & Hudson, 1995), there is growing agreement that they can (at least sometimes) correspond to actual events (e.g., Andrews et al., 1999; Cheit, 1997; Chu, Frey, Ganzel, & Matthews, 1999; Dalenberg, 1996; Duggal & Stroufe, 1998; Kluft, 1998; Lindsay & Briere, 1997; Schacter, 1996; Schooler, 1994, 2000b; Schooler, Bendiksen et al., 1997; Williams, 1995). There remains, however, little consensus regarding the frequency with which recovered memories are authentic or the mechanisms that could lead one to characterize a generally veridical memory as recovered. Indeed, one of the major impediments towards more general acceptance of this phenomenon has been the dearth of compelling theories that might explain how individuals could seemingly lose track of such significant components of their autobiographical memory. The development of theoretical accounts has in turn been hampered by the modest number of well-documented cases, the unique difficulties in corroborating prior forgetting, and the variability of those cases that have been documented. Given these constraints, it is simply infeasible at present to provide an airtight account of the processes that lead individuals to report discovering long forgotten recollections of actual abuse. What is possible, and indeed needed, is an analysis of current evidence within the context of a theoretical account that could (at least in principle) explain how such remarkable discoveries might arise. Towards this end, the present article describes a recent line of case-based research that I and my colleagues (Schooler, 1994, 2000b; Schooler, Ambadar, & Bendiksen, 1997; Schooler, Bendiksen et al., 1997) have been developing to further flesh out the evidence for, and conditions surrounding recovered, or (as will be explained, what I prefer to term) "discovered" memories of abuse. I then introduce two theoretical constructs that may contribute to the process by which individuals conclude that a traumatic memory had previously been entirely forgotten. These include: (a) dissociations between consciousness and meta-awareness, the notion that individuals can be conscious of an experience without being explicitly aware of their appraisal of that experience; and (b) discovery misattribution, the notion that individuals may confuse the source of the phenomenological experience of discovery. Finally, I revisit the previously described cases within the context of these theoretical constructs. The bottom line argument is that the perception that one has remembered a forgotten memory of abuse may result from the sense of discovery that results from changes in individuals' meta-awareness of the abuse experience.

DISCOVERED MEMORIES

Before proceeding, it is necessary to define the term used to describe traumatic memories that are characterized as having been completely forgotten and then later remembered. Such memories are most commonly referred to as either "repressed" or "recovered"; however, both labels are problematic. The term "repressed" confounds a phenomenon (remembering seemingly forgotten trauma) with a mechanism (a dynamic unconscious defense mechanism that is hypothesized actively to keep the memory from consciousness). The term "recovered" though clearly preferable, implies that the memory had been completely lost and was then subsequently found. However, as will be argued, there are both empirical and theoretical reasons to believe that individuals may have profound discovery experiences in which a new understanding of the memory and/or appreciation of the emotion surrounding it is confused with a discovery of the memory itself. Such confusions regarding what exactly has been discovered may lead individuals to conclude erroneously that the memory had previously been entirely inaccessible. I therefore prefer the term "discovered memory," which keeps open the possibility that individuals could have discovery experiences for memories that were not, at least in some sense, entirely forgotten. The term "discovered" also maintains agnosticity regarding the precise mapping between what is discovered and what actually occurred (i.e., individuals could, in principle, discover memories that are entirely veridical, entirely false, or somewhere in between).

The notion that individuals may discover memories that were never entirely forgotten also has important implications for conceptualizing the type of corroboration that can substantiate discovered memories. Specifically, it suggests that individuals may reasonably be characterized as having authentic discovered memories if they can be shown to: (a) be in possession of memories corresponding to actual events, and (b) sincerely believe that they had discovered long lost memories. Importantly, this definition de-emphasizes the importance of documenting actual forgetting. This is helpful because documentation of forgetting is very difficult if not impossible for a number of reasons. Since remembering is often a personal process, it is simply not clear how one could ever document that a memory had never come to mind. Moreover, theoretically, even if a memory had not come to mind for some period, it is still difficult to distinguish whether it was truly unavailable, or, like many memories from our distant past, simply did not have occasion to be remembered. Although it is quite difficult to find evidence retrospectively to confirm forgetting, it is possible to find evidence that can challenge individuals' accounts of their forgetting. Indeed, in several cases that we have investigated, individuals believed that they had been amnesic for their abuse during a period of time in which others reported that they had talked about it. Importantly, despite their apparent errors in characterizing their forgetting, these individuals still very much perceived their memories as profound discoveries.

With respect to corroborating the actual abuse and the perception of a discovery, it is important to emphasize that for both components, corroborate does not mean to prove. Just as a particular experimental result can support a scientific hypothesis without "proving" it, so, too, corroborative evidence can strengthen historical claims without providing incontrovertible documentation. There are a variety of types of evidence that can corroborate reported memories of abuse, including medical records, confessions, witnesses to the fact, etc. In the cases that my colleagues and I have investigated, the corroboration of the abuse has come from independent interviews with other individuals who reported either (a) learning about the victims' abuse soon after it occurred, (b) having also been abused by the accused individual, or (c) having personally heard a confession from the alleged perpetrator. Of course, the memories of corroborators might also be in error. However, if such corroborative reports involve longstanding memories, then they are less vulnerable to the concern that they were the products of a recent suggestion. Indeed, even those who are generally skeptical of recovered memories do not question the abuse recollections of individuals who report having maintained longstanding intact memories of abuse (Loftus, 1994). In short, if the recollections of individuals who report discovered memories of abuse can be corroborated by others who have maintained intact memories, then we may have greater confidence that the discovered memories correspond to actual events.[1]

With respect to establishing that individuals perceive themselves to have discovered a previously unknown memory, such perceptions can be documented through interviews in which individuals describe their recollections of their discovery experience and their beliefs about their prior forgetting. Of course, particularly in cases where some time has passed since the memory was first "discovered," it is possible that individuals' recollections of their discoveries might evolve. For example, they might come to believe that they were originally more shocked at the discovery than they actually were. At a minimum, however, individuals' self-reports can establish that individuals *now* perceive themselves to be in possession of a discovered memory.

The Cognitive Corroborative Case-Based Approach

With the above definitional and evidentiary considerations, my collaborators and I (Schooler, 1994, 2000b; Schooler, Ambadar et al., 1997; Schooler, Bendiksen et al., 1997) have sought to investigate cases of individuals who reported discovering seemingly forgotten memories of abuse. These cases were identified through modest networking and are not in any sense a representative sample. In each case, we sought to document the individuals' characterization of their memory as discovered, and if they recalled the specific situation surrounding the discovery experience. We also sought independent corroboration of the abuse (usually by contacting other individuals who the victim indicated had prior knowledge of either the abuse itself or the abusive tendencies of the alleged perpetrator), and when possible, evidence that might speak to the nature of the intervening forgetting. Six of these cases, or subsets thereof, have been described previously (Schooler, 2000b; Schooler, Ambadar et al., 1997; Schooler, Bendiksen et al., 1997). Case 7 is a new and especially compelling case that has not been reported before.

Case 1: JR (a 39-year-old male) reported discovering a memory of being fondled by a priest during a camping trip at age eleven and subsequently discovering memories of additional incidents of abuse that took place over the next several years. He reported discovering the initial memory at age 30 while lying in bed one night after seeing a movie involving sexual abuse. His characterization of the discovery was as follows: "I was stunned, I was somewhat confused you know, the memory was very vivid and yet . . . I didn't know one word about repressed memory." The corroboration: Another individual reported that the same priest had abused him. Although this individual only made his accusation after JR had discovered his memory, he indicated that he had maintained an intact memory of being abused by this priest.

Case 2: MB (a 40-year-old female) reported discovering a recollection of being raped while hitchhiking at age seventeen. She reported that the discovery experience occurred when she was thirty-four years old after she heard a friend refer to a young woman as "certainly not a virgin." Her recollection of the discovery experience was that she experienced "complete chaos in my emotions. . . . I was overwhelmed, rather than surprised, surprised is too neutral a feeling for what I felt." The corroboration: An individual who was told about the rape the day it occurred confirmed MB's original recounting of the experience.

Case 3: TW (a 51-year-old female) reported discovering a memory at the age of twenty-four of being fondled by a family friend at age nine. She reported that the recollection was triggered after a friend suggested that they hear a talk on sexual abuse. Her characterization of the discovery was as follows: "When I first remembered it I was surprised. Completely taken back by it. Then I . . . I don't even remember speaking . . . I was completely out of it." The corroboration: TW's former husband reported that she had talked about the abuse several times prior to this memory discovery experience.

Case 4: DN (a 41-year-old female) reported discovering a memory of being raped in a hospital at the age of nineteen and then taking the case to court. She discovered the memory at age thirty-five, while driving home several hours after her group therapist remarked that survivors of childhood abuse, which DN had maintained an intact memory of being, often are victimized as adults. Her characterization of the discovery experience was as follows: "I had to just sit there for a while because it was just this extreme emotion of fear and total disbelief. Disbelief that it happened, disbelief that I could have forgotten something that traumatic." The corroboration: DN's former lawyer confirmed that the case had gone to court and that the perpetrator was found guilty.

Case 5: JN (31-year-old female) reported discovering a memory of being molested at age five. The discovery experience occurred when she was eighteen, soon after she became sexually active. JN recalled describing her discovery to her boyfriend soon after discovering the memory: "I just have a recollection of talking about it with him, and talking about the fact that I didn't . . . I remembered this thing happening but I had never remembered it." The corroboration: JN's mother confirmed that this event, as relayed by her older sister at the time, did happen.

Case 6: CV (a 52-year-old female) reported discovering a memory of being molested and exposed to masturbation by her stepfather at age ten. This memory discovery experience occurred during several cleanings of her bathroom at the age of twenty-seven. On one occasion CV described it as "a horrible picture [that] popped into my mind . . . it was like a photo. . . . I felt sickened and shocked that I would think of such a disgusting thing." Although CV reported dismissing the initial recollection, during a subsequent cleaning the memory reportedly returned and this time she could not dismiss it: "That horrible picture came into my mind but this time it did not go away . . . a whole reel of pictures started running through my head . . . . I was terrified." The corroboration: Her sister stated that she had also been abused by the stepfather and had maintained intact memories of the abuse, although she had never discussed it with CV.

Case 7: DJ (a 28-year-old female) reported discovering memories of being regularly sexually abused by a neighbor over a period of 3 years, from ages 5-7. The alleged abuse included genital fondling, genital rubbing, and attempted although unsuccessful sexual intercourse. As DJ described it, "He would perform sexual acts in front of me, or ask me to perform sexual acts to him . . . it was not normal sex, it wasn't just sexual, it was very kind of sick." DJ reported that the memory discovery experience occurred when she was 16 and saw the person at a dinner party. She characterized the memory discovery as follows: "I was very shocked by the memory, I was very overwhelmed I think would be the word. That's a lot to remember." The corroboration: The mother described a meeting in which the alleged perpetrator was confronted and he admitted the abuse, as well as abusing six or seven other girls.

The above cases demonstrate that it is at least sometimes possible to corroborate the abuse associated with memories that are clearly perceived to have been discovered. Indeed, one of the striking qualities of the characterizations of these memory discoveries is how much they share the phenomenological properties of major personal discoveries. Like classic insight experiences (see Schooler & Melcher, 1995), the phenomenology of the discovery of abuse is characterized by suddenness, immediate unpacking, and an emotional onrush. With respect to the suddenness of the experience, JR described the discovery as occurring "fairly suddenly." WB described a "sudden and clear picture." TW noted that "the whole thing was evident and immediate to me." DN observed that "all at once I remembered." As DJ observed, "It came all of a sudden." With respect to the immediate unpacking, TW observed, "It was like . . . a package of some sort . . . something there that's completely unwound instantly, and not only the experience but the sequel of the experience." DN recounted, "All at once I remembered . . . not only that I had been a victim, but that I had to go to court." CV described this unpacking as occurring visually, noting, "Suddenly a whole reel of pictures started running through my mind." DJ distinguished it from other recollection experiences noting, "Most memory I've had when I recalled . . . there is sort of a layering system . . . and this was literally like all of those layers of memory hitting me at once."

The emotional impact of the experience was also observed in the majority of cases. JR described his experience as being "stunned." WB noted "complete chaos in my emotions." DN characterized her reaction as "just this extreme emotion of fear and disbelief," and DJ observed, "It was literally like a brick wall just hit me. . . . I just started crying and screaming uncontrollably." Admittedly this is only a small sampling of cases, and it is certainly likely that other cases may be associated with different phenomenological reports. Nevertheless, the consistent role of discovery that we have found in the set of corroborated cases we have investigated supports the contention that the sense of discovery can be an important element of the phenomenon.

Underlying the sense of discovery is the perception that one had no knowledge of having been abused before the memory discovery experiences. In six of the seven cases, individuals were absolutely confident that they had no knowledge whatsoever of having been abused. As already noted, JR believed that if he had been asked, prior to his discovery, whether he had ever been abused, he would "have absolutely, flatly, unhesitatingly said 'no'." Similarly, TW described the state of her memory before the discovery as "none . . . non-existent." ND remarked, "It's like how could I forget this. As horrible as it was having to go to court . . . and having to tell what happened and everything how could I forget that. I had no idea when I did forget it but I really feel that it had been totally forgotten until that night." And DJ observed, "I am absolutely sure that I forgot about it. . . . I remember feeling some intuitive weirdness about like sex. . . . I definitely never linked it to a memory."

In one case WB (who was raped while hitchhiking) largely believed that she had been entirely amnesic although she did vacillate on this point a bit. When asked whether there was ever a time in which she would have honestly believed that she had not been raped had she been asked directly, she replied, "I actually think this is the case. When I wrote my story about rape I can honestly say I had absolutely no connection to the fact that it had been a personal experience. I was writing it 'on behalf of others.' I thought this is what it must be like for those who experience rape." Nevertheless, she also added the cautionary note "I am really uncertain how I would have responded if someone had asked me directly" [whether she had ever been raped].

Although it was generally believed in all of the cases that the memories had been forgotten, in two cases there was rather compelling evidence of a misconstrual of prior forgetting. In both the cases of TW and WB the victim's ex-husband reported discussing the event with the victim during times in which each had believed that the memory had been forgotten. In both of these cases the individuals were truly shocked to discover that they had been aware of and had talked about the abuse. TW described her reaction upon learning that she had previously told her husband about the abuse in the following manner: "I felt like falling over. Absolutely shocked and floored that it happened. And I still am . . . I can't remember telling him, I can't think of anything about the memory before [the recovery], and it's very disturbing, actually." Similarly, when asked if she was surprised to learn that she had talked about the abuse experience with her husband years after it had occurred, WB exclaimed, "Very much so!"

The fact that individuals can believe that they had forgotten abuse at a time at which they are known to have been aware of it suggests that individuals may, at least sometimes, become confused about exactly what they are discovering. Rather than discovering the existence of the memory itself, these individuals may be discovering the emotionally disturbing understanding of the experience. Nevertheless, because of the profound sense of discovery, individuals may conclude that they must have just remembered a long inaccessible memory. We have previously termed this phenomenon of underestimating prior knowledge of an experience as the "forgot-it-all-along effect," in deference to the related "knew-it-all-along effect" in which individuals over-estimate their prior knowledge (Fischhoff, 1982). As will be seen, the notion that discovered memories may represent changes in individuals' awareness of the meaning of the experience may provide a core premise by which to understand memory discovery experiences more generally. I now turn to a discussion of such an approach.

A META-AWARENESS THEORY
OF DISCOVERED MEMORIES

As noted, one central impediment to the general acceptance of discovered memories has been the absence of cognitively-grounded mechanisms that could explain such discoveries. Clearly, given the limitations of the currently available evidence, any account of discovered memories must be considered tentative at this time. Nevertheless, in the following discussion I will offer a basic framework for understanding discovered memories that although speculative, is consistent with the available data and current cognitive theories (broadly conceived). Towards this end, I first introduce two theoretical constructs: (1) the dissociation between experiential consciousness and meta-awareness, and (2) discovery misattribution, which may help to provide a foundation for understanding discovered memories. I then consider how these constructs may help to account for the various types of discovered memories that have emerged from case analyses such as the ones described above.

DISSOCIATIONS BETWEEN EXPERIENTIAL CONSCIOUSNESS AND META-AWARENESS

A central element of most characterizations of discovered memories is the notion that an event that was experienced with great intensity becomes completely inaccessible to consciousness, only later to re-emerge abruptly. If we take this claim seriously, then we need to explain how events of such significance could seem to slip in and out of consciousness. Although clearly fundamental, this question may presuppose an overly simplistic dichotomy between conscious and nonconscious knowledge. Specifically, there is a third level of consciousness that may be especially important in the context of discovered memories, namely, one's awareness of what he or she is conscious about. Variations on the distinction between one's ongoing conscious experience and one's explicit understanding of that experience have been made by countless philosophers and a number, although perhaps somewhat fewer, psychologists. Although subtle differences in distinctions abound, what I am terming *experiential consciousness* generally corresponds to what others have referred to as "phenomenal consciousness" (Block, 1992); "phenomenological awareness" (Allport, 1988); "perceptual consciousness" (Armstrong, 1981); or "transitive consciousness" (Rosenthal, 1990). What I am terming *meta-awareness* roughly corresponds to what others have referred to as "introspective consciousness" (Armstrong, 1981); "intransitive consciousness" (Rosenthal, 1990); "representation redescription" (Karmiloff-Smith, 1995); and, most commonly in the psychological literature, "self-awareness" (Duval & Wicklund, 1972; Gibbons, 1990; Lewis, 1991; Stuss, 1991); and "reflective awareness" (Bradley, Hollifield, & Foulkes, 1992; Zoltan, 1999).

Given the existence of these various prior distinctions, the reader may reasonably ask whether it is helpful to introduce yet further terminology, and if so, why I have introduced the specific term "meta-awareness." The two closest, commonly-used terms are probably "reflective awareness" and "self-awareness." However, self-awareness has the additional connotation of awareness of one's personal identity, and reflective awareness has the additional connotation of engaging in active deliberation. In addition, the term meta-awareness naturally fits within the broader cognitive construct of meta-cognition (one's knowledge of one's knowledge), and naturally links to related constructs such as meta-memory (one's knowledge of one's memory). In prior discussions (Schooler, 2000a; Schooler, Loewenstein, & Ariely, 2000), I used the term "meta-consciousness" to refer to one's explicit awareness of conscious experience. The terms "awareness" and "consciousness," although possessing slightly different denotations, are typically used interchangeably, largely depending on which "sounds better" in a particular context. In the future, it may prove useful to formally delineate a distinction between the terms "meta-consciousness" and "meta-awareness," or it may suffice to continue to use them interchangeably. In the present context, however, I have found that the term "meta-awareness" seems better suited, and have used it accordingly.

Although the distinction between the basic experience of consciousness and one's explicit awareness of the contents of that experience is sometimes made, it is more often forgotten. Typically, cognitions are classified as either conscious or unconscious. We tend to overlook the many instances in which we are conscious of a thought, yet not meta-aware that we are having it. This dissociation is well illustrated by an all too familiar example. Imagine that you are reading a very important and difficult paper that you must understand completely. Despite your best intentions at some point during the reading you realize that for the last several minutes (or more!) you have not been attending to the text but rather have been engaged in a vivid daydream of an upcoming vacation. Your experience of the daydream conjures up detailed perceptual images of hot sand, blue waters, and cool breezes. In short, you are clearly experientially conscious of the contents of your daydream. Nevertheless you are not meta-aware of the fact that you are daydreaming. Otherwise, you would not have continued to read the very important paper that you know you are responsible for completely understanding. Although readers surely vary in the frequency with which they catch themselves in these flights of fancy, everyone to whom I have mentioned this phenomenon has conceded (typically with a sheepish grin) that they are all too familiar with the experience.

A critical component of the daydreaming-while-reading example is the jolt of meta-awareness that one experiences upon discovering the lapse. It is much like waking up from sleep, except it is a shift to meta-awareness rather than consciousness. In this moment, one becomes both meta-aware of one's current state of consciousness (i.e., typically a sense of annoyance at having to go back) and retrospectively meta-aware of one's prior state of conscious-

ness (i.e., vivid daydreaming). The daydreaming case is a particularly illus-
trative example of a pervasive fact of everyday life, namely, that although our
sentient experience is continuous, our awareness of our awareness is discontinuous. Sometimes we are explicitly attending to what we are doing, but
often we are not. In the daydreaming case, we are fully engaged in our
musing, and yet we fail to realize that we are daydreaming, as evidenced by
the fact that we continue to read. In other cases, the dissociation between
consciousness and meta-awareness may be less poignant, but perhaps no less
pronounced. For example, in social situations, we often engage in exchanges
without explicitly reflecting on our interpretation of the interaction. Indeed,
our ability to suspend meta-awareness (or self-consciousness as it is referred
to in such situations) is the hallmark of comfortable social situations. Unfortunately, such suspensions of reflections can also lead to awkward sudden
resumptions of meta-awareness (the "foot-in-the-mouth" effect).

The notion that we are often not explicitly aware of the contents of our
thought is consistent with a growing body of research on implicit cognition
and automaticity that has documented the surprising degree to which we are
not explicitly aware of our goals (Bargh & Chartrand, 1999), interpretations
(Wilson, Lindsey, & T. Schooler, 2000), or the bases of our actions (Wegner &
Wheatley, 1999). Critically, however, and in contrast to many characterizations of automaticity, the distinction between experiential consciousness and
meta-awareness does not necessarily imply that we carry out automatic mental activities unconsciously. Rather, we may experience our own internal
states like drivers experience the road, with sentience but without reflection
(Bower, 1990), only taking stock of our thoughts when things get difficult.

Lapses in our carrying out of our intended goals (Reason & Mycielska,
1982), as when we discover that we are not thinking about what we intended
to be thinking about (e.g., the daydreaming example), are perhaps the most
common trigger for meta-awareness. However, the most striking elicitors of
meta-awareness occur when we realize the consequentiality of truly significant events, such as births, deaths, and traumas. Such experiences typically
force us to take stock of our emotional state, to reflect on our interpretation of
the experience, and to communicate our impressions of our reactions to
others. Indeed, the propensity of really significant experiences to elicit meta-
awareness may explain why traumatic experiences tend to be remembered
rather well (Brown & Kulik, 1977), though far from perfectly (e.g., McCloskey, Wible, & Cohen, 1988), and why we find it so surprising that such
experiences could ever be forgotten. Interestingly, although serious events
typically elicit meta-aware reflection, they do not always do so at the time the
event is occurring. Often during very demanding serious events such as
avoiding a car accident or engaging in rescue efforts, individuals report that
they just acted on the moment, and did not explicitly think about their reac-

tion to it until afterwards. For other less significant experiences we may be even more likely to consider only "what the experience was like" in retrospect, if we consider it at all. Of course, our recollections of the past are not necessarily reflective. Our episodic memories allow us to engage in the equivalent of mental "time travel" (Wheeler, Shess, & Tulving, 1997), whereby we can virtually relive prior experiences, albeit less vividly. In principle, such re-experiencing could, like our original experiences, also lack explicit reflection about how we were feeling, thinking, or interpreting the experiences. But, particularly, when we must communicate our experiences to others, we tend to take explicit stock of what our experience was like. Such reflective and typically verbal narrative analysis of the past is at the heart of the process by which we construct meaning from our life experiences (Fivush & Reese, 1992; Nelson, 1993). Critically, however, if we derive our explicit appraisals of experiences after the fact, then we may develop a retrospective meta-awareness that differ in significant ways from the implicit interpretations that we held at the time.[2] Such new understandings may fold naturally into our recounting of the experience, leading us to believe that we always perceived the experience in this manner (Fischhoff, 1982). Or, if the new retrospective meta-awareness is very different from our original implicit interpretation, it may produce a sense of profound discovery that may be confused with the discovery of the memory itself.

DISCOVERY MISATTRIBUTION

Strikingly, given how central assessments of prior forgetting are to the recovered memory debate, very little research has specifically examined how individuals come to decide whether or not a recently recalled memory had been previously forgotten. Nevertheless, through analysis of the problem we can identify several factors that may be important. First, assessments of prior forgetting will depend in part on whether or not one can *recall specific prior episodes of remembering* the experience. If one can do so, then the memory is clearly not going to be characterized as having been entirely forgotten. If one cannot recall specific incidents of prior remembering, then more inferential processes may be required. A second essential factor in assessing prior knowledge of a memory is likely to involve *lay theories about memory* (e.g., Ross, 1989). Individuals will presumably consider how likely it is that they would have encountered a situation that would or should have triggered the memory, and how likely it is that they would currently recall such a remembering occasion. If the experience seems very important and they cannot recall previously remembering it, then they are likely to conclude that it had been forgotten. If, however, the experience seems rather obscure, then an inability to recall prior episodes of remembering may not be taken as very significant, and they may simply conclude that previous occasion to think about the event had not arisen. Although individuals may engage in such deliberative ruminations about the prior degree of forgetting, it also seems likely that people's immediate *phenomenology at the time of recollection* may also serve as an important factor in their assessment of their prior forgetting. If individuals experience a marked sense of "aha" or surprise when they recall an event (as virtually all of the individuals in the cases described above reported), they are likely to attribute this surprise to having just discovered a previously forgotten memory. In contrast, a more matter of fact recollective experience may lead individuals to believe that the memory had been generally accessible.

If individuals do in fact use their sense of discovery at the time of recollection as a marker for whether or not the memory had previously been forgotten, then the possibility of "discovery misattribution" becomes very real. Considerable research indicates that individuals are remarkably prone to misattributions of the source of their phenomenological experiences. In the social psychological literature, there are the classic examples of misattributions of arousal, such as attributing arousal actually stemming from a shot of adrenaline to the antics of a confederate (Schacter & Singer, 1962), or attributing the arousal resulting from standing on a suspension bridge to the attractiveness of the person standing nearby (Dutton & Aron, 1974). Other social psychological research indicates that misattributions are not limited to arousal. For example, Schwartz and Clore (1983) find that individuals can misattribute feelings of happiness stemming from the current day's weather to their general state of well-being, and Zajonc (1968) reports that the experience of familiarity resulting from subliminal presentations can be misattributed to feelings of liking.

Recent cognitive research has demonstrated that misattributions can also occur for judgments that are not explicitly affective in nature. For example, various studies have demonstrated that individuals can confuse the source of familiarity. Familiarity stemming from prior presentation of an unknown name can cause participants to think the name was famous (Jacoby, Kelley, Brown, & Jasechko, 1989), and familiarity stemming from the repetition of a statement can increase individuals' belief that a statement is true (Hasher, Goldstein, & Toppino, 1977). More recent findings indicate that it is not merely the amount of familiarity but the disparity between expected and actual familiarity that causes misattributions. For example, in a study by Whittlesea and Williams (1998) participants studied both words and non-words, and then were given a test including both words and non-words. The twist was that some of the non-words were psuedohomophones (e.g., FROG spelled as PHRAWG). Although the new pseudohomophone non-words were read slower than the new real words (i.e., they were less perceptually fluent), they were nevertheless significantly more often classified as "old." Whittlesea and Williams suggest that the tendency to call the pseudohomophones old may have resulted from a misattribution of the surprise that occurred when an unfamiliar letter string suddenly sounded like a real word.

The notion that individuals can misattribute sources of surprise raises the likely possibility that they may also misattribute sources of discovery. Recent research by Schooler, Dougal, and Johnson (1998) addressed this issue by following a list-learning procedure with a word recognition test in which the previously seen items were first presented as anagrams. Consistent with the notion of discovery misattribution, Schooler et al. found that individuals were more likely to call a word old if they had just successfully identified that word in an anagram, compared to when they did not successfully solve the anagram. Schooler et al. suggested that the "self discovery effect" resulted from participants' confusion of the discovery of the solution of the anagram with the discovery of the memory for the word. As will be seen, a similar process may happen in the context of discovered memories, in which individuals may confuse the discovery of their meta-awareness of the experience with the discovery of the memory itself.

APPLYING THE META-AWARENESS THEORY
TO THE VARIETIES
OF MEMORY DISCOVERY EXPERIENCES

Having reviewed the distinction between experiential consciousness and meta-awareness and the notion of discovery misattribution, we can now turn to the application of these constructs to the various specific mechanisms that may be involved in discovered memories. At its simplest level, my basic premise is that *memory discoveries result from an abrupt change in individuals' meta-awareness of their abuse.* For individuals who had previously thought about the event, this discovery may either involve a new meta-awareness of the event, or a re-accessing of an old meta-awareness that had been avoided for some time. For individuals who previously had not developed a meta-awareness of the experience, this discovery represents the full coming to terms of the previously unprocessed meaning of their experience. In either case, the intensity of the discovery may lead individuals to conclude that they are recalling a memory that had been previously entirely forgotten. In the following discussion I will outline the three general types of meta-awareness discoveries that I hypothesize may take place: (1) changing meta-awareness, (2) re-accessing a meta-awareness that had not been visited for a while, and (3) gaining meta-awareness for the first time.

CHANGING META-AWARENESS OF AN EXPERIENCE

In several of the cases reviewed here it is apparent that individuals were initially meta-aware about the occurrence of their abuse experiences, as clearly evidenced by the fact that they described their experiences to others. TW described her molestation experience while on a vacation to her mother soon after they returned. WB confided her rape experience to her boyfriend the day after it happened, and DN actually took her case to court, and thus, must have engaged in elaborate reflection on her experience. Nevertheless, it seems quite likely that shifts in individuals' meta-awareness of the experience over time may have fundamentally contributed to the discovery experiences. In several of these cases it seems quite plausible that the critical shift involved a fundamental change in their interpretation of the experience. For example, TW reported that, although she originally experienced the fondling abuse at age nine as unpleasant, the sexual inappropriateness of the experience was not the most salient aspect of it at the time. As she notes, the most notable unpleasantness of the experience was her feeling that the person had become angry: "I remember this guy was making some kind of disgusted sound . . . then he pushed me away. And my immediate interpretation was that I had done something wrong, and that I was some how at fault." In contrast to her original meta-awareness of the experience as an awkward social situation, her memory discovery experience occurred specifically in the context of seeing a talk on sexual abuse. At this time she may have developed a new meta-awareness of the meaning of the experience, realizing that this childhood event was actually sexual abuse. The sense of surprise and emotion associated with this new meta-awareness of the meaning and implications of the experience may have then been misattributed to the discovery of the memory itself, leading her to think the memory had been previously completely forgotten. This belief may have been further reinforced because in the context of recalling the memory in an affectively upset meta-aware state, she may have had difficulty accessing prior retrievals that occurred in an affectively flat non-meta-aware state. (Interestingly, her husband indicated that when she had referred to the event previously, she had described it matter-of-factly, with little affect.)

A similar scenario seems appropriate for WB. At the time that the event first occurred, although realizing that the experience was negative, she framed it as a sexual experience gone awry. In effect, her original meta-awareness of the experience was that she had had "bad sex" which she had "made such a mess out of . . . by resisting what I thought was supposed to be a sexual experience." However, when subsequently cued by the notion that a woman was no longer a virgin, she re-appraised her own experience, realizing that she had lost her virginity to a rape. Now, rather than thinking of the experience as a sexual experiment gone awry, she viewed it as a rape. With this new meta-aware perspective her first thoughts were "My god . . . I had been raped!. . . . That's a crime! I was 16, just a kid! I couldn't defend myself!" This sudden change in understanding and the consequent experience of discovery that it entailed may have led her to believe, or at least perceive the likelihood, that the memory had been previously entirely forgotten. Moreover, as in the prior case, the striking disparity between the manner in which she recalled the experience now, vs. in the interim where she had described it in an affectively flat way to her husband, may have precluded her recollection of those prior retrieval episodes, thereby further encouraging the conclusion that the memory had been entirely forgotten.

Although these are only two examples, it seems likely that many cases of discovered memories may have operated in a similar fashion. In such cases, individuals have had an important memory discovery, not necessarily of the memory itself so much as the meaning of the experience and its implications for the individuals' view of themselves. Nevertheless, individuals may attribute their strong sense of discovery to the finding of a forgotten memory, a conclusion that is further supported by their inability to recall prior episodes of remembering that lacked their current meta-aware perspective.

RE-GAINING ACCESS TO META-AWARENESS

Although some cases of discovered memories might be accounted for based on a change in the original meta-awareness of the experience, in other cases this account falls short. For example, DN, who was raped as an adult and went to court, clearly possessed at the time a comparable meta-awareness of what had happened to her. Nevertheless, it still seems quite plausible that such cases may involve fluctuations in meta-awareness. DN mentioned that she specifically recalled having maintained an intact memory for the experience for at least several years after the events took place. After that, however, she moved to a new location and had fewer opportunities to be specifically cued regarding the experience. It seems likely that during this time, she avoided thinking about the experience by controlling her meta-monitoring system.[3] Like meditators who can allow thoughts to come and go without "engaging them," when the thought of her rape experience crossed DN's mind, she may have simply let it pass without explicitly attending to it. By not taking stock of the memory, it may have ceased to jar her, making the recollections less memorable, and failing to reinforce her meta-awareness of the experience. In short, although the experience may never have actually been truly forgotten in the sense of being entirely unavailable, by consistently avoiding reflecting on the event, she may have gradually lost a meta-awareness of the experience. Consistent with this view, when she was specifically encouraged to think of specific incidents of adult sexual abuse, the memory (being, in fact, available) was relatively quickly accessed. However, by thinking about the experience specifically in the context of abuse, she was now forced to re-gain meta-awareness of it. And once again the shock at the discovery of the meta-awareness of the experience may have led her to conclude that she previously had lost all knowledge of the experience.

CV's case of being raped and molested once by her stepfather may also fit with the notion of avoidance of meta-awareness. In this case, her abuse was actually alluded to by a family friend a number of years after the experience. However, rather than trying to think through what the friend was referring to she recalls specifically avoiding giving it much thought. As she observed "I had absolutely no idea what she was talking about. . . . I didn't understand anything about the experience and I didn't want to." Similarly, her memory discovery experience was initially preceded by several earlier recollective events in which she imagined images of her stepfather exposing himself to her in the bathroom, but failed fully to take stock of what she was recalling. She notes that the image "left my mind immediately, without me even attempting to understand it." Here again it seems that she may have simply been avoiding reflecting on the information that was available to her. Finally, she had a recollective experience that was too strong to ignore, and she was forced to re-gain a meta-awareness of the unpleasant events.

In sum, although clearly speculative, it seems quite plausible that even the memory discovery experiences of individuals who were initially aware of the full egregiousness of their abuse may involve a discovery of meta-awareness. However, in such cases, rather than discovering a new interpretation of the event, individuals may be re-discovering a meta-awareness that they had let slip from consciousness. Indeed, the notion that individuals could learn simply not to take notice of unwanted thoughts provides a reasonable account of defense mechanisms without having to assume that unwanted thoughts are forcefully kept from entering consciousness. Rather than being repressed, some unwanted thoughts may simply be ignored (for similar suggestions, see Bower, 1990; Bowers & Farvolden, 1996; Brewin, 1997; Erdelyi, 1996).

GAINING META-AWARENESS
FOR THE FIRST TIME

Typically when individuals experience traumatic events, especially novel ones, it seems likely that meta-awareness will be activated either during the episode or soon thereafter. This meta-awareness of the consequentiality of traumatic experiences may account for why such experiences are typically remembered so well (Koss, Tromp, & Tharan, 1995). And indeed, this is one reason why researchers have had such difficulty believing that discovered memories could ever really have been truly forgotten. However, if meta-awareness of traumatic experiences was (somehow) prevented, this could certainly contribute to the failure of that experience to be integrated into one's narrative autobiographical memory. Indeed, the notion that individuals could possess purely experiential traumatic memories that are not integrated into ones' life narrative is central to several accounts of discovered memories (Freyd, 1996; van der Kolk, 1994). Moreover, if individuals had memories that were encoded exclusively at an experiential level, without reflection, then they might not be categorized in a manner that would allow deliberate access. Rather, they might only come to mind when characteristics of the environment sufficiently overlapped with the characteristics of the original memory. In fact, this distinction between verbally accessible memories (VAMs) and situationally accessible memories (SAMs) has specifically been proposed to distinguish those traumatic memories that are integrated with auto-biographical memories from those memories that remain fragmented and only come to mind given appropriate situational cues (Brewin, Dalgleish, & Joseph, 1996). The obstacle is explaining how it could be that memories that should be the most likely to trigger meta-awareness could instead be encoded without it. In the following discussion, I will consider five possible mechanisms that could prevent initial meta-aware encoding: (1) lack of discussion, (2) age, (3) stress, (4) dissociation, and (5) nocturnal occurrence.

Lack of discussion. A necessary, though probably not sufficient, condition for a memory to exist without ever having been examined in the light of self-awareness is that it must never be explicitly described to anyone else. Self-awareness is centrally associated with social interactions, and articulation of experiences by necessity demands that one reflect (at least to some degree) on the experience. Moreover, there is some evidence that experiential memories may qualitatively change when they are articulated (Freyd, 1983; Schooler & Engstler-Schooler, 1990). Because of the unique dynamics of sexual abuse situations (i.e., they are embarrassing and often are perpetrated by an individual who does not want the experience to be disclosed), they may be more likely than other traumatic experiences to go without discussion. Indeed, the particular propensity for sexual abuse experiences to go without disclosure may be one reason why, at least anecdotally, sexual abuse is more likely to be associated with discovered memories than with other types of traumas. Nevertheless, although a lack of discussion may be a pre-condition for the formation of a memory that occurs without meta-awareness, it clearly does not insure such memories. I suspect we all have experiences on which we privately reflected but never communicated to others. Thus, we must look elsewhere to identify factors that may actually preclude meta-aware processing.

Age. One factor that perhaps is the most plausible for preventing the initiation of meta-awareness of traumatic experiences is age. A large body of research indicates that self-awareness does not arise until nearly two years of age, which, perhaps not coincidentally, is precisely the time at which individuals' earliest enduring memories tend to occur (see Wheeler et al., 1997). Although self-awareness can occur as early as two, the regularity with which children engage in self-reflection seems likely to increases with age. Accordingly, if younger children are generally less inclined to engage in meta-reflection, then they may be more apt to experience disturbing events without necessarily explicitly reflecting on them. Moreover, because of their age, such children may not view abuse experiences as seriously as do adults, thus further increasing the possibility that meta-awareness of the experience may be avoided.

JN, who was fondled at age five, may well provide an example of a situation in which age may have prevented meta-awareness of the experience, which in turn may have enabled the memory to have been forgotten and then discovered. In contrast to the other cases analyzed so far, JN did not engage in one of the central processes that encourage meta-awareness: the recounting of an experience to others. In her case, her older sister reported the occurrence of the experience, and the issue was never broached with her. Thus, she had the opportunity to allow the experience to pass without reflection. Moreover, given the ambiguity of a fondling situation, it seems quite plausible that JN may not have fully appreciated the seriousness of the events at the time. Indeed, although JN reported that she perceived the experience as negative at the time, she conceded that she probably did not view it as negatively as she does today. Thus, it seems quite plausible that JN's age may have led her to experience the abuse without much meta-awareness, which in turn may have prevented the experience from becoming integrated into her autobiographical memory. Instead, it awaited situational cues that were not present until she was much older and became sexually active. Strikingly, although apparently dormant for 13 years, the memory came flooding back very soon after the cues became present. Moreover, the recollection was experiential (she recalled the memory quite vividly), but without any sense of integration into her life narrative (i.e., she was not sure whether it was real). In short, JN's memory discovery experience is entirely consistent with the view that, due to her age at the time of the event, she created an experiential memory of which she did not become meta-aware until it was situationally cued as an adult.

Stress and Brain Activation. Stress is known to have a number of profound effects on the brain and cognition (LeDoux, 1994). Animal models suggest that extremely high levels of stress both increase activation of the amygdala and decrease activation of the hippocampus (e.g., LeDoux, 1992; Nadel & Jacobs, 1998). Stress is also likely to reduce the activation of the frontal cortex, which is highly susceptible to cognitive load (of which stress is a major source). Since the frontal cortex is hypothesized to be important for both self-awareness (Stuss, 1991) and the integration of memories into readily retrievable autobiographical memories (van der Kolk, 1994; Wheeler et al., 1997), it seems quite plausible that non-meta-aware traumatic memories could be formed by highly stressful situations that prevent the frontal cortex and hippocampus from integrating and imposing self-awareness on the experience.

Dissociation. Another, albeit controversial, factor that could in principle result in the formation of a memory that lacks meta-awareness is dissociation. Dissociation is typically defined as a "lack of normal integration of thoughts, feelings, and experiences into the stream of consciousness and memory" (Bernstein & Putnam, 1986, p. 727). As noted earlier, one plausible account of dissociation is that it specifically involves lapses of meta-awareness, which arguably provides the glue by which stream of consciousness is held together. Accordingly, when in situations in which the comprehension of an experience is simply too daunting, some individuals may be able to suspend meta-awareness processing. By eliminating self-reflection, individuals may in effect be able to feel detached from their experience. One possible interpretation of these dissociative experiences is that they result from a fundamental elimination of meta-awareness. Although tentative, the suggestion that dissociative tendencies involve a profound lack of meta-awareness would also be consistent with the items found on the Dissociative Experience Scale (DES) (Bernstein & Putnam, 1986) such as, "Some people have the experience of driving a car and suddenly realizing that they don't remember what has happened during all or part of the trip," or "Some people find that sometimes they are listening to someone talk and they suddenly realize that they did not hear part or all of what was said." Such items suggest that dissociative individuals may in fact go for extended periods without meta-awareness of what they are doing, which is precisely what one would expect if dissociation involves an abandonment of standard meta-aware processes.

Although there seems to be good reason to think that dissociation may involve a breakdown in meta-aware processing of experiences, the question remains how individuals achieve this. One possibility is that individuals may be meta-aware of the efforts in which they are engaging to detach themselves from their experience, while at the same time succeeding in suspending meta-awareness about the actual meaning of what is happening to them. Such a partitioning of meta-awareness is broadly consistent with individuals' phenomenological reports. For example, DJ described recalling herself having "the ability to literally detach myself from my body and look at myself, down, like I was on top of the roof. . . . I remember thinking to myself 'hey I'm on top of this ceiling looking down, that's not really me.'" Such accounts suggest the paradoxical possibility that individuals may use meta-aware strategies in order to suspend their meta-awareness of what is happening to them. Alternatively, individuals may actually have no meta-awareness whatsoever during dissociative episodes. Rather, the meta-aware experiences that individuals report (such as DJ's claim that she can "remember thinking to myself") may in fact be retrospective reconstructions. It may be that people are simply not capable of reconstructing what the experience of a total lack of meta-awareness is like. Accordingly, the notion that one was explicitly aware of becoming detached from one's body during an episode of abuse may represent an illusion resulting from the attempt to impose a retrospective meta-aware understanding on an experience that was originally inherently void of meta-awareness.

Regardless of the precise mechanism by which dissociation may allow for the suspension of meta-awareness about an experience, it seems quite plausible that such a suspension may occur. Like the driver who is conscious of the driving experience, but entirely non-reflecting on what s/he is doing, so too the dissociative individual may experience the abuse, and yet somehow manage not to reflect on it. The conscious experience of the abuse may be laid down in memory, but in the absence of reflection, access to the memory may be limited to experiential cues that correspond to the specific conditions in which the memory actually occurred. Consistent with this latter claim, in the case of DJ it was indeed a very specific environmental cue (actually seeing the perpetrator again) that apparently elicited the memory.

Nocturnal Occurrence. One final factor that may contribute to the suspension of meta-awareness during abuse has been surprisingly absent from consideration in discussions of discovered memories, namely the fact that many reported incidents of sexual abuse occur at night. Arguably one of the key characteristics of nocturnal cognition is an absence of meta-awareness. A lack of meta-awareness can explain why individuals fail to notice the remarkable discrepancies that occur in dreams. It also explains why dreams can be so completely and utterly forgotten. Indeed, dreams seem only remembered if individuals specifically reflect on them soon after awakening (Hobson, 1998). Further evidence for the critical role of meta-awareness in mediating the qualities of nocturnal consciousness comes from research on lucid dreaming, which specifically involves becoming self-aware during dreaming (LaBerge, 1985). One of the best ways to encourage the occurrence of lucid dreaming is to encourage regular meta-aware reflection about one's environment during waking hours (LaBerge, 1985). The striking qualitative differences between lucid dreaming and normal dreaming, both with respect to the control that individuals have over the dream environment and with regard to the dream's subsequent memorability illustrate the fundamental lack of meta-awareness that is typically associated with the nocturnal cognition that occurs during dreams.

Although tentative, it seems at least plausible that the absence of meta-aware reflection associated with dreaming cognition may carry over to other nocturnal experiences that immediately precede or follow sleep. We have probably all heard (or participated) in anecdotes of nocturnal conversations that are completely forgotten by morning. And indeed there is a small amount of literature on the significant amnesia associated with events that occur following awakenings in the middle of the night (Bonnet, 1983). It thus seems quite plausible that such amnesias may stem from the lack of meta-aware reflection that is associated with nocturnal cognition.

The fact that meta-awareness may be more apt to be completely suspended at night may help to explain some of the more severe claims of precipitous forgetting that some individuals with discovered memories have reported. For example, JR reported that by the time he woke up in the morning he had forgotten the abuse that happened the night before: "When I woke up in the morning I didn't have any knowledge of what had happened the night before, which is why I could continue to go on trips with him and enjoy it."

In one of the best documented public cases, Ross Cheit, who discovered memories of nocturnal molestation by a camp counselor (which were corroborated by a tape-recorded confession by the perpetrator) similarly characterized his experiences as having been entirely forgotten by morning. As Cheit described in the *Providence Sunday Journal* (Stanton, 1995, May 8, p. A-19), "When morning came, life at Camp Wallace Alexander would slide back into its familiar grooves, the nocturnal ritual would fade into the shadows." " In the daytime," Cheit says, "he was my friend." In a personal communication, Cheit further substantiated this characterization, saying, "I am confident as I can be that I did not think of the abuse in the daytime" (personal communication, R. Cheit, November 1997).

A similar claim of precipitous forgetting of nocturnal abuse also characterizes another one of the best-corroborated claims of authentic discovered memories, that of the former Miss America, Marilyn Van Derbur. Van Derbur discovered memories of years of sexual abuse by her father, which were corroborated by her sister who reported having maintained intact memories of similar abuse. Like JR and Cheit (as cited in Stanton, 1995), Van Derbur indicated that the abuse exclusively occurred at night and that by morning the memories had evaporated. She described her forgetting as follows: "During the days . . . I, the 'day child', had no conscious knowledge of my traumas and the terrors of the 'night child'. . . . I believed I was the happiest person who ever lived" (as cited in Terr, 1994, p. 124). Van Derbur attributed her forgetting of her nocturnal experiences to a splitting between "a day child" and a "night child." However, perhaps a more parsimonious explanation is that at night when the abuse took place, Van Derbur, like Cheit and JR, may have lacked the meta-awareness processes that typically enable such experiences to be integrated into memory.

Clearly, we must be very cautious at this time in drawing any strong conclusions regarding the possible role of nocturnal occurrence of abuse and its possible ramifications for meta-awareness and memory consolidation. Nevertheless, it is certainly striking that in three of the best documented cases of discovered memories of extensive abuse for which precipitous forgetting was claimed, all occurred at night and all were alleged to have been entirely forgotten by morning. Given that disturbing dreams can be lost in a similar fashion, and that dream consciousness is typified by a lack of meta-awareness, it seems quite plausible that the alleged precipitous forgetting of abuse in these cases may have resulted from the severe disruptions of meta-awareness associated with nocturnal consciousness.

Prevention of post-experience retrospective meta-awareness. One challenge to all of the above accounts of how individuals could fail to develop meta-aware understandings of their experiences is: Why aren't the experiences retrospectively assessed in the light of meta-awareness? As noted earlier, we all have had stressful experiences in which it seemed that we just acted without reflecting on the experience at the time. Typically, however, as soon as the experience ends, we put it into perspective. So why does this not also happen in the cases alluded to above? Several essential factors may contribute to individuals' sustained failure to become meta-aware of abuse experiences that are not initially processed with meta-awareness. As already noted, age and lack of rehearsal may be important in this regard. In addition, it is possible that some inhibition of monitoring processes (outlined in the context of temporarily losing meta-awareness) may also be important in some of these situations–particularly in the case of dissociation, where it seems possible that individuals may deliberately inhibit meta-awareness of the experience both during and after its occurrence. In the context of nocturnal experiences, a variety of factors may conspire to prevent retrospective meta-awareness. First, various physiological nocturnal processes that have been associated with dream forgetting (Hobson, 1985) may also contribute to the forgetting of nocturnal abuse. Second, if individuals awake with some vestige recollections of the atrocities that happened to them the night before, they may fail to believe that these bizarre events were real, dismissing them instead as very "bad dreams" (see Johnson, Kahan, & Raye, 1984).

A final factor that may play an important role in the sustained lack of retrospective meta-awareness of abuse experiences is schematicity and connectivity with other life events. When a disturbing experience occurs without meta-awareness, but nevertheless fits into the continuous framework of one's life experiences, it may be relatively easy to "work one's way back" to the event and reconstruct the experience in the light of meta-awareness. However, if an experience is completely bizarre and somehow disconnected to any other understandable life experience, it may be very difficult to reconstruct deliberately the experience retrospectively. This seems especially clear in the context of nocturnal abuse experiences perpetrated by a known caregiver. They are bizarre, occur in isolation, often in the dark, and may be difficult to reconcile with pre-existing schemata (e.g., the perpetrator may be an otherwise loving and kind individual). In the absence of meta-aware processes that enable individuals to take special note of the distinctive experience, like bizarre dreams these aschematic experiences may be very difficult to reconstruct and recall in retrospect. In short, when experiences connect in some natural way to the events that precede and follow them, then it may be straightforward to impose meta-awareness on the experiences retrospectively. If, however, meta-awareness is, for the various reasons mentioned above, prevented during an experience, and if that experience is fundamentally disjointed from the other experiences in one's life, then it may be more difficult to retrieve retrospectively the memory and to impose meta-awareness on it. In such cases, the memory may await experiential cues to return. Moreover, by the virtue of the unique quality of the experience, it may take some time before the appropriate cues are encountered.

CONCLUSION

In sum, the present article has attempted to document and explain how individuals can come to discover seemingly forgotten memories of actual abuse. Although the extent of this phenomenon remains to be determined, the case studies presented here suggest that individuals can have sincere memory discovery experiences corresponding to actual incidents of abuse. An analysis of the possible mechanisms that might lead to such memory discoveries suggests the potential importance of two theoretical constructs: (1) experiential consciousness/meta-awareness dissociations–the notion that individuals can have an experience (experiential consciousness) without being explicitly aware of their interpretation of the experience (meta-awareness), and (2) discovery misattribution–the notion that individuals can confuse the experience of discovering a meta-awareness of a prior experience with the discovery of the memory itself. In this context, discovered memories can be understood as involving changes in individuals' meta-awareness of the abuse. In some cases, such changes may involve the gaining of a new meta-awareness of the meaning of the experience, leading to a profound sense of discovery that persuades individuals, rightly or wrongly, that they are accessing the memory for the first time. In other cases, the change may involve regaining meta-awareness of an event that, through either the deliberate or non-deliberate manipulation of the monitoring system, has not been reflected on for some time. In still other cases, the memory may not have been encoded with any meta-awareness in the first place, as a consequence of a variety of encoding factors, ranging from the very straightforward (e.g., age, lack of discussion, stress) to the more esoteric (e.g., dissociation, nocturnal cognitive processing). Such purely experiential memories, particularly when they are disjunctive with other experiences, may continue to elude retrospective meta-awareness, thereby making them difficult to retrieve deliberately. Instead, they may await unique contextual cues that overlap with the original experiences. Ultimately, such experiential memories of trauma may, in principle, be no different from other, more everyday non-reflected memories that are similarly triggered by experiential cues, but with one central difference. Whereas most memories that are processed without reflection are relatively mundane in nature, non-reflected abuse experiences pack a hidden charge (their unrecognized personal significance), which, like psychological time bombs, literally explode when exposed to the light of meta-awareness.

In closing, it seems appropriate to consider some of the issues left open by the present analysis. Although the present account of discovered memories must be viewed as speculative, many of the suggestions made here are testable. For example, if dissociations between consciousness and meta-awareness are common, then it should be possible to induce them in the lab. (In fact we probably do so all the time, but simply do not appreciate the fact that our participants have caught themselves zoning out.) If individuals make errors in their assessments of forgetting based on discovery misattribution, then experimentally induced "aha" experiences may alter estimations of forgetting. If nocturnal cognition has unique qualities that make individuals especially prone to the formation of memories that can be both precipitously forgotten and yet still recoverable, then such patterns may well be demonstrable in sleep laboratories. While some of the claims suggested in this article may be amenable to laboratory investigation, others will need to rely on the theoretically rich but methodologically thorny corroborative case-based approach outlined here. With larger samples, and a greater variety of characterizations of forgetting, important key hypotheses raised in this analysis could be tested. For example, if a change in meta-awareness of the experience is a key component of the phenomenon, then the sense of discovery that such changes are likely to entail should prove to be a distinguishing feature of discovered memories (particularly ones that are corroboratable). If discoveries of one's meta-awareness of an experience can be confused with discoveries of the memory itself, then instances of such "forgot-it-all-along" errors in estimated forgetting should be found more widely. Finally, if nocturnal abuse is particularly likely to lead to precipitous forgetting, then there should be a relationship between the time at which abuse is alleged to have occurred and the manner in which it is characterized as having been forgotten. Importantly, although many issues (arguably most) of the claims made here remain to be tested, this analysis paves the way for theoretically driven laboratory and field research that may either substantiate the present theory, or provide the basis for a better one.

In addition to raising many issues that require additional testing, the present analysis has also left a number of difficult issues unaddressed, in particular, the controversial legal and therapeutic implications surrounding discovered memories. Having training in neither clinical practice nor jurisprudence, I am wary of treading these dangerous waters. Nevertheless, a few cautious observations may be in order. From a therapeutic perspective, a central question is whether it is helpful to expose abuse memories to the light of meta-awareness. Ultimately this is an empirical question, upon which the jury is still out. One clear risk, however, is that the new found meta-awareness of abuse may not only reactivate old traumas but may also produce new ones as individuals come to appraise their experience in a way they never did before. From a legal perspective, a central issue is establishing the degree to which true "discovery" was involved (see Schooler, 1999). On the one hand, the present analysis suggests that individuals may be accurate in their characterization of the abuse, without necessarily being accurate in their characterization of the forgetting. On the other hand, the present analysis also suggests that individuals with discovered memories of authentic abuse might well have a newfound understanding of the harm they incurred. Finally, from both perspectives, the fact that there are viable theoretical ways to account for the experienced discovery of even extended and severe abuse means that the theoretical inconceivability of such discoveries cannot be used as grounds for dismissing them.

Although much of this article has explored the implications of meta-awareness and discovery misattribution for accounting for discovered memories of real events, it may also have important theoretical implications for discovering false memories. For example, if individuals can confuse the source of discoveries, then one might confuse the discovery of new insights about oneself (e.g., that one feels ambivalence towards a parent) with a discovery about their past (e.g., that one was abused by that parent). If some traumatic experiences are encoded without meta-awareness, and if meta-awareness is necessary for weaving experiences into coherent integrated narrative memories, then traumatic memories that have avoided the light of meta-awareness may be especially prone to distortions, substitutions, and source monitoring errors. Finally, if nocturnal cognition impairs meta-awareness, which in turn dulls the line between reality and fantasy, then whereas sometimes real abuse may be forgotten like dreams, other times dreams may be remembered as real abuse.

Ultimately, of course, the arguments underlying much of the speculations in this article rest on the distinction between experiential consciousness and meta-awareness. If this distinction fails, then many of the arguments made here will undoubtedly fail as well. If, however, it is possible for one to be conscious during an experience without being meta-aware of that experience, then we potentially gain a whole new locus for dissociations of thought. Such dissociations may not only help to clarify discovered memories, but may also illuminate a variety of other domains, such as automaticity (Bargh & Chartrand, 1999), awareness of emotions (Zajonc, 1980), mental control (Wegner, 1994), implicit attitudes (Wilson, Lindsey, & T. Schooler, 2000), and addictive behaviors (Tiffany & Carter, 1998), to name but a few. Whereas many cognitive distinctions may continue to be best characterized in terms of the standard division between conscious and unconscious thought, others may now be better conceived as straddling the typically ignored line between consciousness and meta-awareness.

NOTES

1. Of course, if a discovered memory cannot be corroborated, this does not imply that the memory is necessarily false. By the very nature of abuse, many cases may occur without any incriminating evidence to subsequently corroborate it. Indeed, as will be mentioned later, one form of abuse that may be particularly difficult to corroborate (i.e., that which occurs surreptitiously in the home at night) may also be especially prone to forgetting.

2. Of course, tacit interpretations of experiences are obligatory at all levels of processing, from assigning figure and ground to determining whether a situation requires approach or avoidance. However, just as animals are assumed to interpret their environment without explicit awareness of their interpretations, so too it is assumed that we may routinely interpret our experiences without explicitly reflecting on those interpretations.

3. The fact that meta-awareness comes and goes suggests the existence of some type of meta-monitoring system that determines when meta-awareness is needed. Wegner (1994) has proposed an elegant theory of the monitoring of unwanted thoughts that might provide the basis for such a meta-monitoring system. Wegner postulates the existence of two processes: a control process that searches for anything but the unwanted thought, and an automatic process that monitors the success of the control process by remaining vigilant for the unwanted thought. In contrast to the present discussion, Wegner suggests that the automatic monitoring process searches the contents of thoughts that are in pre-consciousness (i.e., activated but not in consciousness). However, he does not explicitly consider the distinction between consciousness and meta-awareness, and thus does not address the likely case in which an individual may consciously entertain unwanted thoughts without being explicitly aware of doing so. Nevertheless, his model clearly handles such cases by simply assuming that the monitoring system can also monitor the contents of consciousness in order to alert one that s/he is ruminating on an unwanted thought. In effect, the monitor may bring to meta-awareness the basic message "there you go again."

REFERENCES

Allport, A. (1988). What concept of consciousness? In A. J. Marcel & E. Bisiach (Eds.), *Consciousness in contemporary science* (pp. 159-182). New York: Oxford University Press.

Andrews, B., Brewin, C. R., Ochera, J. M., Bekerian, D. A., Davies, G. M., & Mollon, P. (1999). Characteristics, context and consequences of memory recovery among adults in therapy. *British Journal of Psychiatry, 175*, 141-146.

Armstrong, D. (1981). What is consciousness? *The nature of mind*. Ithaca, NY: Cornell University Press.

Bargh, J. A., & Chartrand, T. L. (1999). The unbearable automaticity of being. *American Psychologist, 54*, 462-479.

Bernstein, E., & Putnam, F. (1986). Development, reliability, and validity of a dissociation scale. *Journal of Nervous and Mental Disease, 174*, 727-735.

Block, N. (1992). Begging the question against phenomenal consciousness. *Behavioral and Brain Sciences, 15*, 205-206.

Bonnet, M. H. (1983). Memory for events occurring during arousal from sleep. *Psychophysiology, 20*, 81-87.

Bower, G. H. (1990). Awareness, the unconscious, and repression: An experimental psychologist's perspective. In J. L. Singer (Ed), *Repression and dissociation: Implications for personality theory* (pp. 209-231). Chicago: University of Chicago Press.

Bowers, K. S., & Farvolden, P. (1996). Revisiting a century-old Freudian slip–From suggestion disavowed to the truth expressed. *Psychological Bulletin, 119*, 355-380.

Bradley, L., Hollifield, M., & Foulkes, D. (1992). Reflection during REM dreaming. *Dreaming: Journal of the Association for the Study of Dreams*, Vol. 2, 161-166.

Brewin, C. R. (1997). Psychological defenses and the distortion of meaning. In M. Power & C. Brewin (Eds.), *The transformation of meaning in psychological therapies: Integrating theory and practice* (pp. 107-123). Chichester, England, UK: John Wiley & Sons.

Brewin, C. R., Dalgleish, T., & Joseph, S. (1996). A dual representation theory of posttraumatic stress disorder. *Psychological Review, 103*, 670-686.

Brown, R., & Kulik, J. (1977). Flashbulb memories. *Cognition, 5*, 73-99.

Cheit, R. (1997) Consider this, skeptics of recovered memory. *Ethics and Behavior, 8*, 141-160.

Chu, J. A., Frey, L. M., Ganzel, B. L., & Matthews, J. A. (1999). Memories of childhood abuse: Dissociation, amnesia, and corroboration. *American Journal of Psychiatry, 156*, 749-755.

Dalenberg, C. J. (1996). Accuracy, timing and circumstances of disclosure in therapy of recovered and continuous memories of abuse. *Journal of Psychiatry and the Law, 24* (2), 229-275.

Duggal, S. & Stroufe, A. L. (1998). Recovered memory of childhood sexual trauma: A documented case from a longitudinal study. *Journal of Traumatic Stress, 2*, 301-320.

Dutton, G. G, & Aron, A. P. (1974). Some evidence for heightened sexual attraction under conditions of high anxiety. *Journal of Personality and Social Psychology, 30*, 510-517.

Duval, S., & Wicklund, R. A. (1972). *A theory of objective self-awareness*. New York: Academic Press.

Erdelyi, M. H. (1996). *The recovery of unconscious memories: Hypermnesia and reminiscence*. Chicago: University of Chicago Press.

Fischhoff, B. (1982). For those condemned to study the past: Heuristics and biases in hindsight. In D. Kahneman, P. Slovic, & A. Tversky (Eds.), *Judgment under uncertainty: Heuristics and biases* (pp. 335-351). New York: Cambridge University Press.

Fivush, R. & Reese, E. (1992). The social construction of autobiographical memory. In M. A. Conway, D. C. Rubin, H. Spinnler, & W. A. Wagenaar (Eds.), *Theoretical perspectives on autobiographical memory* (pp. 115-132). Netherlands: Kluwer Academic Publishers.

Freyd, J. J. (1983). Shareability: The social psychology of epistemology. *Cognitive Science, 7*, 191-210.

Freyd, J. J. (1996). *Betrayal trauma: The logic of forgetting childhood abuse*. Cambridge: Harvard University Press.

Gibbons, F. X. (1990). Self-attention and behavior: A review and theoretical update. *Advances in Experimental Social Psychology, 23*, 249-303.

Hasher, L., Goldstein, D., & Toppino, T. (1977). Frequency and the conference of referential validity. *Journal of Verbal Learning and Verbal Behavior, 16*, 107-112.

Hobson, J. A. (1988). *The dreaming brain*. New York: Basic Books.

Hunt, H. T., & Ogilvie, R. D. (1988). Lucid dreams in their natural series. In J. Gackenbach & S. LaBerge (Eds.), *Conscious mind, sleeping brain: Perspectives on lucid dreaming* (pp. 389-417). New York: Plenum Press.

Jacoby, L. L., Kelley, C. M., Brown, J. & Jasechko, J. (1989). Becoming famous overnight: Limits on the ability to avoid unconscious influences of the past. *Journal of Personality and Social Psychology, 5*, 326-338.

Johnson, M. K., Kahan, T. L., & Raye, C. L. (1984). Dreams and reality monitoring. *Journal of Experimental Psychology: General, 113*, 329-344.

Karmiloff-Smith, A. (1992). *Beyond modularity: A developmental perspective on cognitive science*. Cambridge, MA: MIT Press.

Kluft, K. P. (1998). Reflections on the traumatic memories of dissociative identity disorder patients. In S. J. Lynn & K. M. McConkey (Eds.), *Truth in memory* (pp. 304-322). New York: Guilford Press.

Koss, M. P., Tromp, S., & Tharan, M. (1995). Traumatic memories: Empirical foundations, clinical and forensic implications. *Clinical Psychology: Research and Practice, 2*, 111-132.

LaBerge, S. (1985). *Lucid dreaming*. New York: Putnam.

LeDoux, J. E. (1992). Emotion as memory: Anatomical systems underlying indelible neural traces. In S.-A. Christianson (Ed.), *The handbook of emotion and memory: Research and theory* (pp. 269-288). Hillsdale, NJ: Erlbaum.

LeDoux, J. E. (1994, June) Emotion, memory and the brain. *Scientific American, 270*, 50-57.

Lewis, M. (1991). Ways of knowing: Objective self-awareness or consciousness. *Developmental Review, 11*, 231-243.

Lindsay, D. S., & Briere, J. (1997). The controversy regarding recovered memories of childhood sexual abuse: Pitfalls, bridges, and future directions. *Journal of Interpersonal Violence, 12*, 631-647.

Lindsay, D. S., & Read, J. D. (1994). Psychotherapy and memories of child sexual abuse: A cognitive perspective. *Applied Cognitive Psychology, 8*, 281-338.

Loftus, E. F., & Ketcham, K. (1994). *The myth of repressed memory: False memories and allegations of sexual abuse.* New York: St. Martin's Press.

McCloskey, M., Wible, C. G., & Cohen, N. J. (1988). Is there a special flashbulb-memory mechanism? *Journal of Experimental Psychology: General, 117*, 171-181.

Nadel, L., & Jacobs, W. J. (1998). Traumatic memory is special. *Current Directions in Psychological Science, 7*, 154-157.

Nelson, K. (1993). The psychological and social origins of autobiographical memory. *Psychological Science, 4*, 7-14.

Ofshe, R., & Watters, E. (1994). *Making monsters: False memories, psychotherapy, and sexual hysteria.* New York: Scribners.

Pope, H. G., & Hudson, J. L. (1995). Can memories of childhood sexual abuse be repressed? *Psychological Medicine, 25*, 121-126.

Reason, J., & Mycielska, K. (1982). *Absentmindness? The psychology of mental lapses and everyday errors.* Englewood Cliffs, NJ: Prentice-Hall.

Rosenthal, D. M. (1998). A theory of consciousness. In N. Block, O. Flanagan, & G. Guzeldere (Eds.), *The nature of consciousness* (pp. 729-753). Cambridge, MA: Massachusetts Institute of Technology Press.

Ross, M. (1989). Relation of implicit theories to the construction of personal histories. *Psychological Reviews, 96*(2), 341-357.

Schacter, D. L. (1996). *Searching for memory.* New York: Basic Books.

Schachter, S. & Singer, J. E. (1962). Cognitive, social and physiological determinants of emotional state. *Psychological Review, 69*, 370-399.

Schooler, J. W. (1994). Seeking the core: The issues and evidence surrounding recovered accounts of sexual trauma. *Consciousness and Cognition, 3*, 452-469.

Schooler, J. W. (1999). Discovered memories and the "delayed discovery doctrine": A cognitive case based analysis. In S. Taub (Ed.), *Recovered memories of child sexual abuse: Psychological, legal, and social perspectives on a twentieth century controversy* (pp. 121-141). Springfield, IL: Charles C. Thomas.

Schooler, J. W. (2000a, April). Consciousness, meta-consciousness and the value of self-report. Paper presented at the Towards a Science of Consciousness Conference, Tucson, AZ.

Schooler, J. W. (2000b). Discovered memories and the delayed discovery doctrine: A cognitive case based analysis. In S. Taub (Ed.), *Recovered memories of child sexual abuse: Psychological, legal, and social perspectives on a mental health controversy* (pp. 121-141). Springfield, IL: Charles C. Thomas.

Schooler, J. W., Ambadar, Z., & Bendiksen, M. A. (1997). A cognitive corroborative case study approach for investigating discovered memories of sexual abuse. In J. D. Read & D. S. Lindsay (Eds.), *Recollections of trauma: Scientific research and clinical practice* (pp. 379-388). New York: Plenum.

Schooler, J. W., Bendiksen, M. A., & Ambadar, Z. (1997). Taking the middle line: Can we accommodate both fabricated and recovered memories of sexual abuse? In M.

Conway (Ed.), *False and recovered memories* (pp. 251-292). Oxford: Oxford University Press.

Schooler, J. W., Dougal, S., & Johnson, M. K. (1998, November). *The self discovery effect: When solving is confused with remembering.* Paper presented at the Annual Meeting of the Psychonomic Society, Dallas, Texas.

Schooler, J. W., & Engstler-Schooler, T. Y. (1990). Verbal overshadowing of visual memories: Some things are better left unsaid. *Cognitive Psychology, 17,* 36-71.

Schooler, J. W., Loewenstein, G., & Ariely, D. (2000, July). The pursuit of happiness can be self-defeating. Paper presented at the Conference on Psychology and Economics, Brussels, Belgium.

Schooler, J. W. & Melcher, J. M. (1995). The ineffability of insight. In S. M. Smith, T. B. Ward & R. A. Finke (Eds.), *The creative cognition approach* (pp. 97-133). Cambridge, MA: MIT Press.

Schwartz, N., & Clore, G. L. (1983). Mood, misattribution, and judgments of well-being: Informative and directive functions of affective states. *Journal of Personality and Social Psychology, 45,* 513-523.

Stanton, M. (1995, May 8). Bearing witness: A man's recovery of his sexual abuse as a child. *The Sunday Journal* [Massachusetts edition of *The Providence Sunday Journal*], p. A-19.

Stuss, D. T. (1991). Self, awareness, and the frontal lobes: A neuropsychological perspective. In J. Strauss & G. R. Goethals (Eds.), *The self: Interdisciplinary approaches* (pp. 255-278). New York: Springer-Verlag.

Terr, L. C. (1994). *Unchained memories: True stories of traumatic memories, lost and found.* New York: Basic Books.

Tiffany, S. T., & Carter, B. L. (1998). Is craving the source of compulsive drug use? *Journal of Psychopharmacology, 12,* 23-30.

van der Kolk, B. A. (1994). The body keeps score: Memory and the evolving psychobiology of posttraumatic stress. *Harvard Review of Psychiatry, 1,* 253-265.

Wegner, D. M. (1994). Ironic processes of mental control. *Psychological Review, 101,* 34-52.

Wegner, D. M., & Wheatley, T. (1999). Apparent mental causation: Sources of the experience of will. *American Psychologist, 54,* 480-492.

Wheeler, M. A., Stuss, D. T., & Tulving, E. (1997). Toward a theory of episodic memory: The frontal lobes and autonoetic consciousness. *Psychological Bulletin, 121,* 331-354.

Whittlesea, B. W. A., & Williams, L. S. (1998). Why do strangers feel familiar, but friends don't? A discrepancy-attribution account of feelings of familiarity. *Acta Psychologica, 98,* 141-165.

Williams, L. M. (1995). Recovered memories of abuse in women with documented child sexual victimization histories. *Journal of Traumatic Stress, 8,* 649-673.

Wilson, T. D., Lindsey, S., & Schooler, T. Y. (2000). A model of dual attitudes. *Psychological Review, 107,* 101-126.

Zajonc, R. B. (1980). Attitudinal effects of mere exposure. *Journal of Personality and Social Psychology Monograph, 9,* 1-27.

Zoltan, T. (1999). *The crucible of consciousness.* New York: Oxford University Press.

Perspectives on Memory for Trauma and Cognitive Processes Associated with Dissociative Tendencies

Jennifer J. Freyd
Anne P. DePrince

SUMMARY. Cognitive science approaches can inform research in traumatic stress studies by articulating separate scientific issues that may be relevant to understanding alterations in memory and awareness for trauma. This article will first address general issues about disrupted memory and "knowledge isolation" for trauma, as well as introduce specific aspects of "betrayal trauma theory" (Freyd 1994, 1996) that inform our understanding of memory impairment. According to betrayal trauma theory, a potent motivation for knowledge isolation (including amnesia, dissociation, and unawareness) in the face of trauma is to preserve apparently necessary human relationships in which betrayal occurs. Results from three recent laboratory investigations of cognitive processes associated with dissociative tendencies are summarized. These laboratory investigations suggest that the attentional capacities of high dissocators are impaired under conditions of selective attention, but not divided attention. Furthermore, in our laboratory tasks high dissocators have impaired memory for emotionally charged words associated with sexual assault and abuse (e.g., "incest") but not neutral words, as compared with low dissociators. The findings suggest that

---

Address correspondence to: Jennifer J. Freyd, Department of Psychology, 1227 University of Oregon, Eugene, OR 97403-1227 (E-mail: jjf@dynamic.uoregon.edu).

Sections of this paper are based on Freyd, J.J. (1999), "Blind to Betrayal: New Perspectives on Memory for Trauma," *The Harvard Mental Health Letter*, 15 (12) 4-6; Copyright Jennifer J. Freyd, 1999, reprinted by permission of the author.

[Haworth co-indexing entry note]: "Perspectives on Memory for Trauma and Cognitive Processes Associated with Dissociative Tendencies." Freyd, Jennifer J., and Anne P. DePrince. Co-published simultaneously in *Journal of Aggression, Maltreatment & Trauma* (The Haworth Maltreatment & Trauma Press, an imprint of The Haworth Press, Inc.) Vol. 4, No. 2, (#8), 2001, pp. 137-163; and: *Trauma and Cognitive Science: A Meeting of Minds, Science, and Human Experience* (ed: Jennifer J. Freyd, and Anne P. DePrince) The Haworth Maltreatment & Trauma Press, an imprint of The Haworth Press, Inc., 2001, pp. 137-163. Single or multiple copies of this article are available for a fee from The Haworth Document Delivery Service [1-800-342-9678, 9:00 a.m. - 5:00 p.m. (EST). E-mail address: getinfo@haworthpressinc.com].

high dissociators use divided attention and multi-tasking as a way to control the flow of information. Such a view is consistent with betrayal trauma theory. Though in its infancy, this research draws on cognitive science and observations of traumatic response and offers much promise. *[Article copies available for a fee from The Haworth Document Delivery Service: 1-800-342-9678. E-mail address: <getinfo@haworthpressinc.com> Website: <http://www.HaworthPress.com> © 2001 by The Haworth Press, Inc. All rights reserved.]*

KEYWORDS. Child abuse, sexual abuse, forgetting, amnesia, betrayal, attention, recovered memory, repressed memory

A cognitive science perspective is inherently analytic. That is, cognitive scientists will attempt to identify and analyze the underlying components of cognitive processes and structures. This perspective offers the promise of bringing clarity and scientific precision to complex phenomena such as memory and attention for trauma, especially if this componential and scientific approach is ultimately used in conjunction with a variety of other approaches and sources of knowledge about trauma. In this article we draw on the conceptual and methodological tools of cognitive science as we examine memory for trauma and the cognitive processes associated with dissociative tendencies.

MEMORY FOR TRAUMA

In 1992, Frank Fitzpatrick's recovered memories of childhood sexual abuse rocked the mental health and legal professions. This was not the first case of recovered memories for sexual abuse by any means, but it was a dramatic one. Dozens of victims of the Reverend James R. Porter began to come forward only after Fitzpatrick, a Rhode Island insurance adjuster, acted on his own newly recovered memories. Most of the victims said they had always remembered the abuse, but others, like Fitzpatrick, had forgotten it for more than 20 years (Fitzpatrick, 1994; Goleman, 1992).

How and why would anyone forget something so seemingly significant as childhood molestation and then remember it decades later? Fitzpatrick's memories were corroborated by the reports of other victims and by Porter's own statements. But in many other cases the truth is difficult to determine. There may be little or no corroboration. The alleged perpetrator often vigorously denies the accusation, and the memory may be declared to be a product of therapeutic suggestion. Are these memories true or false? Fitzpatrick's revelations added fuel to a smoldering controversy that was soon to burst into flames, the now familiar dispute about recovered memories. By the mid-1990s there was a vitriolic and confusing controversy about memory and trauma that extended from professional venues to the popular media (see Beckett, 1996; Bowman & Mertz, 1996; DePrince & Freyd, 1997; Enns, McNeilly, Corkery, & Gilbert, 1995; Freyd, 1996; 1998; Gleaves & Freyd, 1997; Gleaves, 1996; Loftus, 1993; Loftus & Ketcham, 1994; Pope, 1996, 1997; Pope & Brown, 1996; Scheflin & Brown, 1996, Stanton, 1997).

As we approach the end of the century, some of the chaos is dissipating, and all parties to the debate have gained some knowledge and humility. Scholars have reminded us that the study of traumatic stress has a long history. In the 19th century and again after both world wars, psychiatrists and psychologists grappled with many of the issues that are troubling us now (Herman, 1992; van der Kolk, 1987). We have learned that exposure to trauma can profoundly alter both individuals and larger social groups, and that one kind of change affects our attention, perception, and memory (see, e.g., Arrigo & Pezdek, 1998; Elliott, 1997; Freyd, 1996; Herman, 1992; McFarlane & van der Kolk, 1996).

We have learned to step back from the conceptual muddle that emerges under conditions of heated disagreement and instead untangle some separate issues. These are deeply perplexing and slippery topics. What is the nature of memory, and how is it changed by exposure to trauma? How do the awareness and memory of trauma influence the possibility of healing or prevention? To define more precisely what we know and do not know, we must untangle the several issues involved and ask scientifically tractable questions. First, we must distinguish memory phenomena from their underlying motivations and mechanisms (Freyd, 1996). The phenomena are apparent forgetting and later remembering a significant event (or series of events). Why they occur is a question of motivation, and how they occur a question of mechanisms.

In describing the phenomena of recovered memory, it is critical to distinguish between two dimensions: accuracy (how true or false is a memory?) and persistence (how accessible is a memory to explicit recall?). Figure 1 illustrates the two separate dimensions of memory (also see Freyd, 1998). The two dimensions of persistence and accuracy are not necessarily correlated. There is no good evidence that the accuracy of a memory depends on whether it is experienced as continuously available or as recovered after years of forgetting (see Dalenberg, 1996; Pope & Brown, 1996; Scheflin & Brown, 1996; Williams,1995). Furthermore, we can usually measure only perceived persistence, and people are often mistaken about that. They may believe they have always remembered something they have only recently recalled, or believe that they have only recently learned for the first time about an event

FIGURE 1. Schematic Depiction of Two Conceptually Separable Dimensions of Memory That Are Often Confused with One Another in the Context of the Debate About Recovered Memories of Abuse

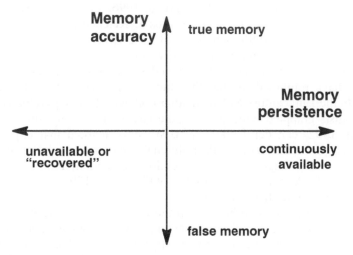

©Jennifer J. Freyd, 1997. Reprinted with permission.

they once described to another person (see Schooler, 2001, in this volume). Therapists should be skeptical about all uncorroborated memories, whether they are newly recovered or not. Any memory, even of good events, can be true or false or a mixture of the two. There are no general rules, and we must live with uncertainty. Much harm can be done by premature efforts to validate or invalidate, judge or label memories.

There is nearly a century of research on nontraumatic memory and its falliability and accuracy. Perhaps the most exciting development to emerge in the second half of the 1990s is the explosion of empirical research on issues of memory malleability, memory persistence, and memory for trauma. The challenge of understanding memory and awareness for trauma requires a truly cross-area approach in which knowledge from various fields is brought to bear on these complex and important issues. Particularly promising in this area is the intersection of traumatic stress studies and cognitive science. As evidenced by this volume, leading trauma researchers and cognitive psychologists are increasingly taking on the very difficult and important task of investigating memory for trauma using research methodologies from cognitive science.

We now have a much clearer picture of the conditions under which human memory is vulnerable to suggestion and distortion (see Oakes & Hyman, 2001, this volume; Pezdek, 2001, this volume). We are beginning to understand the relevance of factors such as event plausibility and social authority. Similarly, we now have access to a substantial number of studies documenting the phenomena of forgetting and remembering trauma, not just the trauma of sexual abuse but a variety of traumas (see Butler, 1996; Cheit, 1998; Corwin & Olafson, 1997; Freyd, 1996; Loftus, Polonsky, & Fullilove, 1994; Kardiner, 1941; McFarlane & van der Kolk, 1996; Sargent & Slater, 1941; Scheflin & Brown, 1996; Schooler, Bendiksen, & Ambadar, 1997; Schooler, 2001, this volume; Williams, 1994; 1995). Additionally, research suggests the rates of forgetting vary for different types of trauma (see Elliott, 1997), and this is very interesting and relevant to the questions of motivations and mechanisms (Freyd, 1996). Through new research in cognitive science and cognitive neuroscience, we are making progress on some of the mechanisms and neuroanatomical structures that play a role in alterations of memory (see Anderson, 2001, this volume; Brewin, 1996; Brewin & Andrews, 2001, this volume; Morton, 1994; Schacter, 1996; Schooler, 2001, this volume; Spiegel, 1997). For example, we have recently found a relationship between basic mechanisms of attention and individual differences in reports of dissociative experiences. Some of our findings and their implications are summarized in the next section of this article.

There are also new perspectives and data on the question of motivations for forgetting traumatic experiences. From psychoanalytic conceptions of avoidance of overwhelming pain or conflict, through innovative theories about our need to believe in a safe world, we have a variety of theories to explore with empirical investigations.

In our own work in this area we have begun to test hypotheses arising from *betrayal trauma theory* (Freyd 1994, 1996), focusing on betrayals of trust such as those that occur in child sexual abuse. According to *The New York Times*:

> Mr. Fitzpatrick's retrieval of the repressed memories began, he said, when "I was feeling a great mental pain . . . ." Mr. Fitzpatrick . . . slowly realized that the mental pain was due to a "betrayal of some kind," and remembered the sound of heavy breathing. "Then I realized I had been sexually abused by someone I loved," said Mr. Fitzpatrick. (Goleman, 1992, p. B5)

Betrayal trauma theory posits that knowledge isolation (including memory repression, dissociation, and unawareness) serves a survival function in necessary human relationships in which betrayal occurs. Human beings are often exquisitely sensitive to betrayal or cheating; we detect the betrayal and then respond with strong negative emotions that guide us away from the betrayer. However, under some circumstances, this very sensitivity can cause us more problems than it solves. It can risk a relationship we may need or believe we need. Child abuse by a caregiver is especially likely to produce such an implicit social conflict for the victim. Withdrawing from a caregiver on whom the child victim depends could further threaten the child's life. For the child who depends upon an abusive caregiver, the situation demands that information about the abuse be blocked from mental mechanisms that control attachment (bonding) behavior. The information that gets blocked may be partial (for instance, blocking emotional responses only), but in many cases the information that gets blocked will lead to a more profound disruption in awareness and autobiographical memory. Consistent with the prediction that the closeness of the victim-perpetrator relationship impacts probability of amnesia, amnesia rates across a variety of studies appear to be higher for parental or incestuous abuse than non-parental or non-incestuous abuse (see Freyd, 1996).

Betrayal also seems to be a central factor in many recovered memory cases involving adults traumatized while in situations of dependence. Vietnam veterans with posttraumatic stress disorder (PTSD) often recall a betrayal by a commanding officer only many years later (Shay, 1994). Battered wives may forget and then remember abuse by their husbands. At the University of Oregon, we are running, in collaboration with colleagues, studies looking at relationship dependence, memory persistence, and other factors in greater detail. Preliminary results support our prediction that the greater the victim's dependence on the perpetrator, the less persistent are memories of abuse (see also Freyd, 1996, for re-analyses of published data sets supporting this premise). Similarly, the data collected by Elliott (1997) on relative rates of delayed recall for different types of trauma are suggestive that memory for trauma varies as a function of the degree of social betrayal.

The role of betrayal in traumatic forgetting has implications for clinical conceptualization and treatment. It suggests that traumas leading to psychic disorders arise from two distinct dimensions of harm: life-threat and social-betrayal (Freyd, in press). From this viewpoint the symptom cluster known as post-traumatic stress disorder may better be understood as arising from two conceptually independent dimensions of trauma (see Figure 2). The dimension of life-threat may be primary for symptoms of fear, anxiety, hyperarousal, and intrusive memories. The dimension of social-betrayal may be primary for symptoms of dissociation, amnesia, numbness, and constricted or abusive relationships. High levels of both life-threat and social-betrayal characterize many of the most severe traumas (e.g., rape, much child abuse, many combat experiences, the Holocaust). With both dimensions present, we expect to see both classes of symptoms present.

Clinicians may be most effective when they understand the separate origins of these different sources of symptoms. We currently have reasonably

FIGURE 2. The Two-Dimensional Model of Trauma

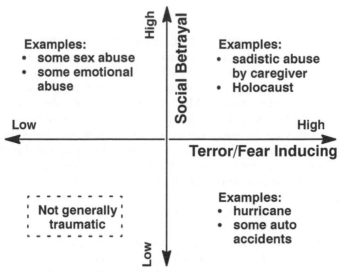

©Jennifer J. Freyd, 1996. Reprinted with permission.

effective methods available for treating the fear, anxiety, and hyperarousal associated with post traumatic stress disorder. Numbing, dissociation, and avoidance have been more difficult to treat. According to betrayal trauma theory, survivors of childhood abuse (and of adult betrayal traumas including battering and some combat situations) have learned to cope with an inescapable social conflict by being disconnected internally. The treatment of these symptoms, according to betrayal trauma theory, will require a focus on social relationships and related cognitive mechanisms used to support such relationships. The treatment goals and methods for promoting internal integration and deeper external connection need not be at odds with the treatment goals and methods for addressing high levels of anxiety, fear, and hyperarousal; however, these goals and methods do have different foci. For instance, clinicians may want to focus on promoting internal integration through the fundamentals of a healthy relationship. Such a relationship supports the explicit verbalization of the traumatic experiences, promoting internal re-coding of disjointed and fragmentary sensory memories. A healthy relationship also can be used by the clinician to encourage the patient's active and appropriate use of trust and reality assessment mechanisms. The potential to heal internal disconnection is almost surely going to be most fully realized in the context of what was so broken in the first place: intimate and trusting relationships.

COGNITIVE PROCESSES ASSOCIATED
WITH DISSOCIATIVE TENDENCIES

We have applied a cognitive science approach to predictions derived from betrayal trauma theory. In particular, we have been interested in the exploration of cognitive processes associated with dissociation. Dissociation has been defined as the lack of integration of thoughts, feelings and experiences into the stream of consciousness. Most people report some dissociative experiences, such as "highway hypnosis" (when one apparently loses conscious awareness of driving for some period of time). However, individual differences in dissociative tendencies have been consistently reported in the literature (see Freyd, 1996, for a review). A number of studies indicate that dissociative tendencies appear to be very high in populations of trauma survivors, including research in which there is external corroboration for the trauma (e.g., see Bremner et al., 1992; Carlson & Rosser-Hogan, 1993; Marmar et al., 1994; Putnam & Trickett, 1997).

Dissociation likely plays a role in various psychiatric disorders, including posttraumatic stress disorder (PTSD) (e.g., Bremner et al., 1992; Carlson & Rosser-Hogan, 1993; Elliott & Briere, 1995; Koopman, Classen & Spiegel, 1994; Marmar et al., 1994; Saxe et al., 1993) as well as the dissociative disorders. Given that higher levels of dissociation are found in trauma populations, and in individuals who meet the criteria for PTSD and the dissociative disorders, understanding dissociation is critical to both research and clinical practice. Despite its clinical importance, dissociation has not been well understood at the cognitive level. While a number of studies provide some hints about the cognitive bases of dissociation and dissociative disorders (e.g., Eich, Macaulay, Lowenstein, & Dihley, 1997; Hilgard, 1986; Kihlstrom & Couture, 1992; Schacter, Kihlstrom, & Kihlstrom, 1989; Litz et al., 1996; Nissen, Ross, Willingham, MacKenzie, & Schacter, 1988), we sought to extend this understanding based on a betrayal trauma theory framework.

Betrayal trauma theory predicts that dissociating information from awareness is mediated by the threat that the information poses to the individual's system of attachment (Freyd, in press, 1994, 1996). Dissociation is implicated as an important factor in removing threatening information from awareness; however, the role of, and mechanisms that underlie, dissociation remain unclear. We posit that basic cognitive processes involved in attention and memory most likely play an important role in dissociating explicit awareness of betrayal traumas. Here we report on three studies from our laboratory that have investigated the role of basic cognitive processes associated with individual differences in dissociative tendencies.

DISSOCIATIVE TENDENCIES
AND SELECTIVE ATTENTION

In the first study (Freyd, Martorello, Alvarado, Hayes, & Christman, 1998) we focused on the basic function of selective attention: the ability to select willfully certain information while inhibiting the selection of other information simultaneously available. Humans generally are impressive at selective attention but it is not an all-or-none ability. While some information may be selected, other information may nonetheless intrude. We hypothesized that dissociative tendencies would be systematically related to selective attentional mechanisms.

We assessed dissociative tendencies using the Dissociative Experiences Scale (DES) (Bernstein & Putnam, 1986). The DES is a 28 item self-report measure that assesses dissociative experiences such as dissociative amnesia, gaps in awareness, derealization, depersonalization, absorption, and imaginative involvement. The DES has been used in over 250 published studies in a wide range of populations. The DES has been shown to have good reliability (internal consistency and test-retest), as well as good convergent validity (see Briere, 1997, for a review). Participants are instructed to indicate the percentage of time for which each item pertains to them. Items include, "Some people have the experience of feeling that other people, objects, and the world around them are not real" and "Some people find that they have no memory for some important events in their lives" (for example, a wedding or graduation). Carlson and Putnam (1993) note that scores above 20 are indicative of highly dissociative experiences about which a clinician would want to gather more information. Scores below 10 are considered in the range of normal dissociative experiences (Carlson & Rosser-Hogan, 1993).

We assessed attentional processes using the Stroop task (Stroop, 1935). The Stroop task is the classic experimental demonstration of our ability to selectively attend and of our inability to completely exclude the unattended stimulus from impacting performance. In the standard Stroop task, participants are asked to name the ink color of a list of words or strings of letters printed in different colors. In its simplest form in the experimental condition, the words are color names (e.g., "blue" or "yellow") and those words are incongruent with the ink colors (thus the word "blue" is printed in yellow ink, while the word "yellow" is printed in red ink). In a control condition, the words are neutral terms (e.g., "book" or "river") or non-word stimuli such as strings of identical letters (e.g., "xxxxx") and the ink colors are randomly assigned to the different words or strings of letters. Participants attempting to name the ink color take longer when the ink colors are paired with incongruent color words than when the ink colors are paired with neutral words, strings of letters, or congruent color terms.

The fact that participants can name the ink colors and inhibit naming the words themselves illustrates the power of selective attention. However, the fact that the meaning of the color words apparently interferes with ink naming demonstrates the inability to completely exclude information that is not chosen for selection. The Stroop paradigm, one of most widely used methodologies for studying selective attention, seemed a good starting place for exploring the hypothesis that participants varying in dissociative tendencies would show a difference in basic attentional processing.

Using a standard Stroop task, Freyd et al. (1998) compared "Stroop interference" for high versus low dissociators. The standard Stroop interference is the difference in reaction time to name a color that is incongruent with the word meaning (e.g., green appears in red ink) from a baseline condition (e.g., name the ink color for a row of xxx's). Forty high and 40 low dissociators were selected from a sample of 154 college students (see Table 1 for participant statistics).

Participants who scored high on the Dissociative Experiences Scale (DES) showed greater Stroop interference for conflicting color terms than individuals with low DES scores. High DES participants took longer to name the ink colors when the lists were conflicting color terms (such as naming the color "yellow" when the word "red" was printed in the ink color yellow) than did the low DES participants. For all other categories but the conflicting color terms, reaction times for high dissociators were equivalent to or slightly faster than the reaction times of the low dissociators, indicating that the increased interference effect is not accompanied by confounding factors such as generalized slowing among the high DES participants (see Table 2).

The results from Freyd et al. (1998) suggested a basic relationship between selective attention and dissociative tendencies: that people with high dissociative tendencies have disruptions of consciously controlled attentional abilities. Notably, the disruptions in attentional abilities were unrelated to emotional content. However, many questions remained, including whether the disruptions in attentional abilities would occur across attentional contexts with different task demands.

TABLE 1. Descriptive Statistics for the High and Low DES Group (Freyd et al., 1998)

	Low DES Group	High DES Group
Number	40	40
Mean	5.56	32.50
Median	5.98	30.62
Std. Dev.	2.13	7.68

TABLE 2. Mean Ink-Naming Times (in Seconds) and Standard Deviations for Lists of 8 Words Grouped by Word Categories (Freyd et al., 1998)

	low DES group	high DES group
Category	*Time (SD)*	*Time (SD)*
Color	6.50 (1.15)	7.03 (1.51)
X's	4.62 (0.81)	4.51 (0.89)
Kinship	4.11 (0.63)	4.10 (0.74)
Animal	4.80 (0.93)	4.78 (0.86)
Household	4.91 (1.01)	4.65 (0.89)
Space	4.57 (0.72)	4.59 (0.80)

FIGURE 3. Ink-Naming Times for 40 High- and Low-DES College Students in the Stroop Task (Freyd et al., 1998)

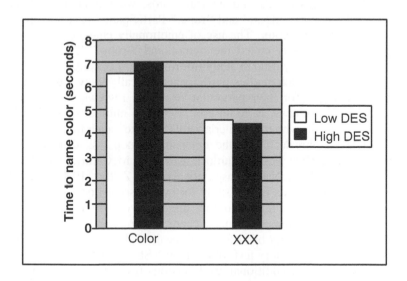

DISSOCIATIVE TENDENCIES,
SELECTIVE AND DIVIDED ATTENTION, AND MEMORY

Freyd et al. (1998) found that individuals with high dissociative tendencies appear to be at a disadvantage when selective attention is required in the

Stroop task. How would high dissociators perform under divided attention conditions? Given the definition of dissociation as a fragmentation of thoughts, feelings, and experiences, we suspected that high dissociators might actually be at a cognitive advantage in tasks where they had to divide (or fragment) their attention. Therefore, we predicted an interaction such that high DES participants might be at an advantage in a divided attention condition and at a disadvantage in a selective attention condition relative to low dissociators. To test this prediction, DePrince and Freyd (1999) designed a study to replicate and extend Freyd et al. that employed both selective and divided attention conditions. Memory was tested for words presented in both the selective and divided attention conditions of the Stroop task.

The Stroop experimental trials involved two separate blocks of trials. In the first block of trials, participants heard standard instructions to name the color of the word as quickly and accurately as possible, while ignoring the word meaning (a selective attention task). During a second block of trials, participants were instructed to attend to the word meaning as well as word color (divided attention).

In addition to presenting participants with color terms (e.g., "red" in red ink), baseline strings of x's and neutral words, we included emotionally charged words such as "incest" and "rape." Participants' task remained the same: to name the ink color. The use of emotionally charged words in the Stroop task is commonly called the "emotional Stroop." The "emotional Stroop" has been widely used to study information processing in a variety of mental disorders. In such studies participants typically view words that are emotionally charged for their particular fears (for reviews, see MacLeod, 1991; Williams, Mathews, & MacLeod, 1996). A number of studies have shown that individuals who meet criteria for PTSD take longer to name the color of words that are threatening in the emotional Stroop task than individuals without PTSD (e.g., Foa, Feske, Murdock, Kozak, & McCarthy, 1991; McKenna & Sharma, 1995; McNally, Kaspi, Riemann & Zeitlin, 1990). We added emotionally charged words in this study for two reasons: first, we were interested in seeing whether high and low dissociative individuals responded more or less slowly to the emotionally charged words, and second, we were interested in the possibility of differential recall of these words for high and low dissociators in a memory test following the Stroop task.

The study had some additional modifications from its predecessor. First, there were some methodological improvements. Stimuli were presented by computer instead of by hand-held cards and reaction times were recorded for each trial by a voice-activated microphone attached to the computer instead of by hand-held stopwatches for lists of words. In addition, filler Stroop items were included at both the beginning and end of each block of trials to absorb the anticipated primacy and recency effects for the subsequent memory tests.

Another improvement involved the addition of two individual difference measures: the Behavioral Inhibition Scale (BIS) (Carver & White, 1994) and seven questions about trauma history. The published original report of De-Prince and Freyd (1999) does not include the results of the BIS and trauma questions; these results will be reported for the first time in print in the current article.

Methods for DePrince and Freyd (1999) Study

Undergraduate students at the University of Oregon were selected based on their scores on the DES (Bernstein & Putnam, 1986). Fifty-four high and 54 low DES participants were tested from an initial group of three hundred and eighty-eight students who were screened using the DES. Table 3 presents participant statistics.

Both the standard and the new dual-task Stroop color-naming tasks were employed. Participants always had the selective attention condition first, then the divided attention condition. Word order and word-color pairings were randomized for each subject. Colored word and non-word stimuli were presented on a computer screen. The experimental stimulus words came from eight categories. Word lists from six of the categories were replicated from Freyd et al. (1998). These words included baseline (strings of x's in varying lengths matched to the length of the color words), animals (e.g., cat, baboon, horse, tiger), space (e.g., star, rainbow, airplane, planet), kinship (e.g., dad, niece, brother, uncle), household (e.g., hall, cellar, television, kitchen), and incongruent colors (e.g., "red" in blue ink). For the purposes of this study, the four semantic categories were collapsed into one neutral category. Emotionally charged words were taken from McNally et al. (1998) (e.g., assault, shame, incest, victim). Finally, congruent color words were added: red, yellow, green, blue. Congruent trials included, for example, the word "red" in red ink. A practice session and final set of trials involved country names.

TABLE 3. Descriptive Statistics for the High and Low DES Group (DePrince & Freyd, 1999)

	Low DES Group	High DES Group
Number	54	54
Mean DES	5.1	29.6
Mean Age	19.6	19.5
% female	79.6%	61.1%

Each stimulus consisted of a single color word at the center of a white-colored personal computer screen. The stimulus remained on the screen until the participant made a voice response into a microphone with a 100 millisecond inter-trial interval. Word-color pairings and word order presentation were randomized for each participant. For the non-color words, half of the words were viewed during the first part of the experiment and half during the second part; list order presentation was randomized across participants.

A free recall task was administered immediately following both the selective and dual-task Stroop blocks. Participants were instructed to write down any words they could remember from the computer list just viewed. Following the free recall task, a stem completion was administered. The stem completion included 22 stems that could be completed with words viewed on the computer; five additional stems were not related to the computer list. The stem completion results are not yet reported.

Participants were tested one at a time in a room with an experimenter present. Participants were instructed that they would be presented with single words in one of four colors in the center of the computer screen, and were told that their task was to name the color as quickly and accurately as possible. They received instructions to ignore the word meanings and to name the color of the word by speaking into a microphone located directly in front of them. Participants were instructed not to correct themselves if they made errors. They engaged in a practice session, which included two blocks of eight country names. Following the practice, participants viewed the first block of words. The list concluded with the presentation of the eight country names from the practice trials. Country names appeared during practice and at the end of the list to help reduce primacy or recency effects for the experimental words in the memory tasks.

Following completion of the first block, participants were given a surprise free recall memory task. They were instructed to write down all of the words that they could remember from the list they had just seen. Next, participants were given a stem-completion task that included stems from the words seen during the Stroop task, as well as five words not viewed during the block.

Participants were given new instructions for the dual-task Stroop task. They were instructed to name the ink color as quickly and accurately as possible while also remembering the words for a memory test at the end. Practice trials using the country names were administered. Immediately following the practice trials, participants viewed a list that did not include any of the non-color words seen during the standard Stroop block. The eight country names were presented at the end of the list. Participants were again instructed to complete free recall and stem-completion tasks.

The DES (Bernstein & Putnam, 1986), the BIS (Carver & White, 1994), and a trauma questionnaire were administered by computer. The BIS is designed to assess anxiety. It contains seven items to each of which the subject responds on a four-point scale, where a response of 1 indicates strong agreement and a response of 4 indicates strong disagreement. The items include: (1) If I think something unpleasant is going to happen I usually get pretty "worked up"; (2) I worry about making mistakes; (3) Criticism or scolding hurts me quite a bit; (4) I feel worried or upset when I think or know somebody is angry at me; (5) Even if something bad is about to happen to me, I rarely experience fear or nervousness; (6) I feel worried when I think I have done poorly at something; (7) I have very few fears compared to my friends. Items 5 and 7 are reverse scored.

One general and six more specific questions about traumatic experiences were asked. For example, participants read statements such as, "I have experienced physical abuse before age 14" and were asked to indicate yes or no. Six categories of abuse were included (sexual abuse before age 14, unwanted touching before age 14, sexual assault after age 14, physical abuse, emotional/psychological abuse, and abuse not otherwise specified).

Summary of Previously Published Results from the DePrince and Freyd (1999) Study

Table 4 includes the mean of the response times in milliseconds for six categories of words during selective and dual-task attention conditions for the high and low DES participants. Interference scores were calculated by subtracting the mean reaction times for the baseline XX category from the incongruent category for each participant. Group means were computed (see Figure 4). In a 2 (dissociation) by 2 (attention task) ANOVA, main effects for dissociation level and attention task were not significant. The crossover interaction of dissociation by attention task was significant. Among the other neutral and charged categories, no significant differences in reaction time between the groups were found.

TABLE 4. Mean (Standard Deviation) Reaction Time in Milliseconds by Condition (DePrince & Freyd, 1999)

	Selective		Dual-Task	
	Low DES	High DES	Low DES	High DES
Baseline (xxx)	669 (144)	649 (82)	784 (167)	785 (174)
Incongruent	759 (136)	778 (129)	900 (190)	878 (155)
Neutral	699 (121)	700 (101)	836 (156)	831 (151)
Charged	691 (151)	687 (103)	843 (163)	820 (178)
Congruent	605 (112)	609 (85)	735 (145)	724 (157)

FIGURE 4. Mean Interference Scores for High and Low DES by Attention Task (Selective and Dual-Task) (DePrince & Freyd, 1999)

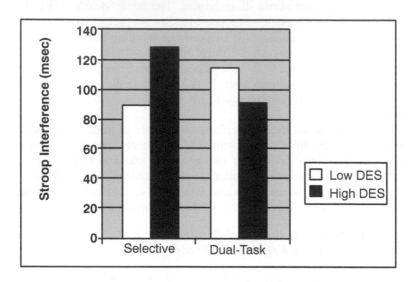

TABLE 5. Mean Percentage of Correctly Recalled Neutral and Charged Words by Condition for High and Low DES (DePrince & Freyd, 1999)

	Selective		Dual-Task	
	Neutral	Charged	Neutral	Charged
Low DES	4.18	9.73	18.05	28.70
High DES	4.40	6.95	18.13	19.45

The two groups did not differ significantly in the total number of words written (correct or not) during the free recall task. The mean percentage of words correctly recalled for neutral and emotionally charged words are presented in Table 5. Using a 2 (dissociation) × 2 (attention task) × 2 (word category) repeated measures mixed design ANOVA, significant effects were found for attention task and word category. The main effect of dissociation was marginally significant. A significant interaction of dissociation by word category revealed that low DES participants recalled fewer neutral words and more emotionally charged words compared to high DES participants.

FIGURE 5. Percentage of Words Recalled by Word Category (Charged or Neutral) for Low and High DES Participants (DePrince & Freyd, 1999)

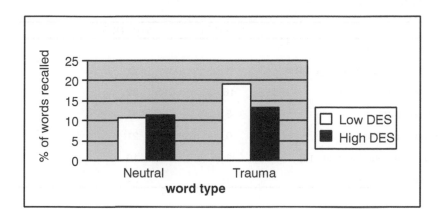

New Results from the DePrince and Freyd (1999) Study

In addition to the DePrince and Freyd (1999) reported data, we now report results from the BIS and trauma questions. Scores on the BIS were computed by adding up the responses for the seven items (Items 5 and 7 reverse scored), for a possible range of 7 to 28, with higher scores representing higher anxiety. We are missing data on the BIS for one subject. Low DES participants had an average BIS score of 14.6 and high DES participants had an average BIS score of 13.9. The groups did not differ on anxiety as measured by the BIS, $t(105) = .993; p = .32$

Table 6 indicates the number of "yes" responses endorsed when asked about six types of trauma: sexual abuse before age 14, uncomfortable touching, physical abuse, emotional abuse, sexual assault after age 14, and other trauma not specified. Participants could endorse more than one type of trauma. Overall we found that high DES participants reported three times as much trauma in their history as did low DES participants. The data were submitted to a logistic regression in order to test whether experiences of trauma could predict high and low dissociation groupings. Six variables were entered as predictors: sexual abuse before age 14, uncomfortable touching, physical abuse, emotional abuse, sexual assault after age 14, and other trauma not specified in the questionnaire. The model was significant (Chi^2 (6, n = 108) = 41.358, p = .0001); the overall success rate of predictions was 70.37%.

TABLE 6. Number of "Yes" Endorsements to Traumatic Experiences in the Order Questions Were Presented to Participants by DePrince and Freyd (1999)

	Low DES	High DES
Type of Trauma		
Sexual Abuse (before age 14)	3	8
Uncomfortable Touching	16	22
Physical Abuse	3	9
Emotional Abuse	0	21
Sexual Assault (after age 14)	2	10
Trauma Not Specified	19	34

DIRECTED FORGETTING, ATTENTIONAL CONTEXT, AND MEMORY

We employed a directed forgetting paradigm in order to further investigate the DePrince and Freyd (1999) memory finding that high DES participants remembered fewer charged words and more neutral words relative to low DES participants. Directed forgetting is a laboratory task in which participants are presented with items and told after each item (or a group of items) whether to remember or forget the material. Subsequent memory is tested for both the "forget" and the "remember" items. We tested high and low DES participants in a directed forgetting paradigm that included both charged and neutral words, as well as both a selective and divided attention condition (DePrince & Freyd, in press). At the onset of the study, we were particularly interested in whether we would see evidence, as in DePrince and Freyd (1999), that high DES participants show impaired memory for the emotionally charged words relative to low DES participants. Additional predictions were tested and will be reported in future publication (DePrince & Freyd, in press).

Method for DePrince and Freyd, in Press

Twenty-eight high DES participants (DES score > 20; mean DES = 26.8; SD = 4.7) and 28 low DES participants (DES score < 10; mean DES = 5.19; SD = 2.8) were tested using a directed forgetting paradigm which replicated and extended a study conducted by McNally and his colleagues (McNally et al., 1998). Participants were asked to read words that appeared on a computer screen for two seconds. Following each word, participants saw instructions to either remember or forget the word they had just read; the memory instruction appeared for three seconds. Participants were told that they would be tested on all words followed by the remember instruction at the end of the experiment. Words were drawn from three categories used in the McNally et al. (1998) study: positive, neutral and emotionally charged for sexual assault.

Participants viewed words under three different attention conditions: selective attention, divided attention with color, and divided attention with numbers. During the selective attention blocks, participants were told that they would see a word and then receive the instruction to either remember or forget that word. In the divided attention color blocks, the color of the word and instruction changed at random intervals between red and blue. In the divided attention color blocks, participants were instructed to press a key each time the color changed while also following the instructions to read and remember words. In divided attention number blocks, participants were asked to count out loud by three's while following instructions to read and remember words. We included two types of divided attention conditions to investigate how different types of divided attention task manipulations affected performance (e.g., one condition required verbal responses, another key press responses).

The stimuli were divided into three lists. Each list was paired with an attention condition and counterbalanced across participants (e.g., List A paired with the selective attention condition, List B paired with the divided attention color condition, List C paired with the divided attention number condition). Each block was repeated three times, thus participants viewed nine blocks in total. The block order was randomized for each participant. At the beginning of each block of stimuli, participants were given instructions for that particular block. Filler words appeared at the beginning and end of each block in order to prevent primacy and recency effects in free recall.

After viewing the nine blocks of stimuli, participants were asked to write down all of the words they could remember from the experiment (free recall task). Participants were instructed to write down words regardless of the remember or forget instructions presented during the experiment. Following the free recall task, participants were given a recognition test. Participants viewed words one at a time on the computer screen. Half of the words were taken from the experiment. The other half were new words, not previously viewed during the experiment, that were matched for word category (e.g., neutral, charged for sexual assault) and part of speech. Participants were instructed to make a key press for each word to indicate whether that word had been previously viewed during the experiment or was new.

Preliminary analyses of the free recall data revealed a 2 (DES, high or low) × 2 (word category, charged or neutral) interaction within the divided attention color condition, $F(1,54) = 5.074$, $p = .028$. Within this interaction, high DES participants remembered fewer charged words and more neutral words than low DES participants who remembered more charged and fewer neutral words. Table 7 displays the mean number of words per condition.

DISCUSSION OF SUMMARIZED RESEARCH INVESTIGATING COGNITIVE PROCESSES ASSOCIATED WITH DISSOCIATIVE TENDENCIES: COGNITIVE ENVIRONMENTS TO CLINICAL IMPLICATIONS

In summary, we found that high DES participants show more interference on the basic Stroop color-naming task than low DES participants (Freyd et al., 1998; DePrince & Freyd, 1999). In contrast, we found an interaction between DES and attention condition such that the high DES group exhibited less interference when they were asked to divide their attention and accomplish two tasks at once (DePrince & Freyd, 1999). We also found that the high DES group remembered fewer emotionally charged words than the low DES group overall (DePrince & Freyd, 1999), as well as in a divided attention condition (DePrince & Freyd, in press), findings suggestive of the adaptive value of dissociation.

Furthermore, we found, in line with other studies, that individuals with high DES scores report significantly more trauma in their histories (DePrince & Freyd, 1999, study; data reported here). The self-reported trauma histories are limited in that they were not corroborated, and there is some reason to be concerned that highly dissociative people may be more inclined to confabulate (e.g., see Hyman & Billings, 1998). However, it seems likely that the substantially higher rates of reported trauma for the high DES participants has some basis in real traumatic exposure, given the evidence that retrospec-

TABLE 7. Mean Number of Words (std. dev.) Recalled in the Divided Attention Color Condition of the Directed Forgetting Experiment (DePrince & Freyd, in preparation).

	Charged	Neutral
Low DES (n = 28)	.93 (.81)	.50 (.75)
High DES (n = 28)	.54 (.74)	.75 (.93)

tive reports of early childhood events are reasonably reliable (Brewin, Andrews & Gotlib, 1993) and the evidence that dissociation is found to be higher in populations with corroborated trauma histories (e.g., Bremner et al., 1992; Carlson & Rosser-Hogan, 1993; Marmar et al., 1994; Putnam & Trickett, 1997).

The current findings suggest that dissociative tendencies and basic cognitive processes of memory and attention are interconnected. The cross-over interaction for Stroop interference suggests that, at least for some tasks requiring the selection of information, dissociative people may perform better when dual-tasking, as compared with non-dissociative people who may perform best when focusing their attention. As a corollary, this finding suggests that although highly dissociative individuals are generally considered impaired, in some contexts they may have a cognitive edge. The interaction between word-category and DES group that we found with the free recall data hints that this dissociation may be adaptive in keeping emotionally charged information out of consciousness (DePrince & Freyd, 1999). The interaction between word-category and DES in the divided attention condition of the directed forgetting study suggests that divided attention conditions may aid high DES participants in keeping threatening stimuli from awareness (DePrince & Freyd, in press).

We currently understand these results as consistent with a "cognitive environments" conceptualization for dissociation. This conceptualization assumes that individuals who are high dissociators have developed ways to cope in life that allow for their dissociation without apparent problems under many circumstances. This lack of integration of experiences, memories, and thoughts creates an environment that requires constant divided attention. Individuals who habitually dissociate information may come to be best able to function in multi-tasking, divided attention, divided control structure environments. Individuals who do not habitually dissociate may be best able to function in relatively more focused attention, task, and control environments.

From a "cognitive environments" viewpoint, traumatized individuals may use dissociation and dual-tasking in order to keep information that is potentially at odds with survival goals away from consciousness and other mental functions. Habitual creation of a divided cognitive environment may lead to both adaptive and maladaptive consequences, depending on the context and functional demands of the situation. In order to make a more concrete connection between the current findings and trauma history, an important replication should include a sample with corroborated trauma histories. In addition, studies that manipulate dissociation will be important in determining whether attentional differences are related to state or trait dissociation.

Finally, we offer the following speculation for future consideration: If some individuals are better able to function under conditions of divided attention, they may take actions to increase the extent of "chaos" in their environment. If so, some of the commonly reported chaos in the lives of clients who are highly dissociative (e.g., trauma survivors, individuals diagnosed with dissociative disorders or PTSD) may be understood as serving a particular cognitive function. If chaos serves a cognitive function, such as creating and maintaining divided cognitive environments, understanding this function may aid clinicians in their therapeutic approaches.

Future Research

The question of causality remains to be addressed. Does trauma lead to dissociative coping strategies which in turn cause changes in attentional mechanisms (and thus memory encoding)? Do these changes in mechanisms, in turn, lead to chronically high levels of dissociation? Longitudinal studies with victims who have corroborated their traumatic experiences would be particularly valuable in addressing this issue (although a challenge here is that corroborated trauma victims are not representative of the majority of incest victims, in which the very dynamics that make corroboration unlikely may make dissociation functional in that family context).

Research questions also rise out of the potential clinical applications of these findings. If dissociative tendencies have implications for basic cognitive mechanisms, then perhaps clinical interventions should take this into consideration. How permanent are attentional changes? Does attentional performance change as an individual becomes more or less dissociative over time? Future studies may attempt to manipulate dissociative level within an individual to see the extent to which attentional function varies.

If additional research replicates and expands upon our findings, this research will have clinical implications. While high dissociators do sometimes make chaos in their lives, they may have certain cognitive "deficits" and "strengths" depending on the task context. Clinicians might help dissociators find appropriate contexts for their particular skills. Clinicians may be more helpful if they understand cognitive and adaptive forces behind the chaos, and should remain alert to the possibility that certain dissociative responses continue to have some current adaptive value to patients.

CONCLUDING REMARKS

In this article we have summarized both our perspective on memory for trauma and the findings from three studies we have conducted investigating the cognitive processes associated with dissociative tendencies. The theoretical perspective of betrayal trauma theory and our observations and readings about the phenomenology of trauma and traumatic stress have provided us with a framework for generating hypotheses. The conceptual and methodological tools of cognitive science have provided us with a framework for testing these hypotheses. The result has been the discovery of some of the ways that attention and memory differ between high dissociators (who we have reason to believe are on average highly traumatized) and low dissociators (who we have reason to believe are on average less traumatized). This research is fundamentally in its infancy, yet there are already clinical implications inherit the conceptualization and findings. We eagerly look forward to continuing to pursue research in this promising area; so much remains to be uncovered about the deeply important question of human response to trauma.

REFERENCES

Anderson, M. C. (2000). Active forgetting: Evidence for functional inhibition as a source of memory failure. *Journal of Aggression, Maltreatment & Trauma* (This volume).

Arrigo, J. M., & Pezdek, K. (1998). Lessons from the study of psychogenic amnesia. *Current Directions in Psychological Science, 6*, 148-152.

Beckett, K. (1996). Culture and the politics of signification: The case of child sexual abuse. *Social Problems, 43(1)*, 57-76.

Bernstein, E. M., & Putnam, F. W. (1986). Development, reliability, and validity of a dissociation scale. *Journal of Nervous and Mental Disease, 174*, 727-735.

Bowman, C. G., & Mertz, E. (1996). What should the courts do about memories of sexual abuse? Towards a balanced approach. *The Judge's Journal, 35(4)*, 7-17.

Bremner, J. D., Southwick, S., Brett, E., Fontana, A., Rosenheck, R., & Charney, D. (1992). Dissociation and posttraumatic stress disorder in Vietnam combat veterans. *American Journal of Psychiatry, 149*:3, 328-332.

Brewin, C. R. (1996). Clinical and experimental approaches to understanding repression. In J. D. Read & D. S. Lindsay (Eds.), *Recollections of trauma*: *Scientific research and clinical practice* (pp 145-163). New York: Plenum Press.

Brewin, C. R., & Andrews, B. (2000) Questions and answers about traumatic memory. *Journal of Aggression, Maltreatment & Trauma*. (This volume).

Brewin, C. R., Andrews, B., & Gotlib, I.H. (1993). Psychopathology and early experience: A reappraisal of retrospective reports. *Psychological Bulletin, 113*, 82-98.

Briere, J. (1997). *Psychological assessment of adult posttraumatic stress.* Washington, DC: American Psychological Association.

Butler, K. (1996). The latest on recovered memory. *Family Therapy Networker, 20(6)*, 36-37.

Carlson, E. B., & Putnam, F. W. (1993). An update on the Dissociative Experiences Scale. *Dissociation, VI*, 16-27.

Carlson, E. B., & Rosser-Hogan, R. (1993). Trauma experiences, posttraumatic stress, dissociation and depression in Cambodian refugees. *American Journal of Psychiatry, 148*, 1548-1551.

Carver, C. S., & White, T. L. (1994). Behavioral inhibition, behavioral activation, and affective responses to impending reward and punishment: The BIS/BAS scales. *Journal of Personality and Social Psychology, 67*, 319-333.

Cheit, R. E. (1998). Consider this, skeptics of recovered memory. *Ethics & Behavior*, *8*, 141-160.

Corwin, D. L., & Olafson, E. (1997). Videotaped discovery of a reportedly unrecallable memory of child sexual abuse: Comparison with a childhood interview videotaped 11 years before. *Child Maltreatment*, *2*, 91-112.

Dalenberg, C. J. (1996). Accuracy, timing and circumstances of disclosure in therapy of recovered and continuous memories of abuse. *Journal of Psychiatry and Law*, *24*, 229-275.

DePrince, A. P., & Freyd, J. J. (in press). Dissociation and directed forgetting under conditions of divided attention. *Journal of Trauma & Dissociation*.

DePrince, A. P., & Freyd, J. J. (1997). So what's the dispute about? *The Judges' Journal: A Quarterly of the Judicial Division of the American Bar Association*, *36(3)*, 70-72.

DePrince, A. P., & Freyd, J. J. (1999). Dissociative tendencies, attention, and memory. *Psychological Science*, *10*, 449-452

Eich, E., Macaulay, D., Lowenstein, R. J., & Dihley, P. H. (1997). Memory, amnesia, and dissociative identity disorder. *Psychological Science*, *8*, 417-422.

Elliott, D. M. (1997). Traumatic events: Prevalence and delayed recall in the general population. *Journal of Consulting and Clinical Practice*, *65*, 811-820.

Elliott, D. M., & Briere, J. (1995). Posttraumatic stress associated with delayed recall of sexual abuse: A general population study. *Journal of Traumatic Stress*, *8*, 629-648.

Enns, C. Z., C. McNeilly, J. Corkery, and M. Gilbert. (1995). The debate about delayed memories of child sexual abuse: A feminist perspective. *The Counseling Psychologist*, *23*, 181-279.

Fitzpatrick, F. L. (1994). Isolation and silence: A male survivor speaks out about clergy abuse. *Moving Forward*, *3(1)*, 4-8.

Foa, E., Feske, U., Murdock, T., Kozak, M. & McCarthy, P. (1991). Processing of threat-related information in rape victims. *Journal of Abnormal Psychology*, *100*, 156-162.

Freyd, J. J. (in press) Memory for trauma: Separating the contributions of fear from betrayal. In J.R. Conte (Ed) *Child Sexual Abuse: Knowns and Unknowns–A Volume in Honor of Roland Summit*. Thousand Oaks, CA: Sage Publications.

Freyd, J. J. (1994). Betrayal trauma: Traumatic amnesia as an adaptive response to childhood abuse. *Ethics & Behavior 4*, 207-309.

Freyd, J. J. (1998) Science in the memory debate. *Ethics & Behavior*, *8*, 101-113.

Freyd, J. J., Martorello, S.R., Alvarado, J.S., Hayes, A. E., & Christman, J.C. (1998). Cognitive environments and dissociative tendencies: Performance on the standard Stroop task for high versus low dissociators. *Applied Cognitive Psychology*, *12*, S91-S103.

Freyd, J. J. (1996). *Betrayal trauma theory: The logic of forgetting childhood abuse*. Cambridge, MA: Harvard University Press.

Gleaves, D. H. (1996). The evidence for "repression": An examination of Holmes (1990) and the implications for the recovered memory controversy. *Journal of Child Sexual Abuse*, *5*, 1-19.

Gleaves, D. H., & Freyd, J. J. (1997). Questioning additional claims about the "false memory syndrome" epidemic. *American Psychologist, 52*, 993-994.

Goleman, D. (1992, July 21). Childhood trauma: Memory or invention? *The New York Times*, p. B5-B8.

Herman, J. L. (1992). *Trauma and Recovery.* New York: Basic Books.

Hilgard, E. R. (1986). *Divided consciousness: Multiple controls in human thought and action.* New York: John Wiley & Sons.

Hyman, I. E., Jr., & Billings, F. J. (1998) Individual difference and the creation of false childhood memories. *Memory, 6*, 1-20.

Kardiner, A. (1941). *The Traumatic Neuroses of War.* New York: Hoeber.

Kihlstrom, J. F., & Couture, L. J. (1992). Awareness and information processing in general anesthesia. *Journal of Psychopharmacology, 6*, 410-417.

Koopman, C., Classen, C., & Spiegel, D. (1994). Predictors of posttraumatic stress symptoms among survivors of the Oakland/Berkeley, Calif., firestorm. *American Journal of Psychiatry, 151*, 888-894.

Litz, B. T., Weathers, F. W., Monaco, V., Herman, D. S., Wulfsohn, M., Marx, B., & Keane, T. M. (1996). Attention, arousal, and memory in posttraumatic stress disorder. *Journal of Traumatic Stress, 9*, 497-520.

Loftus, E. F. (1993). The reality of repressed memories. *American Psychologist, 48*, 518-537.

Loftus, E. K., & Ketcham, K. (1994). *The myth of repressed memory: False memories and allegations of sexual abuse.* New York: St. Martin's Press.

Loftus, E. F, Polonsky, S., & Fullilove, M. T. (1994) Memories of childhood sexual abuse: Remembering and repressing. *Psychology of Women Quarterly, 18*, 67-84.

MacLeod, C. M. (1991). Half a century of research on the Stroop Effect: An integrative review. *Psychological Bulletin, 109*, 163-203.

Marmar, C. R., Weiss, D. S., Schlenger, W. E., Fairbank, J. A., Jordan, B. K., Kulka, R. A., & Hough, R. L. (1994). Peritraumatic dissociation and posttraumatic stress in male Vietnam theater veterans. *American Journal of Psychiatry, 151*, 902-907.

McFarlane, A., & van der Kolk, B. A. (1996) Conclusions and future directions. In B. A. van der Kolk, A. McFarlane, & L. Weisaeth (Eds.), *Traumatic Stress: The effects of overwhelming experience on mind, body, and society.* (pp. 559-575) New York: Guilford Press.

McKenna, F. P., & Sharma, D. (1995). Intrusive cognitions: An investigation of the emotional Stroop task. *Journal of Experimental Psychology: Learning, Memory and Cognition, 21*, 1595-1607.

McNally, R., Kaspi, S., Riemann, B. & Zeitlin, S. (1990). Selective processing of threat cues in post-traumatic stress disorder. *Journal of Abnormal Psychology, 99*, 398-402.

McNally, R. J., Metzger, L. J., Lasko, N. B., Clancy, S. A., & Pitman, R. K. (1998). Directed forgetting of trauma cues in adult survivors of childhood sexual abuse with and without posttraumatic stress disorder. *Journal of Abnormal Psychology, 107*, 596-601.

Morton, J. (1994) Cognitive perspectives on memory recovery. *Applied Cognitive Psychology, 8*, 389-398.

Myers, C. S. (1940) *Shell shock in France 1914-18*. Cambridge, England: Cambridge University Press.

Nissen, M. J., Ross, J. L., Willingham, D. B., MacKenzie, T. B., & Schacter, D. L. (1988). Memory and awareness in a patient with multiple personality disorder. *Brain and Cognition, 8*, 117-134.

Oakes, M. A., Hyman, I. (2000) The role of the self in false memory creation. *Journal of Aggression, Maltreatment & Trauma*. (This volume).

Pezdek, K. (2000) A cognitive analysis of the role of suggestibility in explaining memories for abuse. *Journal of Aggression, Maltreatment & Trauma*. (This volume).

Pope, K. S. (1996). Memory, abuse, and science: Questioning claims about the false memory syndrome epidemic. *American Psychologist, 51*, 957-974.

Pope, K. S. (1997) Science as careful questioning: Are claims of a false memory syndrome epidemic based on empirical evidence? *American Psychologist, 52*, 997-1006.

Pope, K. S., & Brown, L. S. (1996). *Recovered memories of abuse: Assessment, therapy, forensics*. Washington, DC: American Psychological Association.

Putnam, F. W. & Trickett, P. K. (1997). The psychobiological effects of sexual abuse: A longitudinal study. *Annals of the New York Academy Science, 821*, 150-159.

Sargent, W. & Slater, F. (1941). Amnesic syndromes in war. *Proceedings of the Royal Society of Medicine, 34*, 757-764.

Saxe, G. N., van der Kolk, B. A., Berkowitz, R., Chinman, G., Hall, K., Lieberg, G., & Schwartz, J. (1993). Dissociative disorders in psychiatric inpatients. *American Journal of Psychiatry, 150*, 1037-1042.

Schachter, D. L. (1996). *Searching for memory: The brain, the mind, and the past*. New York: Basic Books.

Schacter, D. L., Kihlstrom, J. F., & Kihlstrom, L. C. (1989). Autobiographical memory in a case of multiple personality disorder. *Journal of Abnormal Psychology, 98*, 508-514.

Scheflin, A. W. & Brown, D. (1996). Repressed memory or dissociative amnesia: What the science says. *The Journal of Psychiatry & Law, 24*, 143-188.

Schooler, J. W. (2000) Discovering memories of abuse in the light of meta-awareness. *Journal of Aggression, Maltreatment & Trauma*. (This volume).

Schooler, J. W., Bendiksen, M., & Ambadar, Z. (1997). Taking the middle line: Can we accommodate both fabricated and recovered memories of sexual abuse? In M.A. Conway (Ed.) *Recovered Memories and False Memories*. (pp. 251-291) Oxford: Oxford University Press.

Shay, J. (1994). *Achilles in Vietnam: Combat trauma and the undoing of character*. New York: Atheneum.

Spiegel, D. (1997) Trauma, dissociation, and memory. In R. Yehuda & A. McFarlane (Eds), *Psychobiology of Posttraumatic Stress Disorder* (pp 225-237). New York: The New York Academy of Sciences.

Stanton, M. (1997, July-August). U-turn on memory lane. *Columbia Journalism Review*, 44-49.

Stroop, J. R. (1935). Studies of interference in serial verbal reactions. *Journal of Experimental Psychology, 18*, 643-662.

van der Kolk, B. A. (1987). *Psychological trauma.* Washington, D.C.: American Psychiatric Press.

Williams, J. M. G., Mathews, A., & MacLeod, C. (1996). The emotional Stroop task and psychopathology. *Psychological Bulletin, 120,* 3-24.

Williams, L. M. (1994). Recall of childhood trauma: A prospective study of women's memories of child sexual abuse. *Journal of Consulting and Clinical Psychology, 62,* 1167-1176.

Williams, L. M. (1995). Recovered memories of abuse in women with documented child sexual victimization histories. *Journal of Traumatic Stress, 8,* 649-674.

A Biological Model
for Delayed Recall
of Childhood Abuse

J. Douglas Bremner

SUMMARY. There is currently scientific controversy related to the validity of delayed recall of memories of childhood abuse. Post-Traumatic Stress Disorder (PTSD), which affects 8% of the general population, is a possible consequence of childhood abuse. Changes in brain structures and systems mediating memory offer a possible explanation for delayed recall of childhood abuse in patients with abuse-related PTSD. Brain areas affected by traumatic stress are involved in memory and the modulation of emotion and include the hippocampus and medial prefrontal cortex. Stress also results in acute and chronic changes in neurochemical systems, including cortisol and norepinephrine, that strengthens or weakens the laying down of memory traces. Patients with PTSD have alterations in a broad range of memory functions, including insertions, deletions and distortions. PTSD patients also show changes in structure and function in brain regions mediating memory, including the hippocampus and medial prefrontal cortex, as well as in brain chemical systems involved in the stress response that influence the laying down and retrieval of memories, including cortisol and nore-

The research reviewed in this article was supported by a NIH-sponsored General Clinical Research Center (GCRC) Clinical Associate Physician (CAP) Award and a VA Research Career Development Award to Dr. Bremner, and the National Center for PTSD Grant.

Address correspondence to: J. Douglas Bremner, MD, VA Connecticut Healthcare System (115a), 950 Campbell Avenue, New Haven, CT 06520 (E-mail: j.bremner@ yale. edu).

[Haworth co-indexing entry note]: "A Biological Model for Delayed Recall of Childhood Abuse." Bremner, J. Douglas. Co-published simultaneously in *Journal of Aggression, Maltreatment & Trauma* (The Haworth Maltreatment & Trauma Press, an imprint of The Haworth Press, Inc.) Vol. 4, No. 2 (#8), 2001, pp. 165-183; and: *Trauma and Cognitive Science: A Meeting of Minds, Science, and Human Experience* (ed: Jennifer J. Freyd, and Anne P. DePrince) The Haworth Maltreatment & Trauma Press, an imprint of The Haworth Press, Inc., 2001, pp. 165-183. Single or multiple copies of this article are available for a fee from The Haworth Document Delivery Service [1-800-342-9678, 9:00 a.m. - 5:00 p.m. (EST). E-mail address: getinfo@haworthpressinc.com].

pinephrine. The effects of stress on the brain highlight the importance of considering PTSD in research on memory that is generalized to questions about the delayed recall of childhood abuse. *[Article copies available for a fee from The Haworth Document Delivery Service: 1-800-342-9678. E-mail address: <getinfo@haworthpressinc.com> Website: <http://www.HaworthPress.com> © 2001 by The Haworth Press, Inc. All rights reserved.]*

KEYWORDS. Trauma, memory, hippocampus, neurobiology, PTSD

INTRODUCTION

Delayed recall of childhood abuse is a controversial topic that has had a major impact on our society. Self-reported childhood sexual abuse affects 16% of women (about 40 million) in this country (including rape, attempted rape, or molestation) at some time before their 18th birthday (McCauley et al., 1997) and one million new cases of childhood abuse are documented each year. Post-Traumatic Stress Disorder (PTSD), a psychiatric disorder associated with exposure to psychological traumas, such as childhood abuse, is characterized by symptoms including intrusive memories, hyperarousal, sleep disturbance, flashbacks, increased emotional responsivity, dissociation, and problems with memory and concentration (Saigh & Bremner, 1999). PTSD affects 8% of the general population at some time in their lives (Kessler, Sonnega, Bromet, Hughes, & Nelson, 1995), and is seen in about 15% of individuals exposed to a severe psychological trauma, such as childhood sexual abuse.

Alterations in memory form an important part of the clinical presentation of patients with childhood abuse-related PTSD (Bremner & Marmar, 1998). As reviewed in this article, PTSD patients report deficits in declarative memory (memory for facts or lists, as reviewed below), fragmentation of memories (both autobiographical and trauma-related), memory distortions, and dissociative amnesia (gaps in memory that can occur for minutes to days and are not due to ordinary forgetting). We have demonstrated significant increases in dissociative amnesia based on structured interviews in combat veterans with PTSD compared to combat veterans without PTSD (Bremner, Steinberg, Southwick, Johnson, & Charney, 1993). Many abuse victims claim to remember only certain aspects of the abuse event, a phenomenon related to dissociative amnesia. The wide range of effects that traumatic stress has on memory complicates questions related to delayed recall of childhood abuse.

There is a limited amount of research on delayed recall of childhood abuse. Cases of individuals who have no memory for childhood sexual abuse and then suddenly remember an abuse event years after the fact have been widely publicized in the popular literature. For example, one man who was listening to a report of a priest who was arrested for molesting children 20 years ago suddenly had a memory of being molested by that particular priest. The validity of this type of delayed recall of childhood abuse has been hotly debated in the scientific literature, as reviewed elsewhere in this volume. Studies show that memories are, in fact, susceptible to insertions, deletions, and distortions, often resulting in a situation where the individual remains convinced of the validity of the memory as experienced in its altered form (Kihlstrom, 1987). A variety of experimental paradigms have demonstrated the capacity for false recall, as reviewed in detail elsewhere in this volume. Findings from these studies have led to criticism of clinical reports of delayed recall of childhood abuse. The clinical and scientific literature related to delayed recall of childhood abuse has become polarized with two conflicting viewpoints related to whether or not delayed recall of childhood abuse are valid.

In the current article, I outline a model for how changes in the brain may mediate delayed recall of childhood abuse. One of the primary criticisms of the viewpoint that delayed recall represents valid memories is the apparent illogicality of forgetting of events that most people would consider impossible to forget. However, studies in animals have demonstrated that stress can impair memory function in some circumstances, acting through stress hormones and brain chemicals that affect the way memories are laid down. In addition, stress can result in lasting changes in the structure and function of brain areas involved in memory. The results of animal studies of stress have been used to direct hypotheses related to the effects of stress on patients with abuse-related PTSD. Many of the findings from animal studies have been replicated in humans, including findings of long-term alterations in brain systems and structures involved in the stress response and memory (Bremner, Southwick, & Charney, 1999). Good research data on the proportion of PTSD patients who experience delayed recall of abuse does not exist; however, clinical experience dictates that fragmentations and alterations in memory for traumatic events are more common in patients with PTSD, and include memories for some events that are continuous, memories for other events that are delayed or fragmented, and other memories that are never retrieved at all.

HIPPOCAMPAL DYSFUNCTION AS A POTENTIAL CAUSE OF DELAYED RECALL OF ABUSE

Stress-induced hippocampal damage represents one possible mechanism for delayed recall of childhood abuse. The hippocampus is a brain area involved in learning and memory (Squire & Zola-Morgan, 1991) that is particularly sensitive to stress (Bremner, 1999; McEwen et al., 1992; Sapolsky, 1996). This function is critical to the stress response, for example, in assessing potential threat during a life-threatening situation, as occurs with exposure to a predator. Work from laboratories such as Sapolsky (1996) at Stanford University and McEwen et al. (1992) at Rockefeller University demonstrated that, in a variety of animal species, high levels of glucocorticoids (cortisol in man) seen in stress are associated with damage to the hippocampus. When male and female vervet monkeys are caged together, the female monkeys attack the males, leading to extreme stress in the males which is often fatal. Monkeys who were improperly caged and died spontaneously following exposure to severe stress had multiple gastric ulcers on autopsy, consistent with exposure to chronic stress, as well as enlarged adrenal cortices, consistent with sustained glucocorticoid release. Stress was found to result in damage to the CA3 subfield of the hippocampus (Uno, Tarara, Else, Suleman, & Sapolsky, 1989) that was related to exposure to glucocorticoids (Sapolsky, Uno, Rebert, & Finch, 1990). Studies showed that direct glucocorticoid exposure to the hippocampus results in decreased dendritic branching (Woolley, Gould, & McEwen, 1990), a loss of neurons, and an inhibition of neuronal regeneration (Gould, Tanapat, McEwen, Flugge, & Fuchs, 1998). Glucocorticoids disrupt cellular metabolism (Lawrence & Sapolsky 1994), thereby increasing the vulnerability of hippocampal neurons to excitatory amino acids like glutamate (Virgin et al., 1991). Other neurochemical systems interact with glucocorticoids to mediate the effects of stress on memory and the hippocampus, including brain-derived neurotrophic factor (BDNF) (Nibuya, Morinobu, & Duman, 1995; Smith, Makino, Kvetnansky, & Post, 1995).

Stress also has effects on functions of new learning and memory that are mediated by the hippocampus. Exposure to the stress of an unfamiliar environment resulted in deficits in working memory indicative of hippocampal dysfunction (Diamond, Fleshner, Ingersoll, & Rose, 1996), while high levels of glucocorticoids seen with stress were associated with both deficits in new learning and damage to the hippocampus (Luine, Villages, Martinex, & McEwen, 1994). Long-term subcutaneous implants of glucocorticoids that mimic the chronic stress situation resulted in deficits in new learning and memory for maze-escape behaviors (Arbel, Kadar, Silberman, & Levy, 1994). Stress was also shown to affect long-term potentiation (LTP), which is used as a model for the molecular basis of new learning and memory (Diamond, Branch, Fleshner, & Rose, 1995).

Stress-mediated hippocampal damage may lead to dysregulation of others aspects of the organism's stress response system. The hippocampus has an inhibitory effect on the corticotropin releasing factor (CRF)/(hypothalamic-pituitary-adrenal (HPA) axis (Jacobson & Sapolsky, 1991). CRF, which is released during stress, has behavioral effects that are characteristic of anxiety or the stress response. Stress-induced damage to the hippocampus results in increased levels of CRF (Herman et al., 1984). Consistent with this, an increase in CRF is seen in patients with PTSD, as measured in cerebrospinal fluid (Bremner, Licinio et al., 1997).

In order to test hypotheses about the effects of traumatic stress on memory function in human subjects based on the animal studies reviewed above, we used neuropsychological testing to measure declarative memory function in PTSD. We selected measures that were validated in studies of patients with epilepsy to be specific probes of hippocampal function. Sass and colleagues (1990) in the Yale Neurosurgery Program administered the Wechsler Memory Scale (WMS)-Logical Subscale (paragraph recall) (Russell, 1978) and verbal Selective Reminding Test (vSRT) (Hannay & Levin, 1985) to patients with epilepsy who subsequently underwent surgical resection of the hippocampus. These investigators found that decreases in percent retention of the WMS paragraph after delayed recall, and deficits on the Long Term Retrieval (LTR) subscale of the vSRT were correlated with decreases in neuronal number of the CA3 region of the left hippocampus. The findings were specific to verbal, and not visual, memory. In an initial study, we (Bremner, Scott et al., 1993) found deficits in verbal declarative memory function in combat-related PTSD. These declarative memory deficits included problems with paragraph recall, as measured by the WMS, for immediate and delayed recall, and percent retention of the paragraph on delay. Patients also had problems with new learning of word lists, as measured by the vSRT. IQ and visual memory were intact. In order to test the hypothesis that traumatic stress results in hippocampal damage, we (Bremner, Randall, Scott et al., 1995) used magnetic resonance imaging (MRI) to quantitate hippocampal volume in living human subjects with a history of traumatic stress and a diagnosis of PTSD. An initial study showed an 8% smaller right hippocampal volume (but not comparison regions) in Vietnam veterans with combat-related PTSD (Figure 1). Decreases in right hippocampal volume in the PTSD patients were associated with deficits in short-term memory, as measured by the WMS-Logical, percent retention subcomponent ($r = .64, p < .05$).

Next, we (Bremner, Randall, Capelli et al., 1995) looked at survivors of childhood physical and/or sexual abuse with a diagnosis of PTSD (n = 18), and compared them to healthy subjects (n = 17) matched for age, sex, race, years of education, and years of alcohol abuse. We found deficits in the ability to recall a paragraph, both immediately and after a 30 minute delay, as measured by the WMS, in patients with abuse-related PTSD. These patients also showed deficits in the ability to learn new words, as measured by the SRT ($p < .01$). Deficits in short-term memory in the childhood abuse patients were significantly correlated with level of abuse, as measured by the composite severity score on the Early Trauma Inventory (Bremner, Vermetten, & Mazure, in press) ($r = -.48, p < .05$) (Figure 2). There was no difference in

FIGURE 1. Magnetic Resonance Imaging (MRI) Scan of the Hippocampus in a Normal Control and a Patient with PTSD. There Is a Visible Reduction in Hippocampal Volume in the PTSD Patient

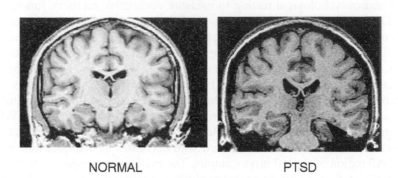

NORMAL   PTSD

FIGURE 2. Deficits in Verbal Declarative Memory Were Correlated with Sexual Abuse Severity in Patients with Abuse-Related PTSD (r = .48, p < .05)

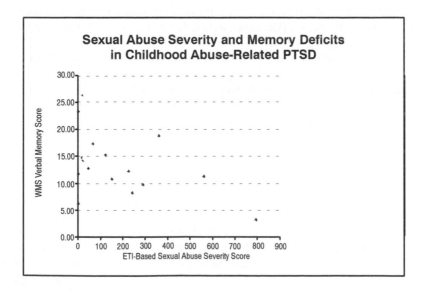

IQ or visual memory. Using MRI we (Bremner, Randall et al., 1997) measured hippocampal volume in 17 male and female adults with a history of severe childhood physical and/or sexual abuse and long-term psychiatric consequences in the form of PTSD, and compared them to 17 case-matched healthy controls. There was a 12% reduction in left hippocampal volume in the patients with abuse-related PTSD in relation to comparison subjects. This reduction was statistically significant ($p < .05$). A 3.8% reduction in volume of the right hippocampus was not significant.

Other studies found reductions in hippocampal volume in clinical populations of traumatized subjects. Stein, Koverola, Hanna, Torchia, and McClarty (1997) found a statistically significant 5% reduction in left hippocampal volume in 21 sexually abused women, relative to 21 nonabused female controls. Most (although not all) of the abused women had a current diagnosis of PTSD. Gurvits et al. (1996) compared hippocampal volume in seven patients with Vietnam combat-related PTSD to seven Vietnam combat veterans without PTSD, and eight healthy nonveteran controls. The authors found a 26% bilateral decrease in hippocampal volume, which was statistically significant for both left and right hippocampal volume considered separately. Although subjects were not case matched for alcohol abuse, there continued to be a significant difference in hippocampal volume after adjusting for years of alcohol abuse using analysis of covariance. In summary, there are several replicated studies in more than one population of traumatized patients showing atrophy of the hippocampus, which appears to be specific to a PTSD diagnosis.

Declarative memory deficits have an important effect on PTSD patients. These patients cannot remember simple things on a daily basis and, for this reason, are often unable to hold regular jobs. The magnitude of memory impairment is a 40% reduction on neuropsychological tests relative to normal controls and is equivalent to patients with epilepsy who have had their hippocampus surgically resected (Lencz ct al., 1992). My patients often describe the debilitating effects of their memory impairments on their social and occupational functioning. For example, one of my abuse-related PTSD patients complained that she felt like she had an early dementia. I frequently counsel my patients not to pursue a career or training that requires memorization.

Empirical studies on memory and the hippocampus may shed some light on the controversy surrounding delayed recall of memories of childhood abuse. The hippocampus plays an important role in integrating or binding together different aspects of a memory at the time of recollection (Squire & Zola-Morgan, 1991). It is felt to be responsible for locating the memory of an event in time, place, and context. We (Bremner, Krystal, Charney, & Southwick, 1996) have hypothesized that atrophy and dysfunction of the hippocampus following exposure to childhood abuse may lead to distortion and fragmentation of memories.

For example, an abused patient who was locked in the closet remembered the smell of old clothes, but had no visual memory of being in the closet, and no affective memory of fear. Perhaps with psychotherapy there is a facilitation of associations to related events that may bring all of the aspects of the memory together. Or, if the patient experiences an event such as being trapped in a dark elevator, the feeling of fear associated with darkness and the enclosed space may be enough to trigger a recollection of the entire memory.

NEUROCHEMICAL MODULATION OF MEMORY

Animal studies of the effects of stress early in development on neurochemical systems have implications for delayed recall of childhood abuse. The cortisol hormonal system is particularly relevant because cortisol released during stress acts over a period of hours to weaken the strength of memory traces laid down at the time of a stressful event (reviewed in De Wied & Croiset, 1991). Stress is associated with an acute increase in cortisol in humans (Rose, Poe, & Mason, 1968). Animal models of childhood abuse and neglect demonstrated that animals exposed to stress early in life subsequently have an increased sensitivity of glucocorticoid responsiveness throughout their lifespan (Fride, Dan, Feldon, Halevy, & Weinstock, 1986; Ladd, Owens, & Nemeroff, 1996; Levine, 1962; Levine, Weiner, & Coe, 1993; Plotsky & Meaney, 1993; Stanton, Gutierrez, & Levine, 1988). PTSD is associated with chronic dysregulation of the cortisol system. The findings are most consistent with elevated levels of cortisol in children in the early aftermath of childhood abuse (Lemieux & Coe, 1995), which may lead to chronic dysregulation and low cortisol levels in adults with chronic PTSD many years after the psychological trauma (Yehuda, Southwick, Nussbaum, Giller, & Mason, 1991). These findings are relevant to the delayed recall controversy, because changes in cortisol levels in childhood abuse survivors will affect how memories are laid down and retrieved.

The adrenaline system (norepinephrine) is another neurochemical system that plays a critical role in the stress response that is relevant to delayed recall of childhood abuse (reviewed in Bremner, Krystal, Southwick et al., 1996). Norepinephrine released during stress has a short period of action to strengthen the laying down of memory traces (reviewed in McGaugh, 1989). Childhood abuse-related PTSD is associated with increased levels of norepinephrine, as measured in 24-hour urine (Lemieux & Coe, 1995). Stimulation of the norepinephrine system with a medication called yohimbine (a noradrenergic alpha-2 receptor antagonist) results in increased symptoms of PTSD in patients with combat-related PTSD, suggesting that increased norepinephrine activity underlies symptoms of PTSD (Southwick et al., 1993). Patients with combat-related PTSD administered yohimbine had differences in brain function compared to healthy subjects that were also consistent with increased norepinephrine release in the brain following administration of this drug (Bremner, Innis et al., 1997). These findings are consistent with long-term alterations in memory function in PTSD. Alterations in noradrenergic activity in PTSD may lead to changes in memory encoding and/or retrieval.

Modulation of memory function by cortisol and norepinephrine may represent a mechanism of delayed recall of childhood abuse. As mentioned above, cortisol acts over a period of hours to weaken the laying down of memory traces, while norepinephrine has a rapid effect to strengthen memory traces. Long-term dysregulation of these systems may result in chronic changes in the way memories are retrieved in abuse survivors with PTSD. For example, exaggerated cortisol release during stress in PTSD may result in an inhibition of memory retrieval. This may account for the finding that rape victims report that memories for the rape trauma are actually less clear than those for neutral memories (Koss, Figueredo, Bell, Tharan, & Tromp, 1996). Exaggerated release of norepinephrine with stress in PTSD would actually be expected to facilitate recall based on the animal studies cited above. Such a mechanism may be responsible for the sudden eruption into consciousness of long-lost memories of childhood abuse during adult stressors that some PTSD patients claim to experience. Both acute and chronic responses of these neurochemical systems to stress need to be considered in order to understand alterations in memory encoding and retrieval that we propose underlie delayed recall of childhood abuse.

DYSFUNCTION OF THE MEDIAL PREFRONTAL CORTEX AS A MECHANISM OF DELAYED RECALL OF CHILDHOOD ABUSE

Abnormalities of frontal lobe function may also underlie delayed recall of childhood abuse. The medial prefrontal cortex is of particular interest because of the role it plays in emotion, social behavior, and inhibition of responses. Human subjects with lesions of medial prefrontal cortical areas (e.g., the famous case of Phineas Gage; Damasio, Grabowski, Frank, Galaburda, & Damasio, 1994) have deficits in interpretation of emotional situations that are accompanied by impairments in social relatedness. Other aspects of prefrontal cortical function may be relevant to PTSD. The prefrontal cortex is involved in selecting responses and planning for execution of action. Patients with lesions of the prefrontal cortex exhibit a variety of abnormalities of cognition, including impairments in ability to select a correct response, as well as insertion, distortions, and confabulations of memory.

These types of memory alterations are seen in patients with abuse-related PTSD. We (Bremner, Shobe, & Kihlstrom, 2000) used a paradigm to assess capacity for false memory that assesses free recall using lists of words that are all highly associated with a single primary associate ("critical lure") (Roediger & McDermott, 1995). For example, for the critical lure *needle*, the list words were *thread, pin, eye, sewing, sharp, point, prick, thimble, haystack, thorn, hurt, injection, syringe, cloth, knitting*. During free recall, about 40% of normal subjects falsely recalled the "critical lure" word *needle*. We used this paradigm to assess the propensity for false memory recall in 63 subjects, including women with a self-reported history of early childhood sexual abuse (with and without a diagnosis of PTSD), and healthy men and women without a history of childhood abuse. Women with abuse-related PTSD had a higher frequency of false recognition recall of critical lures (95%) than women with abuse histories without PTSD (76%), and non-abused non-PTSD women (79%). There were no differences between normal men and normal women. PTSD women also showed a pattern of poorer recall of previously studied words, consistent with previous findings of declarative memory deficits in PTSD, and a greater number of intrusions on nonstudied words other than critical lures. These findings are consistent with a greater propensity for distortions in memory in women with self-reported childhood sexual abuse and PTSD. As noted above, prefrontal cortical dysfunction in abuse-related PTSD is a possible explanation for these phenomena, which would explain the increase in capacity for distortion and source amnesia effects.

Medial prefrontal cortical dysfunction in abuse-related PTSD could explain both cognitive deficits (insertions and distortions), as well as problems regulating mood and emotion. Medial prefrontal cortical areas modulate emotional responsiveness through inhibition of amygdala function, and we have hypothesized that dysfunction in these regions may underlie pathological emotional responses in patients with PTSD (Bremner, Narayan et al., 1999). The development of conditioned fear responses, as in the pairing of a neutral stimulus (bright light–the conditioned stimulus) with a fear-inducing stimulus (electric shock–the unconditioned stimulus), which leads to fear responses to the light alone, is mediated by the amygdala (Davis, 1992; LeDoux, 1993). Repeated exposure to the conditioned stimulus alone normally results in the gradual loss of fear responding. The phenomenon, known as extinction to conditioned fear responses, has been hypothesized to be secondary to the formation of new memories that mask the original conditioned fear memory (Bouton & Swartzentruber, 1991). The extinguished memory is rapidly reversible following reexposure to the conditioned-unconditioned stimulus pairing, even up to one year after the original period of fear conditioning (McAllister & McAllister, 1988), suggesting that the fear response did not disappear, but was merely inhibited. This inhibition may take place through connections between the medial prefrontal cortex and the amygdala (Carmichael & Price, 1995; Devinsky, Morrell, & Vogt, 1995; Vogt, Finch, & Olson, 1992).

Imaging studies of brain function in PTSD are consistent with dysfunction of the medial prefrontal cortex in PTSD. We (Bremner, Innis et al., 1997) stimulated PTSD symptoms with the noradrenergic agent, yohimbine, and found a relative failure of activation in metabolism in parts of the medial prefrontal cortex, as well as decreased function in the hippocampus, as measured by positron emission tomography (PET) assessment of metabolism in combat-related PTSD compared to healthy controls. In a second study of combat-related PTSD, using PET and $[^{15}0]H_20$ measurement of cerebral blood flow, we (Bremner, Staib et al., 1999) studied 10 Vietnam veterans with PTSD and 10 Vietnam veterans without PTSD during exposure to combat-related and neutral slides and sounds. Vietnam veterans with combat-related PTSD demonstrated a decrease in blood flow in the medial prefrontal cortex (Brodmann's area 25, or subcallosal gyrus) and the medial temporal cortex (auditory cortex) during exposure to combat-related slides and sounds. These changes were not seen in the non-PTSD combat veterans. There was also a failure of activation in the anterior cingulate (areas 32 and 24), and increased activation in the posterior cingulate, motor cortex, and lingual gyrus in PTSD (Figure 3). In another study, we (Bremner, Narayan et al., 1999) examined cerebral blood flow correlates of exposure to personalized scripts of childhood sexual abuse in women with histories of childhood abuse, with (n = 10) and without (n = 12) PTSD. PTSD women showed

FIGURE 3. Statistical Parametric Map Overlaid on an MRI Showing Areas of Decreased Blood Flow During Traumatic Reminders in PTSD.

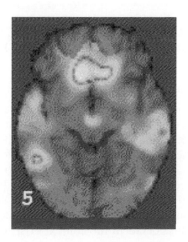

decreased blood flow in the medial prefrontal cortex (area 25), and failure of activation in the anterior cingulate, with increased blood flow in the posterior cingulate and motor cortex (replicating findings in combat-related PTSD), and anterolateral prefrontal cortex. PTSD women also had decreased blood flow in the right hippocampus, parietal and visual association cortex.

Other studies (Rauch et al., 1996; Shin et al., 1997) of traumatic imagery in combat-related PTSD found alterations in the orbitofrontal and temporal cortex in patients with PTSD. These imaging findings are consistent with dysfunction of the medial prefrontal cortex in PTSD. Medial prefrontal cortical/anterior cingulated activation may represent a "normal" brain response to traumatic stimuli that serves to inhibit feelings of fearfulness when there is no true threat. Failure of activation in this area, and/or decreased blood flow in the adjacent medial prefrontal cortex in PTSD, may lead to increased fearfulness that is not appropriate for the context, a behavioral response that is highly characteristic of patients with PTSD. If abuse-related PTSD patients are unable to regulate emotional responses to exposure to cues of the original trauma, this may lead to behaviors in which patients avoid reminders in order to protect themselves, leading to "amnesia" which is only overcome in unusual circumstances that are later identified as "delayed recall." Consistent with this idea, studies do show that PTSD symptoms increase after delayed recall of childhood abuse.

Medial prefrontal cortical dysfunction may also play a role in the increase in intrusions, distortions, and source amnesia seen in patients with PTSD. In addition, considering the role of the medial prefrontal cortex in inhibition of responses, dysfunction in this area may underlie the dysregulation of memory inhibition and access, including childhood abuse memories in PTSD, further facilitating delayed recall of childhood abuse.

RELEVANCE OF THE EFFECTS
OF TRAUMATIC STRESS ON MEMORY SYSTEMS
TO PSYCHOTHERAPY

The model for the effects of traumatic stress on brain systems and structures involved in memory may have clinical relevance for psychotherapy of childhood abuse survivors. Psychotherapy may influence delayed recall of childhood abuse. Psychotherapy naturally involves the facilitation of recall through encouraging the investigation of feelings related to traumatic events. The psychotherapist may provide a supportive environment that allows the patient to experience strong emotions, which s/he may be afraid to experience outside of the therapeutic setting. If brain systems and structures that mediate memory are dysfunctional in patients with abuse-related PTSD, then recall of childhood abuse may only occur in the context of special situations, such as psychotherapy sessions. Psychotherapy may therefore facilitate remembrance in ways other than providing false suggestions or promoting insertions of memories that never, in fact, took place. This may explain why some traumatic events are fully recalled for the first time during psychotherapy, which has fueled the controversy about whether these recalled events are true or false. The fact that traumatic events are recalled during therapy does not necessarily imply that they represent a false memory. Many therapists are nevertheless concerned about how to proceed with psychotherapy in light of the recent controversy concerning the engendering of false memories of abuse. They feel that if they ask directly about abuse, they may be accused of suggesting abuse events to their patients that did not, in fact, take place. Patients should be allowed to tell their own story, not the story of their therapists. Considering the evidence supporting the potential for suggestion to facilitate false memory illusions, it is important to avoid imposing one's own ideas as a therapist on the patient regarding a past history of abuse. Patients with PTSD may be even more susceptible to suggestion than normal persons. However, due to issues of shame and other reasons, they may not report abuse unless asked directly.

CONCLUDING COMMENTS

This article has presented a biological model for delayed recall of episodes of childhood abuse. The model is based on studies in animals and patients with abuse-related PTSD, and is therefore not generalizable to all situations, rather it is presented to stimulate thinking about possible neural mechanisms that may underlie delayed recall of childhood abuse. Evidence is reviewed showing that traumatic stress has lasting effects on brain chemical and structural systems involved in memory, emotion and the stress response, and that this may contribute to delayed recall of childhood abuse, was presented. Cortisol and norepinephrine released during stress can influence memory storage and retrieval, leading to either a weakening or a strengthening of memory traces. Long-term dysregulation of these systems occurs in abuse-related PTSD that may further influence memory retrieval and contribute to delayed recall effects (Figure 4). The hippocampus is particularly sensitive to stress, and stress-induced hippocampal damage may lead to deficits in declarative memory as well as impairments in the ability of the hippocampus to integrate memory elements at the time of retrieval. Hippocampal damage in PTSD may be associated with impairment in normal memory retrieval, leading to delayed recall in abuse survivors with PTSD. Another brain area affected by stress is the medial prefrontal cortex. Functional imaging studies show dysfunction in this area during presentation of traumatic reminders. Medial prefrontal cortical inhibition of amygdala responsiveness is felt to

FIGURE 4. Lasting Effects of Childhood Abuse on the Brain, Showing Long-Term Dysregulation of Norepinephrine and Cortisol Systems, and Vulnerable Areas of the Hippocampus, Amygdala, and Medial Prefrontal Cortex That Are Affected by Abuse

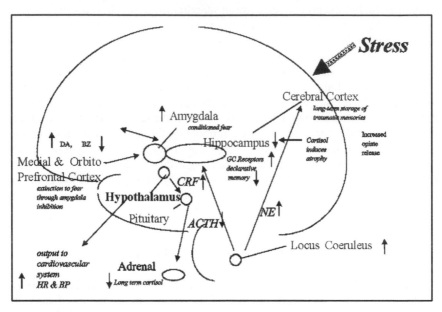

underlie extinction to fear responding. Dysfunction of this area in abuse-related PTSD may lead to problems modulating emotion that result in an avoidance of reminders of the trauma or associations to memories connected to the trauma. Memories of abuse may be "walled off" until they erupt into consciousness at a later time point. Prefrontal cortical dysfunction may also contribute to problems with source amnesia or memory distortion that may actually be more common in abuse-related PTSD, and that further complicate the story related to delayed recall of childhood abuse.

REFERENCES

Arbel, I., Kadar, T., Silberman, M., & Levy, A. (1994). The effects of long-term corticosterone administration on hippocampal morphology and cognitive performance of middle-aged rats. *Brain Research, 657,* 227-235.

Bouton, M. E., & Swartzentruber, D. (1991). Sources of relapse after extinction in Pavlovian and instrumental learning. *Clinical Psychology Reviews, 11,* 123-140.

Bremner, J. D. (1999). Does stress damage the brain? *Biological Psychiatry, 45,* 797-805.

Bremner, J. D., Innis, R. B., Ng, C. K., Staib, L., Duncan, J., Bronen, R., Zubal, G., Rich, D., Krystal, J. H., Dey, H., Soufer, R., & Charney, D.S. (1997). PET measurement of central metabolic correlates of yohimbine administration in posttraumatic stress disorder. *Archives of General Psychiatry, 54*, 146-156.

Bremner, J. D., Krystal, J. H., Charney, D. S., & Southwick, S. M. (1996). Neural mechanisms in dissociative amnesia for childhood abuse: Relevance to the current controversy surrounding the "False Memory Syndrome." *American Journal of Psychiatry, 153*, FS71-82.

Bremner, J. D., Krystal, J. H., Southwick, S. M., & Charney, D. S. (1996). Noradrenergic mechanisms in stress and anxiety: II. Clinical studies. *Synapse, 23*, 39-51.

Bremner, J. D., Licinio, J., Darnell, A., Krystal, J. H., Nemeroff, C. B., Owens, M., & Charney, D. S. (1997). Elevated CSF corticotropin-releasing factor concentrations in posttraumatic stress disorder. *American Journal of Psychiatry, 154*, 624-629.

Bremner, J. D., & Marmar, C. (Eds.). (1998). *Trauma, memory and dissociation.* Washington, DC: APA Press.

Bremner, J. D., Narayan, M., Staib, L. H., Southwick, S. M., McGlashan, T., & Charney, D. S. (1999). Neural correlates of memories of childhood sexual abuse in women with and without posttraumatic stress disorder. *American Journal of Psychiatry, 156*, 1787-1795.

Bremner, J. D., Randall, P. R., Capelli, S., Scott, T., McCarthy, G., & Charney, D. S. (1995). Deficits in short-term memory in adult survivors of childhood abuse. *Psychiatry Research, 59*, 97-107.

Bremner, J. D., Randall, P., Scott, T. M., Bronen, R. A., Seibyl, J. P., Southwick, S. M., Delaney, R. C., McCarthy, G., Charney, D. S., & Innis, R. B. (1995). MRI-based measurement of hippocampal volume in combat-related posttraumatic stress disorder. *American Journal of Psychiatry, 152*, 973-981.

Bremner, J. D., Randall, P., Vermetten, E., Staib, L., Bronen, R. A., Capelli, S., Mazure, C. M., McCarthy, G., Innis, R. B., & Charney, D.S. (1997). MRI-based measurement of hippocampal volume in posttraumatic stress disorder related to childhood physical and sexual abuse: A preliminary report. *Biological Psychiatry, 41*, 23-32.

Bremner, J. D., Scott, T. M., Delaney, R. C., Southwick, S. M., Mason, J. W., Johnson, D. R., Innis, R. B., McCarthy, G., & Charney, D. S. (1993). Deficits in short-term memory in post-traumatic stress disorder. *American Journal of Psychiatry, 150*, 1015-1019.

Bremner, J. D., Shobe, K. K., & Kihlstrom, J. F. (2000). False memories in women with self-reported childhood sexual abuse: An empirical study. *Psychological Science, 11*, 333-337.

Bremner, J. D., Southwick, S. M., & Charney, D. S. (1999). The neurobiology of posttraumatic stress disorder: An integration of animal and human research. In P. Saigh & J. D. Bremner (Eds.), *Posttraumatic stress disorder: A comprehensive text* (pp. 103-143). New York: Allyn & Bacon.

Bremner, J. D., Staib, L. H., Kaloupek, D., Southwick, S. M., Soufer, R., & Charney, D. S. (1999). Neural correlates of exposure to traumatic pictures and sound in Vietnam combat veterans with and without posttraumatic stress disorder (PTSD): A positron emission tomography study. *Biological Psychiatry, 45*, 806-816.

Bremner, J. D., Steinberg, M., Southwick, S. M., Johnson, D. R., & Charney, D. S. (1993). Use of the Structured Clinical Interview for DSM-IV-Dissociative Disorders for systematic assessment of dissociative symptoms in posttraumatic stress disorder. *American Journal of Psychiatry, 150,* 1011-1014.

Bremner, J. D., Vermetten, E., & Mazure, C. M. (in press). Development and preliminary psychometric properties of an instrument for the measurement of childhood trauma: The Early Trauma Inventory. *Depression and Anxiety.*

Carmichael, S. T., & Price, J. L. (1995). Limbic connections of the orbital and medial prefrontal cortex in macaque monkeys. *Journal of Comparative Neurology, 363,* 615-641.

Damasio, H., Grabowski, T., Frank, R., Galaburda, A. M., & Damasio, A. R. (1994). The return of Phineas Gage: Clues about the brain from the skull of a famous patient. *Science, 264,* 1102-1105.

Davis, M. (1992). The role of the amygdala in fear and anxiety. *Annual Review of Neuroscience, 15,* 353-375.

Devinsky, O., Morrell, M. J., & Vogt, B. A. (1995). Contributions of anterior cingulate to behavior. *Brain, 118,* 279-306.

De Wied, D., & Croiset, G. (1991). Stress modulation of learning and memory processes. *Methods and Achievements in Experimental Pathology, 15,* 167-199.

Diamond, D. M., Branch, B. J., Fleshner, M., & Rose, G. M. (1995). Effects of dehydroepiandosterone and stress on hippocampal electrophysiological plasticity. *Annals of the New York Academy of Sciences, 774,* 304-307.

Diamond, D. M., Fleshner, M., Ingersoll, N., & Rose, G. M. (1996). Psychological stress impairs spatial working memory: Relevance to electrophysiological studies of hippocampal function. *Behavioral Neurosciences, 110,* 661-672.

Fride, E., Dan, Y., Feldon, J., Halevy, G., & Weinstock, M. (1986). Effects of prenatal stress on vulnerability to stress in prepubertal and adult rats. *Physiology and Behavior, 37,* 681-687.

Gould, E., Tanapat, P., McEwen, B. S., Flugge, G., & Fuchs, E. (1998). Proliferation of granule cell precursors in the dentate gyrus of adult monkeys is diminished by stress. *Proceedings of the National Academy of Sciences USA, 95,* 3168-3171.

Gurvits, T. G., Shenton, M. R., Hokama, H., Ohta, H., Lasko, N. B., Gilberson, M. W., Orr, S. P., Kikinis, R., Lolesz, F. A., McCarley, R. W., & Pitman, R. K. (1996). Magnetic resonance imaging study of hippocampal volume in chronic combat-related posttraumatic stress disorder. *Biological Psychiatry, 40,* 192-199.

Hannay, H. J., & Levin, H. S. (1985). Selective Reminding Test: An examination of the equivalence of four forms. *Journal of Clinical and Experimental Neuropsychology, 7,* 251-263.

Herman, J. P., Schafer, M. K. H., Young, E. A., Thompson, R., Douglass, J., Akil, H., & Watson, S. J. (1984). Evidence for hippocampal regulation of neuroendocrine neurons of the hypothalamus-pituitary-adrenocortical axis. *Neuroscience, 9,* 3072-3082.

Jacobson, L., & Sapolsky, R. (1991). The role of the hippocampus in feedback regulation of the hypothalamic-pituitary-adrenocortical axis. *Endocrinology Reviews, 12,* 118-134.

Kessler, R. C., Sonnega, A., Bromet, E., Hughes, M., & Nelson, C. B. (1995).

Posttraumatic stress disorder in the national comorbidity survey. *Archives of General Psychiatry, 52,* 1048-1060.

Kihlstrom, J. (1987). The cognitive unconscious. *Science, 237,* 1445-1451.

Koss, M. P., Figueredo, A. J., Bell, I., Tharan, M., & Tromp, S. (1996). Traumatic memory characteristics: A cross-validated mediational model of response to rape among employed women. *Journal of Abnormal Psychology, 105,* 421-432.

Ladd, C. O., Owens, M. J., & Nemeroff, C. B. (1996). Persistent changes in CRF neuronal systems produced by maternal separation. *Endocrinology, 137,* 1212-1218.

Lawrence, M. S., & Sapolsky, R. M. (1994). Glucocorticoids accelerate ATP loss following metabolic insults in cultured hippocampal neurons. *Brain Research, 646,* 303-306.

LeDoux, J. E. (1993). Emotional memory systems in the brain. *Behavioral and Brain Research, 58,* 69-79.

Lemieux, A. M., & Coe, C. L. (1995). Abuse-related posttraumatic stress disorder: Evidence for chronic neuroendocrine activation in women. *Psychosomatic Medicine, 57,* 105-115.

Lencz, T., McCarthy, G., Bronen, R. A., Scott, T. M., Inserni, J. A., Sass, K. J., Novelly, R. A., Kim, J. H., & Spencer, D. D. (1992). Quantitative magnetic resonance imaging studies in temporal lobe epilepsy: Relationship to neuropathology and neuropsychological function. *Annals of Neurology, 31,* 629-637.

Levine, S. (1962). Plasma-free corticosteroid response to electric shock in rats stimulated in infancy. *Science, 135,* 795-796.

Levine, S., Weiner, S. G., & Coe, C. L. (1993). Temporal and social factors influencing behavioral and hormonal responses to separation in mother and infant squirrel monkeys. *Psychoneuroendocrinology, 4,* 297-306.

Luine, V., Villages, M., Martinex, C., & McEwen, B. S. (1994). Repeated stress causes reversible impairments of spatial memory performance. *Brain Research, 639,* 167-170.

McAllister, W. R., & McAllister, D. E. (1988). Reconditioning of extinguished fear after a one-year delay. *Bulletin of the Psychonomic Society, 26,* 463-466.

McCauley, J., Kern, D. E., Kolodner, K., Dill, L., Schroeder, A. F., DeChant, H. K., Ryden, J., Derogatis, L. R., & Bass, E. G. (1997). Clinical characteristics of women with a history of childhood abuse: Unhealed wounds. *Journal of the American Medical Association, 277,* 1362-1368.

McEwen, B. S., Angulo, J., Cameron, H., Chao, H. M., Daniels, D., Gannon, M. N., Gould, E., Mendelson, S., Sakai, R., Spencer, R., & Woolley, C. (1992). Paradoxical effects of adrenal steroids on the brain: Protection versus degeneration. *Biological Psychiatry, 31,* 177-199.

McGaugh, J. L. (1989). Involvement of hormonal and neuromodulatory systems in the regulation of memory storage: Endogenous modulation of memory storage. *Annual Review of Neuroscience, 12,* 255-287.

Morgan, M. A., & LeDoux, J. E. (1995). Differential contribution of dorsal and ventral medial prefrontal cortex to the acquisition and extinction of conditioned fear in rats. *Behavioral Neuroscience, 109,* 681-688.

Nibuya, M., Morinobu, S., & Duman, R. S. (1995). Regulation of BDNF and trkB mRNA in rat brain by chronic electroconvulsive seizure and antidepressant drug treatments. *Journal of Neuroscience, 15*, 7539-7547.

Plotsky, P. M., & Meaney, M. J. (1993). Early, postnatal experience alters hypothalamic corticotropin-releasing factor (CRF) mRNA, median eminence CRF content and stress-induced release in adult rats. *Molecular Brain Research, 18*, 195-200.

Rauch, S. L., van der Kolk, B. A., Fisler, R. E., Alpert, N. A., Orr, S. P., Savage, C. R., Fischman, A. J., Jenike, M. A., & Pitman, R. K. (1996). A symptom provocation study of posttraumatic stress disorder using positron emission tomography and script-driven imagery. *Archives of General Psychiatry, 53*, 380-387.

Roediger, H. L., & McDermott, K. B. (1995). Creating false memories: Remembering words not presented in lists. *Journal of Experimental Psychology: Learning, Memory & Cognition, 21*, 803-814.

Rose, R. M., Poe, R. O., & Mason, J. W. (1968). Psychological state and body size as determinants of 17-OHCS excretion. *Archives of Internal Medicine, 121*, 406-413.

Russell, E. (1978). A multiple scoring method for the assessment of complex memory functions. *Journal of Consulting and Clinical Psychology, 43*, 800-809.

Saigh, P. A., & Bremner, J. D. (Eds.). (1999). *Posttraumatic stress disorder: A comprehensive text*. New York: Allyn & Bacon.

Sapolsky, R. M. (1996). Why stress is bad for your brain. *Science, 273*, 749-750.

Sapolsky, R. M., Uno, H., Rebert, C. S., & Finch, C. E. (1990). Hippocampal damage associated with prolonged glucocorticoid exposure in primates. *Journal of Neuroscience, 10*, 2897-2902.

Sass, K. J., Spencer, D. D., Kim, J. H., Westerveld, M., Novelly, R. A., & Lencz, T. (1990). Verbal memory impairment correlates with hippocampal pyramidal cell density. *Neurology, 40*, 1694-1697.

Shin, L. M., Kosslyn, S. M., McNally, R. J., Alpert, N. M., Thompson, W. L., Rauch, S. L., Macklin, M. L., & Pitman, R. K. (1997). Visual imagery and perception in posttraumatic stress disorder: A positron emission tomographic investigation. *Archives of General Psychiatry, 54*, 233-237.

Smith, M. A., Makino, S., Kvetnansky, R., & Post, R. M. (1995). Stress and glucocorticoids affect the expression of brain-derived neurotrophic factor and neurotrophin-3 mRNA in the hippocampus. *Journal of Neuroscience, 15*, 1768-1777.

Southwick, S. M., Krystal, J. H., Morgan, C. A., Johnson, D., Nagy, L. M., Nicolaou, A., Heninger, G. R., & Charney, D. S. (1993). Abnormal noradrenergic function in posttraumatic stress disorder. *Archives of General Psychiatry, 50*, 266-274.

Squire, L. R., & Zola-Morgan, S. (1991). The medial temporal lobe memory system. *Science, 253*, 1380-1386.

Stanton, M. E., Gutierrez, Y. R., & Levine, S. (1988). Maternal deprivation potentiates pituitary-adrenal stress responses in infant rats. *Behavioral Neuroscience, 102*, 692-700.

Stein, M. B., Koverola, C., Hanna, C., Torchia, M. G., & McClarty, B. (1997). Hippocampal volume in women victimized by childhood sexual abuse. *Psychological Medicine, 27*, 951-959.

Uno, H., Tarara, R., Else, J. G., Suleman, M. A., & Sapolsky, R. M. (1989). Hippocampal damage associated with prolonged and fatal stress in primates. *Journal of Neuroscience, 9*, 1705-1711.

Virgin, C. E., Taryn, P. T. H., Packan, D. R., Tombaugh, G. C., Yang, S. H., Horner, H. C., & Sapolsky, R. M. (1991). Glucocorticoids inhibit glucose transport and glutamate uptake in hippocampal astrocytes: Implications for glucocorticoid neurotoxicity. *Journal of Neurochemistry, 57,* 1422-1428.

Vogt, B. A., Finch, D. M., & Olson, C. R. (1992). Functional heterogeneity in cingulate cortex: The anterior executive and posterior evaluative regions. *Cerebral Cortex, 2,* 435-443.

Woolley, C. S., Gould, E., & McEwen, B. S. (1990). Exposure to excess glucocorticoids alters dendritic morphology of adult hippocampal pyramidal neurons. *Brain Research, 531,* 225-231.

Yehuda, R., Southwick, S. M., Nussbaum, E. L., Giller, E. L., & Mason, J. W. (1991). Low urinary cortisol in PTSD. *Journal of Nervous and Mental Disease, 178,* 366-369.

Active Forgetting:
Evidence for Functional Inhibition
as a Source of Memory Failure

Michael C. Anderson

SUMMARY. Forgetting is often assumed to be a passive process. A program of research in theoretical memory is reviewed that shows how many instances of ordinary forgetting arise from active inhibitory processes that serve a very important attentional function: Selective retrieval. These inhibitory processes have been shown to cause long-lasting forgetting of "distracting" memories that interfere during our attempts to retrieve a particular fact or event. It is argued that these inhibitory processes may form the basis of some instances of traumatic forgetting, and that they provide a mechanistic account of an important phenomenon in the study of amnesia for childhood sexual abuse: the greater incidence of forgetting for betrayal traumas than for abuse perpetrated by strangers. *[Article copies available for a fee from The Haworth Document Delivery Service: 1-800-342-9678. E-mail address: <getinfo@ haworthpressinc.com> Website: <http://www.HaworthPress.com> © 2001 by The Haworth Press, Inc. All rights reserved.]*

KEYWORDS. Inhibitory processes, betrayal trauma, abuse, memory retrieval, selective retrieval

Address correspondence to: Michael C. Anderson, Department of Psychology, University of Oregon, Eugene, OR 97403-1227 (E-mail: mcanders@darkwing.uore gon.edu).

[Haworth co-indexing entry note]: "Active Forgetting: Evidence for Functional Inhibition as a Source of Memory Failure." Anderson, Michael C. Co-published simultaneously in *Journal of Aggression, Maltreatment & Trauma* (The Haworth Maltreatment & Trauma Press, an imprint of The Haworth Press, Inc.) Vol. 4, No. 2 (#8), 2001, pp. 185-210; and: *Trauma and Cognitive Science: A Meeting of Minds, Science, and Human Experience*, (ed: Jennifer J. Freyd, and Anne P. DePrince) The Haworth Maltreatment & Trauma Press, an imprint of The Haworth Press, Inc., 2001, pp. 185-210. Single or multiple copies of this article are available for a fee from The Haworth Document Delivery Service [1-800-342-9678, 9:00 a.m. - 5:00 p.m. (EST). E-mail address: getinfo@haworthpressinc.com].

To most people, forgetting is a negative experience. It is to lose our cherished past, it is to suffer confusion where there was once understanding, or it is to neglect one's responsibilities to oneself or to others. It is something that one rarely does on purpose, but is rather a human frailty to be avoided or to be overcome. Yet, forgetting is often precisely what we want and need to do. Life is filled with unpleasant, even traumatic experiences that we would prefer to forget if we only could. To remember is to remake a past we would rather have not occurred and to disrupt our efforts to live peacefully in the present. More often than we realize, forgetting is the goal and remembering, the human frailty.

The need to forget is not limited to trauma. Indeed, sometimes good memory for once useful knowledge can thwart our goals. Very often, the world changes in ways that require us to adapt, to update our knowledge base. None of us enjoys accidentally walking to yesterday's parking spot three blocks away from today's, or misdialing an old telephone number after it has been changed. Furthermore, we all have occasions when it is difficult to concentrate on a train of thought, because recent events or thoughts (pleasant or unpleasant) call our attention too powerfully. In each of these cases, to not forget is to risk disruptions to the most basic of activities, disruptions that can have unfortunate consequences. To call one's current spouse by the name of a previous one is certainly to remember too well for one's own good.

If we accept that forgetting is sometimes a positive goal, we must ask how people accomplish it, when successful. Two approaches that someone might take to goal-directed forgetting will be briefly outlined, only one of which will be developed in detail. The first approach is to deliberately foster the conditions necessary for passive forgetting mechanisms to take effect. To the extent that someone has a sense of how their memory works, they might engineer their life situation to encourage the operation of these mechanisms. A simple example would be of someone who moves out of an apartment or a city to help them avoid the environmental cues that remind them of something they wish to forget. If the change in environment is substantial, people will be less likely to be spontaneously reminded of the undesired memories. Indeed, the memories may ultimately become more difficult to recall even when they are sought, as suggested by basic research on context-dependent memory (Godden & Baddeley, 1975). Such an approach, though deliberate, makes use of processes that are passive in the sense that they do not involve mechanisms that directly act on the memories themselves.

The second approach involves the more controversial notion that we can forget by suppressing information directly. In this article, a program of research on theoretical memory that suggests that people do indeed have such mechanisms, inhibitory processes that deactivate mental representations and that, as a result, make us forget will be reviewed. In the first part of the article, research on the role of inhibitory processes in episodic forgetting will be reviewed. In particular, the empirical phenomenon of retrieval-induced forgetting, and the methodology by which it is studied in the laboratory will be described. Then the experimental findings that have led to the conclusion that retrieval-induced forgetting arises from active inhibitory processes that suppress intrusive mental representations: cross category inhibition will be described. Finally, several properties of retrieval-induced forgetting will be described that may prove important in appreciating the significance of this phenomenon in understanding traumatic amnesia.

In the second part of this article, some preliminary ideas on how these memory inhibition processes may contribute to some instances of traumatic amnesia are presented. In particular, how retrieval-induced forgetting may be applied to understanding an important phenomenon, the greater incidence of amnesia for betrayal traumas than for abuse by strangers will be described. Far from being a complete theoretical work, this portion of the paper should be regarded as a springboard for new research on how experimental studies of inhibitory processes might inform and be informed by people seeking to understand the causes of traumatic amnesia.

INHIBITORY PROCESSES
AND THE FORGETTING OF EVENTS

Most of the work that I have conducted concerns how human beings retrieve particular events from their past. Our approach to studying episodic retrieval has been to ask people to recall simple events (typically words that were studied in a laboratory procedure) and to later measure any side effects that retrieval may have caused. Of particular concern have been the effects of retrieval on the later ability to recall other memories that may be related to the retrieved event. Studying the side effects of retrieval on other things in memory allows us to make inferences about the basic mechanisms underlying the retrieval process. To illustrate this approach, the theoretical perspective guiding our empirical work will first be discussed. The experimental paradigm used to explore this perspective, as well as some typical results will then be presented.

Theoretical Background

A concept that guides much of the work conducted in the author's laboratory is the idea that retrieval can be regarded as a case of conceptually focused attention. This idea is illustrated in Figure 1, taken from Anderson and Spellman (1995), which contrasts the case of perceptually-focused attention on the left side, with that of conceptually-focused selective attention, or retrieval, on the right side. When we focus attention on the perceptual world, our aim is to focus on or isolate one representation from the many that have been activated by perceptual input. This aim is illustrated in Figure 1. Suppose we are looking at a bowl of fruit, and we wish to focus on the apple. The function of attention is one of isolating the mental representation of the apple from the mental representations of other objects that have been "activated" in parallel by external perceptual input.

A similar situation arises when we try to retrieve a particular thing from long-term memory, a specific event or concept, for instance. Suppose we wish to recall a particular type of fruit that begins with the letter A. When we search for a specific representation in this way (e.g., "Apple"), we typically confront interference, even if momentarily, from the many irrelevant representations (e.g., Orange, Banana) that may be activated by the retrieval cues (e.g., Fruit) guiding memory search. In this situation, the function of attention is to isolate the desired memory from the many distracting items activated by the cues we are using, that is, to overcome interference. The main difference between memory retrieval and the case of perceptually-focused selective attention is that in the latter, interference is initiated by sensory input, and the output of attentional mechanisms is a

FIGURE 1. Relationship Between Externally and Internally Focused Attention. The "A" Represents Attention Being Focused on a Representation. Focusing Attention Externally (Left) onto a Particular Object Requires Us to Ignore Other Objects in the Surrounding Environment (e.g., a Lemon, a Pear). Focusing Attention Internally (Right), to Recall a Particular Fruit (e.g., an Apple) Requires Us to Ignore Highly Similar Items in Memory (Lemon, Pear) That May Be Activated by the Cue "Fruit."

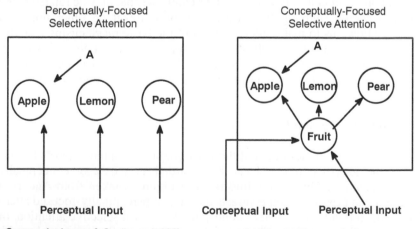

Source: Anderson & Spellman (1995).   ©APA, used by permission.

consciously experienced percept; in the case of retrieval, however, interference is initiated conceptually by thinking of the retrieval cues, and the output of attentional mechanisms is a consciously experienced memory or idea.

If retrieval can be seen as a case of internally focused attention, then we need to ask the question: how does attention come to isolate the desired representation? Is attentional focus achieved by facilitating the desired memory? Or is focus achieved by inhibiting the competing representations? This critical question guides many of the experiments reviewed in this article.

Experimental Approach and Basic Findings

All of the experiments reviewed in this article used variations on the same basic procedure, which is referred to as the retrieval practice paradigm. The retrieval practice paradigm capitalizes on a very simple implication of the attentional focusing view described previously: If recalling something from long-term memory entails the suppression of competing representations, suppressed items should become more difficult to recall on a delayed test. The suppressed competitors should be more difficult to recall, relative to items from a baseline category that was also studied, but none of whose members were repeatedly retrieved. This logic can be illustrated with the example given in Figure 2. If repeatedly recalling the item "Orange" suppresses related items like "Banana," then delayed recall performance on "Banana" should be impaired relative to the recall performance for items in an unrelated category (Drinks) that was also studied, but that was not practiced.

To test this prediction, subjects participated in the retrieval-practice procedure depicted in the bottom half of Figure 2. In this procedure, subjects studied a number of categories (Phase I), typically around eight, like "Fruits" and "Drinks," with six members in each, and were then asked to do "retrieval practice" on some of the items they studied (Phase II). The aim of this retrieval practice phase was to have subjects repeatedly recall some of the items from some of the categories they studied, with the ultimate aim of examining the impact of that repeated practice on the long-term retention of related items, like "Banana." To foster selective retrieval of "Orange," we provided subjects with cues like "Fruit or___," which directed them to recall the particular example they studied before that corresponded to those retrieval cues. Each practiced item was typically practiced three times by the person, to ensure that the retrieval-practice manipulation was fairly strong.

After a 20-minute delay, subjects' memory for all of the items was tested (Phase III). Each category name was provided in turn, and subjects were instructed to recall as many members that they remembered having studied before as they could. Figure 3 illustrates typical results obtained with the retrieval practice procedure. Each of these diagrams represents a category that subjects studied, and the numbers in the circles are the average percentage of items

FIGURE 2. The Retrieval-Practice Paradigm. The Top Panel Represents the Mental Structures Assumed to Be Formed by Subjects After Studying the Pairs "Fruit Banana, Fruit Orange, Drinks Scotch, and Drinks Gin." Category Exemplars (Circles at Bottom) Are Assumed to Be Linked to Their Category (Circle at Top) Through Associations (Lines in Diagram). The Bottom Panel Lists the Three Phases of the Retrieval-Practice Procedure–the Study Phase, During Which Subjects Study Category Exemplar Pairs; The Retrieval-Practice Phase and a Final Category-Cued Recall Phase. Retrieval Practice Is Assumed to Strengthen the Practiced Items (Orange in this Example), Which Is Depicted by a + Next to the Practiced Association.

The Retrieval-Practice Paradigm

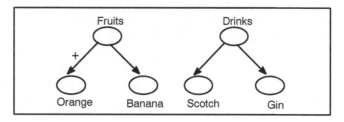

I.   Study Phase
II. Retrieval Practice Phase ----e.g., Fruit or_____

- - - - - - - -
20 Minute Delay
- - - - - - - -

III. Final Category-Cued Recall Phase

correctly recalled by subjects on the final category cued recall test at the end of the experiment (Phase III). The first thing to note about these results is that practicing items like "Orange" significantly facilitated their performance on the final test, relative to performance on baseline items, a sizable effect, though not particularly surprising because practice tends to, in general, improve performance. Of greater interest is the fact that the earlier retrieval practice impaired the long-term retention of semantically related items like "Banana," which are clearly recalled more poorly than items from the baseline condition (Drinks). In other words, repeatedly remembering or recalling some items caused long-lasting forgetting of related items, a phenomenon that we have termed Retrieval-induced forgetting. This finding was first reported by Anderson, Bjork, and Bjork (1994), but has since been replicated on dozens of occasions in my own laboratory and many others across the world.

FIGURE 3. Typical Results Obtained Using the Retrieval Practice Procedure. The Numbers Next to Each Example Are the Percentages of That Type of Item That Were Correctly Recalled on the Final Category-Cued Recall Test at the End of the Experiment. Items That Were Given Retrieval Practice Are on the Far Left (Orange), and Baseline Study Items That Were Unpracticed Are on the Right (Drinks). Inhibition of Nonpracticed Items That Were Related to the Ones That Were Practiced Is Seen by Comparing Performance on Banana to the Baseline on the Right.

Retrieval-Induced Forgetting

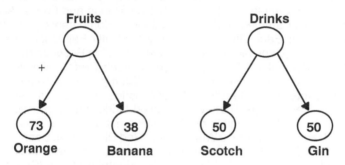

Source: Anderson, Bjork, & Bjork (1994)

Is Retrieval-Induced Forgetting Caused by Active Suppression?

Retrieval-induced forgetting would seem to provide very strong support for the idea that recalling information from long-term memory involves the suppression of competing representations. Although these findings are supportive, the conclusion that retrieval-induced forgetting is caused by inhibitory processes cannot rest on these results alone. The reason is that retrieval-induced forgetting of this sort can be produced by mechanisms that do not involve active suppression (see Anderson & Bjork, 1994; Anderson & Neely, 1996, for reviews). For instance, the impaired recall of "Banana" illustrated in Figure 2 might simply reflect greater interference on the final recall test from strengthened category mates like "Orange." That is, perhaps while trying to recall the item "Banana" on the final test, subjects are only able to think of "Orange" because it has been made hyper-accessible by the earlier retrieval practice manipulation. "Orange" may "get in the way" or block access to "Banana," even if "Banana" is not itself suppressed as we have assumed. Because these sorts of blocking mechanisms can explain retrieval-induced forgetting, we need a different form of evidence to provide unique support for the existence of active suppression processes.

To show that items like "Banana" are truly suppressed, we need a method for separating out the effects of suppression from the effects of other non-inhibitory sources of impairment, such as blocking. In collaboration with my colleague, Barbara Spellman, I devised a method for separating out these factors, called the independent probe method. The basic logic of this method is illustrated in Figure 4. The independent probe method makes use of the retrieval practice procedure outlined previously, but requires different categorical materials with special properties. In this method, subjects study new

FIGURE 4. Stimuli Used to Study Cross-Category Inhibition, and Typical Results. In this Example, Subjects Study Red Things and Foods. Although Each Item Is Only Studied Under One Category, Some Items (e.g., Tomato and Radish) from Each Studied Category Implicitly Fall Under the Other Category as Well (Depicted by Dotted Lines Crossing Between the Categories). After Studying Items Such as These, Subjects Perform Retrieval Practice on Some Exemplars (Red-Blood in this Example, as Depicted by the + Sign). Of Key Interest Is the Effect of that Practice on Subjects' Later Ability to Recall the Red Things That Were Studied Under the Unpracticed Food Category (e.g., Radish). Inhibitory Models Predict that Final Recall Performance on "Radish" Should Be Worse After "Red Blood" Has Been Practiced (Top) than for a Control Condition in which "Food Radish" Is Studied, but the Related Red Items Are Omitted from the Experiment (Bottom) (Compare the Two Recall Percentages Enclosed in the Dotted Box to See Cross-Category Inhibition).

Cross-Category Inhibition

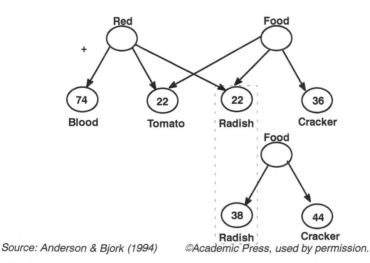

Source: Anderson & Bjork (1994)   *©Academic Press, used by permission.*

categories like Red things and Foods, with examples like "Blood," "Tomato," "Radish" and Crackers (see Figure 4). They then do retrieval practice on some of the examples, as in the standard retrieval practice paradigm. In the example depicted in Figure 4, subjects would practice "Red Blood," which we would expect to impair the later recall of related items like "Tomato," replicating the basic retrieval-induced forgetting phenomenon.

The new question in this method is whether practicing "Red Blood" would not only impair "Tomato," but also other red items like "Radish," which are both studied and tested under an independent category cue, Food. As Figure 4 illustrates, "Radish" is a red thing, although we do not tell subjects this. Rather, we simply assume that they know this on the basis of general knowledge, as illustrated by the dotted line in Figure 4. The crucial question is whether practicing "Red Blood" would impair subjects' ability to recall "Radish" when cued with the category Food?

There is good reason to expect that it would. Because both "Tomato" and "Radish" are members of the Red category, both of these items should become activated when subjects try to recall "Red Blood" during the retrieval practice phase. Activation of "Tomato" and "Radish" should interfere with recalling the practiced item. If inhibitory processes suppress interfering representations, both "Tomato" and "Radish" should be suppressed, harming the ability to recall these items later on. The suppression of "Radish" should be measurable on recall tests that cue subjects with the category cue Food. In other words, "Food Radish" should be recalled less well when "Red Blood" is practiced than it should be in a control condition in which Red things are not studied, and an irrelevant category (e.g., Tools) is studied and practiced instead (bottom of Figure 4).

If practicing "Red Blood" impairs both "Radish" and "Tomato," we have very specific evidence that suppression contributes to retrieval-induced forgetting. Whereas it is possible that the impaired recall of "Tomato" could be produced by blocking from items like "Blood" when subjects are cued with the category "Red" (i.e., subjects just can't think of anything other than blood because it is so strongly practiced), it is very difficult to imagine how "Blood" could block subjects' recall of "Radish" when they are recalling members of the Food category. "Blood" is simply not a food, and should not be elicited by that category cue. It seems that impaired recall of "Radish" on the final test would have to be the result of inhibitory processes acting directly on that item. Thus, final recall performance for "Radish" provides a window into the operation of suppression processes, uncontaminated by non-inhibitory influences, such as blocking.

Figure 4 displays the results of the experiment in which we first used this procedure. As in previous diagrams, the numbers in the circles reflect the percentage of items that subjects recalled on the final category cued recall test at the end of the experiment. The first thing that stands out in these data is that the practiced items (e.g., "Blood" in this example) are recalled extremely well on the final test, about a 30% facilitation effect, relative to performance on baseline items (Baseline is 44%, see Crackers, bottom right of Figure 4), which is substantial, but not surprising, given that practice improves performance.

More important, however, is the finding that retrieval practice on "Red Blood" impaired subjects' later recall of both "Tomato" and "Radish," and to a substantial degree, which you can see by comparing performance on those items to the baseline recall for "Tomato" when Red things were not studied or practiced (Tomato in bottom half of Figure 4), an effect of around 16%. Retrieval-induced impairment did not vary in size, whether recall was tested for "Tomato," given the cue "Red," or for "Radish" given the cue "Food." These findings strongly suggest the operation of an inhibitory process that suppresses "Tomato" and "Radish" during the retrieval practice process. For a blocking process to explain the impaired recall of "Radish," we would have to believe that when subjects are given the cue Food, they accidentally recall the item "Blood" and can't get it off their minds in order to recall "Tomato." It is very difficult to see how such blocking could occur, given that "Blood" is not a food and is unlikely to ever be elicited by that cue. Thus, the impaired recall of "Radish" is likely to reflect the direct suppression of that item. It is important to note, for present purposes, that the impaired recall of these items was induced by a retrieval practice phase that occurred twenty minutes prior to the final retention test, so the effects of these inhibitory processes are not only substantial, but enduring.

What Function Does Inhibition Serve?

I have argued that competing items are suppressed because they interfere with the recall of to-be-practiced items during the retrieval practice phase of our procedure. However, although the preceding experiment supports the existence of inhibition, it does not provide specific evidence for a functional role of inhibition in overcoming interference. It is possible, for instance, that doing any kind of additional processing on the practiced items (e.g., Red Blood) would cause inhibition of related examples. It may not matter whether additional processing involved retrieval practice or simply involved studying the to-be-practiced items again, and it might not matter whether subjects had to overcome interference from related items (e.g., Tomato, Radish). If the amount of inhibition did not vary with the need to overcome interference during retrieval, it would suggest that suppression is not functioning to overcome distraction (interference), as we have argued. This would yield a very different conception of this phenomenon than would be suggested by the attentional perspective discussed thus far.

Recently, this issue has been examined (Anderson & Shivde, 1998, 1999). Anderson and Spellman's (1995) procedure was replicated exactly, except for one crucial variation. One group of subjects performed retrieval practice on the to-be-practiced items (e.g., Red Blood), just as in the Anderson and Spellman experiment. The new aspect of this study came with the addition of a second condition, which we call the Extra Presentations group. Instead of retrieval-practice, subjects in this new condition were given additional exposures to the to-be-practiced pairs (e.g., they would see Red Blood instead of Red Bl___) for exactly the same number of repetitions. We reasoned that if inhibition depended on the need to overcome interference during the recall process, retrieval-practice subjects should be impaired, but extra presentations subjects should not, because in the latter group there is no need to overcome interference during the extra exposures.

The results of this study are displayed in Figure 5. Unlike in previous figures, each number displayed in a circle reflects the difference in recall performance between that condition and its baseline, with positive and negative scores indicating facilitation above and impairment below baseline, respectively. As can be seen in the upper portion of this figure, subjects in the retrieval practice condition showed the pattern observed by Anderson and Spellman (1995): practiced items (Red Blood) were significantly facilitated, and both the within-category (Red Tomato) and cross-category items (Food Radish) were significantly impaired. However, in the extra exposures condition (the lower portion of this figure), practiced items were also facilitated, but neither the within-category nor the cross-category items showed impairment. These findings thus show that extra processing on "Red Blood" by itself does not cause inhibition; rather, inhibition arises specifically from the need to suppress interference caused by competing items during the retrieval practice process, exactly as would be predicted by the attentional suppression perspective.

Does Remembering Always Cause Forgetting?

What the findings of Anderson and Shivde (1998) show is that active recall of the to-be-practiced items during the practice phase is necessary for related items to be suppressed. What is less clear, however, is whether active recall is sufficient to induce inhibition. Might it be possible to do retrieval practice without suppressing related items? According to the attentional suppression approach, it should be possible to perform retrieval practice on a set of target items without impairing related memories, to the extent that related items do not interfere with retrieval-practice. If related items don't interfere, there should be no need for suppression, and so retrieval practice should cause no impairment.

FIGURE 5. A Study by Anderson and Shivde (Under Review) Showing the Active Recall (from Incomplete Cues–e.g., Red Bl___) During the Retrieval Practice Phase Is Necessary to Cause Cross-Category Inhibition. This Figure Simplifies the Presentation of Results by Presenting Difference Scores for Each Item, Relative to its Baseline. A Positive Score Means That an Item Was Facilitated Above Its Baseline; a Negative Score Means an Item Was Inhibited Below Its Baseline. Note: That Retrieval Practice of "Red Blood" (Top Half of Figure) Caused 11% Cross Category Inhibition of "Radish." However, Another Group of Subjects Who Simply Got Extra Exposures of the Same Items Suffered Virtually No Inhibition (2%).

Active Recall Is Necessary

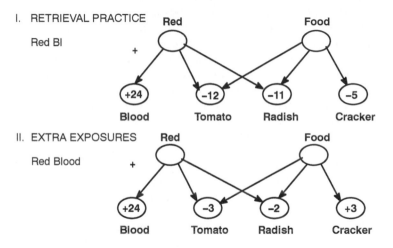

Source: Anderson & Shivde (under review)

One way to make related items non-interfering is to have subjects integrate them with the to-be-practiced target items. Classical research indicates that when items are linked with one another, the competition that one ordinarily sees during retrieval can be eliminated (Horton & Kjeldergaard, 1961; Jenkins, 1963; Kjeldergaard, 1968; see also Radvansky & Zacks, 1991; Smith, Adams, & Schoor, 1978). For instance, although the examples Orange and Banana might normally interfere with each other when the retrieval cue Fruit is presented, this competition will be greatly reduced or eliminated if subjects form direct connections between Orange and Banana (e.g., "they are both fruits that you peel") while studying them. If integrating competing memories reduces competition, it should then be possible to do retrieval practice on these items (e.g., Fruit Orange) without suppressing competitors (e.g., Fruit Banana).

This implication was recently explored using the materials of Anderson, Bjork, and Bjork (1994), in which subjects studied simple categories like fruits and drinks (with no cross-categorizable items) (Anderson & McCulloch, 1999). In this experiment, two groups of subjects were treated identically except for one crucial variation during the initial study phase of the experiment. In the no-integration condition, subjects were given the standard study-phase instructions to study each category exemplar pair for a later test. In the integration condition, however, subjects were given those same instructions, but were also told to form inter-relationships (integrate) between the exemplar themselves. No specific instructions about how to integrate items were given. Following this, subjects did retrieval practice, and ultimately were tested on their memory for all items.

The results of our study are depicted in Figure 6. As can be seen, retrieval practice facilitated performance on practiced items (e.g., Fruit Orange) to exactly the same degree across the no-integration and integration conditions (compare performance on Orange to baseline on right side of figure). Retrieval-induced forgetting was only observed, however, in the no-integration condition. Thus, when subjects integrated the category exemplars with each other, it eliminated inhibition altogether. This result shows that there are clear limits on when suppression will impair related memories and when it will not. This finding regarding integration may prove especially important in understanding the implications of these findings for traumatic amnesia.

Properties of Retrieval-Induced Forgetting: A Summary

Figure 7 summarizes the properties of retrieval-induced forgetting. The first property (point I) is simply the observation that the act of remembering can itself impair later recall of related memories through inhibition. Second, the inhibition caused by retrieval generalizes to a variety of cues with which one might test that inhibited item (point II), as suggested by cross-category inhibition (Anderson & Spellman, 1995). This result strongly favors an inhibitory interpretation of retrieval-induced forgetting over other plausible non-inhibitory ones, such as blocking. Third, whether related items are inhibited depends on whether they interfere during the retrieval-practice of to-be-practiced items (Anderson, Bjork, & Bjork, 1999; Anderson & Shivde, 1998, 1999) suggesting that related items get inhibited for a good functional reason (point III). Finally, inhibition appears to be restricted to those items that are not well integrated with the retrieval target, and that impede selective retrieval of that item (Anderson & McCulloch, 1999) (point IV).

In the context of this summary, two additional properties of retrieval-induced forgetting bear mentioning without going into a lot of detail on the studies that support them, because these properties are also quite important. First, to our great surprise, the inhibitory processes at work in this phenomenon

FIGURE 6. Results of a Study by Anderson and McCulloch Studying the Effects of Integration on Retrieval-Induced Forgetting. The Upper Portion of the Figure Is the Data from a Group of Subjects Who Participated in the Standard Retrieval Practice Procedure. Numbers in the Circles Are the Percentages of Items Recalled on the Final Recall Test. Note that the Earlier Retrieval Practice of Fruit-Orange Facilitated Final Recall of Orange on the Final Test, Relative to the Baseline (Drinks), and Impaired Recall of Banana. Subjects in the Bottom Portion of the Figure Were Instructed to Link the Category Exemplars to Each Other (Represented by the Lines Linking the Examples) During the Study Phase. As Can Be Seen, Integration in the Study Phase Insulated Subjects from Later Retrieval-Induced Forgetting on Banana.

Integration Reduces Impairment

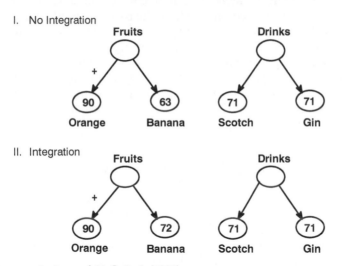

Source: Anderson & McCulloch (1999)

impair the ability to recognize study items as well as the ability to recall them. That is, if subjects are shown studied items on the final test, and are simply asked to decide if they have seen the items before, they will be less likely to recognize the items than if they hadn't been inhibited. Even when they do recognize the study items, they are less confident that they do (Anderson, De Kok, & Child, 1997).

Second, retrieval-induced forgetting has been generalized to non-verbal stimuli. For example, it has been found with arbitrary multidimensional geometric stimuli. People have been induced to forget the location, shape, and color of an object by retrieving information about similar objects (Ciranni & Shimamura, 1999). This work has also shown that impairment is specifically caused by retrieval-practice and not mere presentation of similar objects.

FIGURE 7. A Summary of the Important Properties of Retrieval-Induced Forgetting and the Studies that Support Each Property

Properties of RIF

I.   Retrieval Impairs Related Memories

II. Cue-Independence

III. Interference Dependence

    A. Recall Specific

    B. Taxonomic Frequency Effects

IV. Non-Integrated Events Suffer Most

V.   Recognition Memory Impaired

VI. Generalized to Non-Verbal Stimuli

Furthermore, retrieval-induced forgetting has been found in an eyewitness memory paradigm, with rather more complex stimuli than used here (Shaw, Bjork, & Handel, 1995). By "interrogating" subjects about a mock crime that they witnessed during a slide presentation, subjects can be induced to forget other similar information not included in the initial interrogation. These findings argue that this effect is not restricted to memory for previously studied words, but generalizes to memories varying widely in content and complexity.

INHIBITORY PROCESSES
AND TRAUMATIC AMNESIA

In the first portion of the article, the phenomenon of retrieval-induced forgetting, and the evidence suggesting that this form of memory impairment is caused by active inhibitory processes was reviewed. These inhibitory processes are thought to suppress competing mental representations in the interest of attentional control during memory search. If cognitive control employs such mechanisms in these more mundane (though necessary) circumstances, it seems reasonable to wonder whether these mechanisms might be applied strategically under more extreme circumstances–as would occur in efforts to forget a traumatic experience (Bjork, Bjork, & Anderson, 1997).

The next portion of the article develops a proposal for how such mechanisms might explain at least a part of the findings on traumatic amnesia. While far from being a finished theory, my hope is that this proposal, if nothing else, will generate the discussion necessary for such a theory to evolve.

Focus of the Proposal

There are several limits on the scope of the current proposal that should be described at the outset. First, this proposal is not meant to address all instances in which a traumatic experience is forgotten. There are many reasons why trauma could be forgotten, having to do with disruption at virtually any stage of processing in the memory system, either with encoding or elaboration, as argued by van der Kolk and Fisler (1995), or with retrieval. This proposal will address the latter variety of forgetting, in which an experience has been adequately encoded, and for which the difficulty lies primarily with retrieval.

Second, this proposal is limited to forgetting of the declarative representation of the experience, and does not address other forms of knowledge such as conditioned responses or procedural knowledge. By declarative representation, I do not mean to restrict the account to verbal representation, rather to propositional representations (linguistic or not) that may be consciously experienced by the rememberer (Squire, 1992; Cohen & Eichenbaum, 1993). The present account is focused on declarative representations because, to date, all studies of retrieval-induced forgetting have studied declarative knowledge, and because it is entirely possible that nondeclarative representations are not affected in the same way by the processes discussed thus far. For instance, it may be possible to suppress the declarative representation of trauma without altering a person's conditioned emotional responses to trauma-related stimuli (see Bechara, Tranel, Damasio, & Adolphs, 1995, for evidence on the potential independence of declarative representations and fear conditioning).

Finally, the proposal focuses on trauma for interpersonal experiences, specifically childhood sexual abuse. Of particular interest is the striking finding that people reporting childhood sexual abuse are much more likely to report a period of forgetting if the abuse was perpetrated by a family member than if by a non-family member. I first encountered this finding in Jennifer Freyd's book, *Betrayal Trauma: The Logic of Forgetting Childhood Abuse*, in which she develops a compelling argument about why traumatic amnesia may come about (Freyd, 1996). Freyd argues that many instances of amnesia for sexual abuse reflect adaptive responses of a child who has been abused by a trusted caregiver. A child who has been abused by a parent or relative often has very few options about how to respond. Freyd (1996) argues that it is in the child's best interests to not know about or to forget the abuse if remembering it would disrupt their ability to maintain significant attachment relationships with the caregiver. If this view is correct, one would expect to see a greater incidence of amnesia for abuse perpetrated by family members than by strangers, for whom no significant attachment relationships exist. This is exactly the pattern that has been observed empirically. In a reanalysis of several existing data sets on traumatic amnesia (Cameron, 1993; Feldman-Summers & Pope, 1994; Williams, 1994), Freyd (1996) found much greater rates of forgetting when the perpetrator was a family member.

Figure 8, adapted from Freyd (1996), gives several examples of this finding, only one of which I will discuss for the sake of illustration. In a study reported by Feldman-Summers and Pope (1994), over 300 psychologists filled out a survey regarding sexual abuse. Of these psychologists, 25% reported having been abused themselves as children. Freyd categorized these individuals by whether or not they reported having had a period during which they could not recall the experiences, and by whether or not the abuse was perpetrated by a family member.

One can see from these data that when people were abused by a family member, they were more likely to have had a period of forgetting of the experience than to have had continuous memory for it. However, respondents who reported having been abused by strangers were more likely to have had continuous memory for the abuse. These findings are mirrored in the reanalyses of other studies by Williams (1994) and Cameron (1993), that used different methodologies and different subject populations. Although caution

FIGURE 8. Three Studies That Have Found Evidence for Heightened Incidence of Forgetting for Betrayal Traumas as Compared to Stranger Abuse. Subjects Are Classified According to Whether They Were Abused by a Family Member or Not, and by Whether They Ever Had a Period During Which They Had Forgotten the Abuse. The Numbers in the Table Are the Percentages of Subjects Who Fell into the Relevant Classifications.

**Heightened Incidence
of Forgetting for Betrayal Trauma**

Feldman-Summers & Pope (1994)

Family Member	Abuse Ever Forgotten?	
	Yes	No
Yes	53%	47%
No	30%	70%

Williams (1994)

Family Member	Abuse Reported	
	Yes	No
Yes	53%	48%
No	69%	31%

Cameron (1993)

Family Member	Abuse Ever Forgotten?	
	Yes	No
Parent	72%	28%
Non-Parent	19%	81%

needs to be exercised in interpreting people's self assessments of prior retriev-ability (see Schooler, 1996), taken at face value these findings lend support to betrayal trauma theory. The current proposal attempts to explain how the circumstances of a betrayal trauma ultimately cause these incidents of forget-ting through the normal operation of memory inhibition mechanisms.

The Selective Retrieval Hypothesis

What mechanisms might underlie greater forgetting for betrayal traumas? The proposal offered here is that betrayal traumas are much more likely to create circumstances conducive to retrieval-induced forgetting, and thus sup-pression, than are cases of stranger abuse. This will be referred to this as the selective retrieval-hypothesis. The suggestion will be posed that betrayal traumas and stranger abuse will tend to be forgotten by somewhat different memory mechanisms.

Cognitive Differences Between Betrayal-Trauma and Stranger Abuse. To appreciate how betrayal traumas may be more likely to create conditions conducive to retrieval-induced forgetting, it is important to consider the many systematic differences between these situations that are likely to create differ-ences in representation and processing in the child. Several significant differ-ences are illustrated in Figure 9, which describes the situation of betrayal trauma on the left, and that of stranger abuse on the right.

First, as is obvious, in betrayal trauma, the abuse is committed by a trusted caregiver about whom the child already knows much, there is extensive knowledge and prior experience that has already been encoded about the caregiver prior to the encoding of the abuse. This situation contrasts with stranger abuse, in which (by definition) little is known about the stranger. Indeed, the abuse may be the only thing that is known about the person, making it highly retrievable. This contrast is depicted in Figure 9 as a greater number of associated memories linked to the central cues for the abuse in betrayal traumas (i.e., the caregiver, left side) than in stranger abuse (i.e., the stranger, right side).

Second, in betrayal trauma, the cues that would remind the child about the abuse are not escapable, the child must live with the parent, and in the location of the abuse despite the fact that these stimuli will tend to cue the memory powerfully. In stranger abuse, however, cues are at least potentially avoidable and escapable, the child need not encounter the stranger again, and may be able to avoid the location in which the abuse occurred.

Third, as a result of the prior difference, children suffering betrayal trau-mas will encode more subsequent experiences with the caregiver because the child is forced to live and interact with them. These new experiences only add to the knowledge available in memory to compete with the abuse memory (imagine more associated memories in the diagram on the left of Figure 9). In

FIGURE 9. Systematic Differences in Representation and Processing Across Betrayal Traumas and Stranger Abuse. Diagrams Represent Simplified Versions of the Memory Structures Assumed to Be Represented in the Case of Betrayal Trauma and Stranger Abuse.

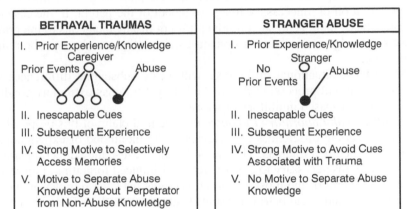

Differences Between Betrayal Trauma and Stranger Abuse

the case of stranger abuse, there will be less subsequent experience concerning the abuser (for the reasons cited above), which will only preserve the unique and thus highly accessible status of the memory as an association to the most potent cues, the perpetrator or the location of the abuse.

Fourth, as argued by Freyd (1996), the child suffering a betrayal trauma has a powerful motive for selectively accessing some of the knowledge about the caregiver. Because the child cannot escape the retrieval cue, the caregiver, they must develop a way to selectively retrieve knowledge about the caregiver that will ensure their survival and that will be relevant to supporting essential attachment relationships with the parents. If retrieving abuse-related knowledge undermines these objectives, retrieval of that knowledge should be avoided. In the case of stranger abuse, however, there is no such motive because there is no attachment relationship with the stranger. Furthermore, because no other knowledge has been stored about the stranger and because the cue itself (the stranger) is avoidable, selective retrieval is both impossible and, in any event, unnecessary. Rather, the main tool for forgetting abuse perpetrated by a stranger will likely be to avoid the cues altogether.

Finally, in betrayal traumas, the child has a motive to separate out knowledge associated with the abuse from other knowledge about the perpetrator.

In everyday interactions with the caregiver, it may be difficult for a child to behave normally if memories, thoughts, and feelings about the abuse were not set aside in some fashion. Indeed, conclusions and feelings compelled by thoughts of the abuse may be in a fundamental conflict with basic assumptions concerning the caregiver, assumptions which underlie much of the child's physical and emotional responses to that person (Horowitz, 1986). The ability to separate out abuse from nonabuse knowledge may thus allow the preservation of a necessary image or model of the parent. In the case of stranger abuse, there is no such motive; it is not disadvantageous to integrate abuse knowledge with whatever nonabuse information was known about the perpetrator.

All of these situational differences will create substantial differences in representation and processing that make betrayal traumas extremely conducive to retrieval-based inhibitory processes.

Parallels with Laboratory Phenomena. A central claim of this proposal is that the foregoing differences are relevant to the likelihood of experiencing amnesia for betrayal traumas. They are relevant because they directly pertain to the conditions necessary to observe retrieval-induced forgetting. Figure 10 highlights several of the most important parallels between retrieval-induced forgetting (left side) and betrayal-trauma (right side). In the retrieval practice paradigm, the subject's aim is to selectively recall a particular target item (e.g., Orange) in response to a retrieval-practice cue (e.g., Fruit or___), and to not retrieve other intrusive items (e.g., Banana). In the case of betrayal trauma, the child needs to selectively retrieve nontraumatic information about the caregiver, to the exclusion of the traumatic knowledge. The similarities between these two situations are depicted graphically in the center of Figure 10, in which it can be seen that both situations require the progression from a retrieval cue to a particular memory, despite the presence of many competing memories. Thus, both situations demand selective retrieval.

Consider several other significant parallels. First, in the retrieval practice paradigm, alternative memories intrude and interfere with access to the retrieval practice target, triggering their suppression. In the case of betrayal trauma, traumatic memories intrude and must be suppressed to sustain behaviors and thoughts consistent with the goal of maintaining the current attachment relationships with the caregiver. Second, as highlighted earlier, unintegrated memories are hardest hit by retrieval-induced forgetting; integrated information is often unimpaired by the selective retrieval of related knowledge. In betrayal trauma situations, the victim often keeps traumatic information from being integrated with nonabuse knowledge. This segregation of abuse knowledge has two effects: it keeps the information out of awareness while attachment behavior proceeds, but it also renders the abuse knowledge more vulnerable to the suppression.[1,2,3]

FIGURE 10. Parallels Between the Representation and Processing Demands Typical of Retrieval-Induced Forgetting and Those Likely to Be True in Cases of Betrayal Trauma. Diagrams in the Center Represent Simplified Versions of the Memory Structures Presumed to Be Formed in Each Case. In the Retrieval Practice Paradigm, There Is a Cue (a Category Typically) Associated to Many Exemplars. In Betrayal Trauma, the Memory Retrieval Cue Is the Caregiver, and the Associated Memories Are of Personal Experiences with or Knowledge About the Caregiver.

RIF and Traumatic Forgetting:
Some Parallels

RETRIEVAL-INDUCED FORGETTING		FORGETTING OF BETRAYAL TRAUMA
I. Need to Selectively Retrieve a Memory	Cue  Targets	I. Desire to Selectively Retrieve Non-Traumatic Knowledge
II. Related Memories Intrude, Triggering Inhibition		II. Traumatic Memories Impede Attachment Behaviors
III. Unintegrated Responses Get Inhibited		III. Trauma Kept from Being Integrated
IV. Repeated Access of Target Causes More Impairment	Caregiver Targets	IV. Repeated Occasions to Retrieve Non-Traumatic Knowledge Over Years
V. Inhibited Material Is Forgotten When Recalled, Less Confident		V. Inhibited Material Is Forgotten When Recalled, Less Confident

Fourth, in the retrieval-practice paradigm, practiced memories are repeatedly retrieved throughout the practice phase, causing greater inhibition of related items. Recently, the degree of retrieval induced forgetting has been shown to increase with the number of retrievals of practiced items (Anderson & Shivde, 1999). If inhibition increases with the number of times that a related item is retrieved, this would make betrayal traumas powerfully conducive to suppression. Even if a child fails to suppress memories of the trauma initially, many years of experience with the caregiver following the incident will provide more than enough opportunities to master the task of selective retrieval. As the child becomes more skilled at "thinking the right thoughts" about the caregiver, suppression of the trauma seems a natural consequence. Indeed, studies of abused children indicate that abusers may encourage this process by grooming the child to have a particular (positive) understanding of the abuser (Veldhuis & Freyd, 1999).

Perhaps the most important parallels between these situations lie in the qualitative characteristics of the phenomena themselves. In laboratory studies, inhibition causes the interfering information to be forgotten. Importantly, even when the inhibited item is remembered, subjects are much less confident about having experienced it (Anderson et al., 1997). In betrayal traumas, as in retrieval-induced forgetting, the result of suppression is long lasting amnesia for the abuse event, followed by a period of uncertain memory for the experience, if it is ever recalled at all.

Research on retrieval-induced forgetting also suggests new explanations for observations in traumatic amnesia that might otherwise seem paradoxical. For instance, Terr (1991) has observed that, contrary to what one might expect, victims of repeated abuse have a higher incidence of amnesia than do victims who have been abused a single time. Freyd (1996) speculated that this pattern may arise because multiple-abuse cases tend to be betrayal traumas. If Freyd is correct, victims of multiple instances of abuse may suffer more amnesia because betrayal traumas foster retrieval-induced forgetting. In addition, if victims encode multiple abuse-related memories that are highly similar to one another, as might be the case if the abuse took place in the same location and at the same time of day, betrayal traumas may foster memories that are particularly sensitive to suppression. First, as a rule, the memories that are most likely to be suppressed are those that interfere with attempts to selectively retrieve target items during retrieval practice (Anderson et al., 1994; Anderson et al., 1999; Anderson & Shivde, 1998; 1999; Anderson and Spellman, 1995). Factors that increase the accessibility of a memory (e.g., repetition) should also make it highly interfering, and potentially more susceptible to suppression. Second, recent work has shown that more suppression occurs when to-be-suppressed memories are highly similar to one another (Anderson, McCulloch, & Green, 2000). Thus, to the extent that betrayal traumas foster highly intrusive abuse memories that are similar to each another, people suffering from them might be particularly susceptible to retrieval-induced forgetting.

Although there are clearly many differences between the this simple laboratory procedure and betrayal traumas, the preceding parallels make it clear that the conditions of betrayal trauma encourage the sorts of inhibitory processes studied in the retrieval-practice paradigm, indeed, much more so than cases of stranger abuse. This may provide a useful starting point for understanding the mechanisms underlying the greater incidences of amnesia for betrayal traumas (Freyd, 1996).

Differences in Mechanisms Underlying Forgetting of Stranger Abuse and Betrayal Trauma. The foregoing analysis does not imply that traumatic amnesia will be restricted to cases of betrayal trauma. It merely argues that the conditions of betrayal trauma are particularly conducive to retrieval-based inhibitory processes. The present analysis does suggest, however, that different mechanisms may underlie forgetting of betrayal traumas and stranger abuse. Unlike in betrayal trauma, the retrieval cues that are most likely to reinstate memory for the abuse event, the location of the abuse and the abuse, are typically more avoidable in the case of stranger abuse. By deliberately avoiding situations in which these cues would arise, a person who was abused by a stranger can learn to forget by the mechanisms of context dependent memory rather than by direct suppression. Although it is difficult to know what implications this mechanistic difference may have for the ability to recover those prior experiences, it seems plausible that forgetting by this mechanism may be more reversible than it is for betrayal traumas, given reinstatement of the cues. This seems likely because the avoidance of cues ensures that those cues remain uniquely associated to the abuse event, and thus effective at eliciting the abuse event.

It remains possible, however, that some instances of traumatic amnesia from stranger abuse may be caused by memory inhibition processes. Although victims may be able to avoid the abuser and the location of the abuse, sexual experiences later in life may also serve as cues to the abuse event. One response to such remindings would be to avoid sexual encounters altogether, in much the same way as the location of the abuse is avoided. Alternatively, if a person chooses not to avoid sexual experiences, the potency of such experiences as cues to the recalling the abuse event (or at least its declarative representation) may diminish as more sexual experiences are stored in memory. By learning to focus on more recent experiences, a person may initiate the suppression processes described previously.

CONCLUDING REMARKS

Although forgetting is often an undesirable outcome, there are many cases in which it is desirable. It is equally clear that people often make deliberate efforts to forget things (at least temporarily), even in relatively simple non-traumatic circumstances. To the extent that such forgetting is possible, we must explain the mechanisms that underlie it. In this article, a program of research in theoretical memory that shows that people use inhibitory control processes to "push aside" interfering representations in memory has been reviewed. These mechanisms are adaptive because they help to focus cognition in the face of internal distraction from the abundance of representations that may become active as we perform a cognitive act. These inhibitory processes render the inhibited representations less accessible in the long run.

If inhibitory processes cause forgetting in these more mundane circumstances, it is reasonable to ask to what extent they may underlie the forgetting of concern to those studying traumatic amnesia. Although there is no direct evidence linking this simple phenomenon to traumatic amnesia, I have argued that retrieval-induced forgetting provides a highly plausible laboratory model of the processes that may lead to traumatic amnesia, particularly so in the case of betrayal trauma. Retrieval-induced forgetting arises whenever a person must learn to selectively retrieve some memories associated to a cue and not others. A child suffering from a betrayal-trauma is often confronted with precisely the same problem: To learn to recollect some memories (positive, attachment related memories) about an abuser and not others (the abuse event/s), if he or she is to maintain attachment relationships with the caregiver. Although matters are clearly more complex than this simple analogy suggests, the selective retrieval hypothesis is consistent with reports of the greater incidence of forgetting for betrayal trauma than for stranger abuse. If correct, the selective retrieval hypothesis suggests that different mechanisms may underlie the forgetting of betrayal traumas and stranger abuse. If so, it becomes important to separate these two situations in research aimed at understanding the characteristics of memory for childhood sexual abuse.

NOTES

1. The preparation of this article was supported by startup funds from the University of Oregon. The author would like to thank Jennifer Freyd and Anne DePrince for useful comments on an early version of this paper.

2. In laboratory studies, the particular pattern of integration between the exemplars of a category plays a crucial role in whether integration will prevent retrieval induced forgetting. For integration to prevent impairment, the information that receives retrieval practice should be directly integrated with the related material that would otherwise be suppressed. Integration *between the practiced exemplars themselves*, or between the *related items* will not prevent the retrieval of those practiced items from suppressing the related exemplars. Similarly, neither integration of nonabuse memories with each other, nor abuse memories with each other should be sufficient to prevent traumatic amnesia.

3. It is unclear whether the segregation of abuse knowledge from nonabuse knowledge is a conscious, goal directed activity. Although the present account does not require any commitment on this point, we suspect that knowledge segregation may be an indirect consequence of attempts to keep abuse knowledge out of awareness during attachment related activities. Because integration requires *simultaneous processing* of the items of knowledge being integrated, such a practice would prevent integration.

4. It should be emphasized that the current assumptions about the situation of betrayal trauma represent the author's analysis of that situation and does not necessarily reflect the assumptions of betrayal trauma theory (Freyd, 1996).

REFERENCES

Anderson, M. C., & Bjork, R. A. (1994). Mechanisms of inhibition in long-term memory: A new taxonomy. In D. Dagenbach & T. Carr (Eds.), *Inhibitory processes in attention, memory, and language* (pp. 265-325). San Diego, CA: Academic Press.

Anderson, M. C., Bjork, R. A., & Bjork, E. L. (1994). Remembering can cause forgetting: Retrieval dynamics in long-term memory. *Journal of Experimental Psychology: Learning, Memory, and Cognition, 20,* 1063-1087.

Anderson, M. C., Bjork, E. L., & Bjork, R. A. (in press). Retrieval-induced forgetting: Evidence for a recall-specific mechanism. *Psychonomic Bulletin and Review.*

Anderson, M. C., De Kok, D., & Child, C. (1997, November). Retrieval-induced forgetting on a test of recognition memory. *Abstracts of the Psychonomic Society, 2,* Volume 2.

Anderson, M. C., & McCulloch, K. C. (1999). Integration as a general boundary condition on retrieval-induced forgetting. *Journal of Experimental Psychology: Learning, Memory, and Cognition, 25,* 608-629.

Anderson, M. C., McCulloch, K.C., & Green, C. (submitted). What doesn't inhibit "banana" makes it stronger: Why similarity can both increase and decrease retrieval-induced forgetting.

Anderson, M. C., & Neely, J. H. (1996). Interference and inhibition in memory retrieval. In E. L. Bjork & R. A. Bjork (Eds.), *Memory. Handbook of perception and cognition* (2nd ed.) (pp. 237-313). San Diego, CA: Academic Press

Anderson, M. C., & Shivde, G. (May, 1998). Inhibition in episodic memory: Evidence for a retrieval-specific mechanism. *Poster presented at the 10th Annual Conference of the American Psychological Society,* Washington DC, May, 1998.

Anderson, M. C., & Shivde, G. (November, 1999). The functional role of inhibitory processes in retrieval: Evidence from a parametric study of retrieval-induced forgetting. *Abstracts of the Psychonomic Society,* Volume 4.

Anderson, M. C., & Spellman, B. A. (1995). On the status of inhibitory mechanisms in cognition: Memory retrieval as a model case. *Psychological Review, 102,* 68-100.

Bechara, A., Tranel, D., Damasio, H., & Adolphs, R., Rockland, C., & Damasio, A.R. (1995). Double dissociation of conditioning and declarative knowledge relative to the amygdala and hippocampus in humans. *Science, 269*(5227), pp. 1115-1118.

Bjork, E. L., Bjork, R. A., & Anderson, M. C. (1997). Varieties of goal directed forgetting. To appear in J.M. Golding & C.M. McCleod (Eds.), *Directed Forgetting: Interdisciplinary Approaches.* (pp. 103-138). Lawrence Erlbaum Associates.

Cameron, C. (1993). *Recovering memories of childhood sexual abuse: A longitudinal report.* Paper read at the Western Psychological Association convention, Phoenix, Arizona, April.

Ciranni, M. A., & Shimamura, A. P. (in press). Retrieval-induced forgetting in episodic memory. *Journal of Experimental Psychology: Learning, Memory, and Cognition.*

Cohen, N. J., & Eichenbaum, H. (1993). *Memory, amnesia, and the hippocampal system.* MIT Press, Cambridge, MA.

Feldman-Summers, S., & Pope, K. S. (1994). The experience of forgetting childhood abuse: A national survey of psychologists. *Journal of Consulting and Clinical Psychology, 62,* 636-639.

Freyd, J. J. (1996). *Betrayal trauma: The logic of forgetting childhood abuse.* Cambridge, MA: Harvard University Press.

Godden, D., & Baddeley, A. D. (1975). Context dependent memory in two natural environments: On land and under water. *British Journal of Psychology, 66,* 325-331.

Horowitz, M. J. (1986). *Stress response syndromes* (2nd ed.). New York: Jason Aronson.

Schooler, J. W. (1996). Seeking the core: The issues and evidence surrounding recovered accounts of sexual trauma. In K. Pezdek & W.P. Banks (Eds.), *The recovered memory/False memory debate.* (pp. 279-296). Academic Press.

Shaw, J. S., Bjork, R. A., & Handal, A. (1995). Retrieval-induced forgetting in an eyewitness-memory paradigm. *Psychonomic Bulletin & Review, 2,* 249-253.

Squire, L. R. (1992). Memory and the hippocampus: A synthesis from findings with rats, monkeys, and humans. *Psychological Review, 99,* 195-231.

Terr, L. C. (1991). Childhood trauma: An outline and overview. *American Journal of Psychiatry, 148,* 10-20.

van der Kolk, & Fisler (1995). Dissociation and the fragmentary nature of traumatic memories: Overview and exploratory study. *Journal of Traumatic Stress, 8,* 505-525.

Veldhuis, C. B., & Freyd, J. J. (1999). Groomed for silence, groomed for betrayal. In M. Rivera (Ed.), *Fragment by fragment: Feminist perspectives on memory and child sexual abuse* (pp. 253-282). Charlottetown, PEI Canada: Gynergy Books.

Williams, L.M. (1994). Recall of childhood trauma: A prospective study of women's memories of child sexual abuse. *Journal of Consulting and Clinical Psychology, 62,* 1167-1176.

Experiential Avoidance
and Post-Traumatic Stress Disorder:
A Cognitive Mediational Model
of Rape Recovery

Laura E. Boeschen
Mary P. Koss
Aurelio José Figueredo
James A. Coan

SUMMARY. Does experiential avoidance predict PTSD severity among rape survivors? We tested a hypothesized model where causal attributions, cognitive schemas, and memory characteristics mediated the relationship between experiential avoidance and PTSD. Experiential avoidance was measured as a cognitive coping strategy; women scoring high on this measure did not try to integrate or make meaning of their rape experiences, but rather attempted to block out memories of

The study was supported by a Research Career Development Award from the National Institute of Mental Health (NIMH) and research funding from the Violence and Traumatic Stress Studies Branch of NIMH and from the Women's Health Office of the National Institutes of Health.

This study fulfilled part of the dissertation requirements of Laura E. Boeschen. The authors gratefully acknowledge the contributions of two members of our research group, Janine Goldman-Pach and Ron Prince, for their assistance in preparing these data. Caroline von Thompson of the University of Kostanz, Germany, is thanked for her contributions to the development of the qualitative scoring.

Address correspondence to: Mary P. Koss, PhD, Arizona Prevention Center, 2223 E. Speedway Boulevard, Tucson, AZ 85719 (E-mail: *mpk@u.arizona.edu*).

[Haworth co-indexing entry note]: "Experiential Avoidance and Post-Traumatic Stress Disorder: A Cognitive Mediational Model of Rape Recovery." Boeschen, Laura E. et al. Co-published simultaneously in *Journal of Aggression, Maltreatment & Trauma* (The Haworth Maltreatment & Trauma Press, an imprint of The Haworth Press, Inc.) Vol. 4, No. 2 (#8), 2001, pp. 211-245; and: *Trauma and Cognitive Science: A Meeting of Minds, Science, and Human Experience* (ed: Jennifer J. Freyd, and Anne P. DePrince) The Haworth Maltreatment & Trauma Press, an imprint of The Haworth Press, Inc., 2001, pp. 211-245. Single or multiple copies of this article are available for a fee from The Haworth Document Delivery Service [1-800-342-9678, 9:00 a.m. - 5:00 p.m. (EST). E-mail address: getinfo@haworthpressinc.com].

their rapes or minimize or rationalize their rape experiences in some way. Data were cross-sectional. Participants were rape survivors (N = 139; 23% with current PTSD). Results included a measurement model of social cognitive factors and PTSD and the structural model. Two sets of pathways were delineated, both exacerbated PTSD. Overall, 60% of the variance in PTSD was explained. The results suggested that the effects of experiential avoidance on psychological outcomes were detrimental, but small. Re-experiencing was the only memory characteristic to mediate the rape-PTSD relationship. Causal attributions and maladaptive belief changes were far more powerful than any other predictors in explaining prolonged distress. Neither was strongly affected by levels of avoidance. *[Article copies available for a fee from The Haworth Document Delivery Service: 1-800-342-9678. E-mail address: <getinfo@haworthpressinc. com> Website: <http://www.HaworthPress.com> © 2001 by The Haworth Press, Inc. All rights reserved.]*

KEYWORDS. Trauma, mediators, sexual assault, experiential avoidance, PTSD, rape, recovery

Post Traumatic Stress Disorder (PTSD), characterized by intrusive recollections and cycles of avoidance and arousal, has been diagnosed in as many as 94% of rape victims assessed immediately after an assault (Rothbaum, Foa, Riggs, Murdock, & Walsh, 1992). This statistic suggests that almost all rape survivors experience some serious form of stress reaction following a sexual assault. Only the minority, one-third, go on to develop chronic PTSD, however (Solomon & Davidson, 1997). What causes one survivor to develop PTSD while another survivor does not? Certainly, no two rapes are exactly the same. But even people who encounter the identical traumatic event, such as two people who are in the same floor of a building during a natural disaster, often perceive and mentally experience it in different ways. In searching for predictors of PTSD, attention has focused on individual differences including demographic characteristics, preexisting psychopathology, social support, attitudes, crime descriptors, and cognitions such as perceptions of imminent death or bodily harm (e.g., Kilpatrick et al., 1989; Norris, 1992; Resnick, Kilpatrick, Dansky, Saunders, & Best, 1993). The intent of the present study is to test an expanded conceptualization of solely cognitive mediators of rape-induced PTSD in an effort to understand the process by which one survivor, but not another, would develop such debilitating symptoms.

To begin our discussion of experiential avoidance and PTSD, we first provide a definition of experiential avoidance. This definition is followed by an overview of the theories that influenced the conceptualization of our model and a description of the hypothesized model itself. A literature review of experiential avoidance is then presented which includes a general discussion of the current problems with research on avoidance. Finally, several brief reviews of the empirical findings that connect each of the mediating cognitive factors and describe their associations with psychological distress conclude the introductory section of this article.

DEFINITION OF EXPERIENTIAL AVOIDANCE

Because intrusive memories can be disruptive and painful, many survivors go to great lengths to avoid reminders of the trauma.

> Experiential avoidance is the phenomenon that occurs when a person is unwilling to remain in contact with particular private experiences (e.g., bodily sensations, emotions, thoughts, memories, behavioral predispositions) and takes steps to alter the form or frequency of these events and the contexts that occasion them. (Hayes, Wilson, Gifford, Follette, & Strosahl, 1996, p. 1154)

Experiential avoidance thus refers to cognitive, emotional, and behavioral avoidance strategies. Cognitive avoidance can include such strategies as not choosing to, or not being able to, think about the event, and rationalizing or minimizing the event. Behavioral avoidance involves avoiding places and people that remind a survivor of the experience, or refusing to do anything about the situation. Emotional avoidance generally refers to a survivor's efforts to avoid associated feelings (e.g., anger, guilt, sadness) when she is reminded of the rape.

Model Conceptualization

The intent of the present study is to expand the existing PTSD literature by testing an integrative model of the relationships between several different cognitive, social, and psychological elements, instead of examining each single category of variables separately. Our model focuses specifically on cognitive coping mechanisms, social cognitions, and reconstructed memories in an attempt to describe and understand the pathways by which cognitive factors mediate the relationship between rape and subsequent PTSD.

Several rich conceptualizations about the process by which rape leads to PTSD symptoms informed our model. We looked to both social cognitive theories that emphasize the impact of trauma on survivor's individual belief systems and preexisting views of the world (e.g., Harvey, 1996; Horowitz, 1986; Janoff-Bulman, 1992), as well as information-processing theories of PTSD that focus more on how trauma-related information is cognitively represented and processed (e.g., Foa & Riggs, 1995). Brewin, Dalgleish, and Joseph's (1996) dual representation theory of PTSD was also influential in the construction of our model. Their theory not only explains the different types of memory that are associated with PTSD, but also takes elements of social-cognitive theories into account. According to Brewin and his colleagues, emotional processing of traumatic events refers to the manipulation of representations of past and future events and associated bodily states in working memory. This process involves both the activation of unconscious detailed sensory and physiological information about the trauma, and the conscious attempt to accommodate information that is incompatible with preexisting beliefs by searching for meaning and making attributions about cause. Recovery occurs when memories of the trauma have been fully processed and integrated with the survivor's other memories and beliefs about the self and world.

The model also benefited from discussions of mechanisms of remembering and forgetting. Christianson (1997) pointed to two seemingly contradictory mechanisms of emotional memory. The first makes traumatic memory persistent, a function that has evolved to assist humans in identifying and remembering threatening situations. Though persistent and unpleasant, traumatic memories are not always accessible, however. Thus, it can be inferred that a second mechanism operates to assist in "forgetting" unpleasant memories from conscious awareness.

Although the present study does not attempt to construct a comprehensive model of PTSD, these theoretical conceptualizations were critical to our process of determining the serial ordering of the model. We used these theoretical leads to hypothesize an a priori cognitive mediational model of rape recovery, and looked to the past empirical findings (described in the literature review) to ground each hypothesized link.

The mediational model (illustrated in Figure 1) proposes the following causal sequence. First, experiential avoidance, as measured as a cognitive coping strategy ("blocking"), influences social cognitions about rape. The social cognitions included in this model are causal attributions (behavioral and characterological self-blame and external blame) and cognitive schemas (beliefs and personal constructs). Second, both cognitive coping strategy and social cognitions influence the qualities of reconstructed rape memory. Third, the operation of these mediators substantially predicts PTSD symptom severity.

The causal relationships hypothesized between the attribution variables were not based on previous work on these particular variables, but were based on more general theories of causal attribution. Looking at the entire pattern of social cognitions tested, our causal order goes from Behavioral Self-Blame to Characterological Self-Blame to External Blame to Beliefs (about the world and one's place in it). This sequence implicitly goes from local, specific, and unstable attributions (thought to be the least damaging) to more global, general, and stable attributions regarding blame for the event (the rape experience). First a survivor blames the rape on one particular action, then she blames her character, then she blames others, and finally she blames the nature of the world in general or at least her social place within it.

In Figure 1, the solid arrows below the diagonal that connect the successive categories indicate the major sequential pathways that were assigned causal priority according to the mediational hypothesis. The dashed arrows above the diagonal indicate alternative hypotheses that there were residual direct effects between the categories, even after the direct and indirect effects of the hypothesized sequence were completely accounted for. The objective was to restrict as many of these dashed paths as was consistent with the data to achieve a fully mediated model.

FIGURE 1. Conceptual Model for Cognitive Mediation of the Impact of Experiential Avoidance on PTSD

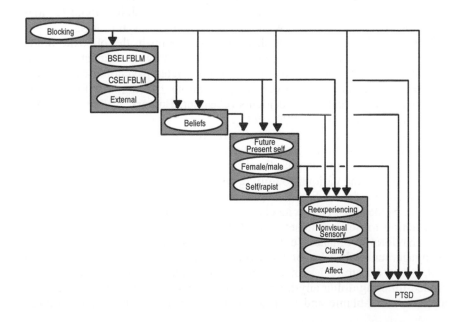

LITERATURE REVIEW

Experiential Avoidance

Researchers have both theoretically and empirically attempted to predict the effects of using such experiential avoidance coping strategies. The approach-avoidance theory of coping predicts experiential avoidance to play an adaptive role immediately following a traumatic event but a maladaptive one in the long-run. According to theory, avoidance coping permits victims to confront their traumatic experiences in manageable doses immediately after an event, but ultimately interferes with the integration process necessary for recovery over the long term (e.g., Horowitz, 1986; Lazarus & Folkman, 1984; Roth & Cohen, 1986). Some studies in which avoidance coping was measured immediately after an assault support the immediate adaptive role of avoidance. Not thinking or doing anything about the problem, and keeping busy and suppressing negative thoughts were associated with less psychological distress immediately following a rape (Frazier & Burnett, 1994; Frazier, Klein, & Seales, 1996). Evidence also supports the maladaptive effects of avoidance in the long term. Several studies of adult survivors of child sexual abuse and rape survivors interviewed at least one year post rape found avoidance coping to predict psychological distress (e.g., Coffey, Leitenberg, Henning, Turner, & Bennett, 1996; Santello & Leitenberg, 1993; Ullman, 1996). Alternatively, Arata's (1999) more approach-oriented expressive coping, which includes behaviors such as expressing and talking about feelings around others, was associated with fewer psychological symptoms.

Other experiential avoidance data, however, point in the opposite direction. Prospective studies of avoidance as measured by the Impact of Events Scale (Horowitz, Wilner, & Alvarez, 1979) predicted psychological disorder early on, but not later in recovery in populations of trauma witnesses and survivors of life-threatening accidents (Creamer, Burgess, & Pattison, 1992; Joseph, Yule, & Williams, 1994, 1995).

The inconsistencies in the coping literature can at least partially be attributed to variability in how experiential avoidance has been conceptualized and measured. Most of the standardized avoidance measures tap into different combinations of the various cognitive, emotional, and behavioral elements of experiential avoidance. For example, the Avoidance subscale of the Impacts of Events Scale (IES; Horowitz et al., 1979) taps into both emotional (e.g., "I avoid letting myself get upset when I think about it or am reminded of it") and behavioral avoidance (e.g., "I stay away from reminders of it"). The Disengagement subscales of the Coping Strategies Inventory, on the other hand, focus on strategies of cognitive and behavioral avoidance (e.g., "I avoided thinking/doing anything about the situation") as well as statements directed at self-blame and wishful thinking that the event would go away

(Tobin, Holroyd, Reynolds, & Wigal, 1989). Although it is not possible to describe every measure of experiential avoidance here, the examples presented illustrate the heterogeneous way in which this construct has been conceptualized and operationalized.

In summary, the inconsistencies in the avoidance coping literature appear to be attributable to both when avoidance was measured (how long after a rape) and how it was operationalized and measured. In addition, it appears that experiential avoidance may play different roles for different groups of trauma survivors. Evidence suggests that avoidance coping may be more adaptive for some types of trauma survivors than for others. As described above, studies of sexual abuse survivors generally find avoidance to be helpful in the short-term but maladaptive over time. In contrast, studies of witness and accident populations report the opposite. It is impossible, however, to separate and determine which of these three issues (time, measurement, or population) best explains the inconsistencies in the literature. Unfortunately, disentangling these confounds and resolving the inconsistencies in the literature are beyond the scope of the present study. Our awareness of these problems, however, influenced the manner in which we chose to measure and define experiential avoidance in this study.

Social Cognitions

Causal Attributions. Causal attributions, including the way in which a rape survivor apportions blame for the event, have been tied directly to post-traumatic functioning. Janoff-Bulman (1979, 1992) hypothesized that behavioral self-blame (blaming the event on one's behavior), as opposed to characterological self-blame (blaming the event on one's character), was adaptive because survivors experience a sense of control and believe they can avoid future sexual assaults. Empirical data, however, have actually associated both forms of self-blame with higher psychological distress in rape survivors (Abbey, 1987; Arata, 1999; Frazier, 1990; Frazier & Schauben, 1994; Hill & Zautra, 1989; Meyer & Taylor, 1986; or see Kushner, Riggs, Foa, & Miller, 1992, for a study of general uncontrollabililty and distress in crime victims).

Although most of the attribution literature has focused on these two types of self-blame, Frazier (1990) found that survivors actually blamed external factors, such as the rapist and society, more often than they blamed themselves for the cause of their rape. Blaming external factors, however, was not found to be as harmful as blaming one's self for the rape. Only behavioral and characterological self-blame were associated with depression in this sample of rape survivors. Regardless, rape survivors who report spending more time thinking about why the rape occurred have been found to suffer more psychological symptoms (Frazier, 1990; Frazier & Schauben, 1994). Thus, spending the mental energy to assign blame, even to someone else, is not predicted to be an adaptive exercise.

Cognitive Schemas. Traumatic experiences such as rape are thought to affect both a survivor's beliefs about the world and her personal schemas or constructs, which are beliefs about herself and the people around her. Kelly (1955) proposed that people form personal constructs in an attempt to understand and predict people and events. Changes in these constructs are thought to be disruptive and stressful and to have consequences on some aspects of recovery (e.g., Janoff-Bulman, 1985; McCann & Pearlman, 1990).

Certain basic assumptions or schemas are thought to be especially vulnerable to trauma. Assumptions about power, safety, and trust, for example are often disrupted by traumatic experiences (e.g., Janoff-Bulman, 1992; McCann & Pearlman, 1990). Maladaptive changes in these types of beliefs have been shown to mediate the relationship between violent crime and psychological distress (Norris & Kaniasty, 1991). Frazier and Searles (1997) found that women raped by strangers, compared to those raped by men they knew, engaged in more behavioral and characterological self-blame and showed more maladaptive change in their core beliefs. Harter, Alexander, and Neimeyer (1988) similarly found that sexual abuse was linked to increased discrepancy in ratings of personal constructs of the self contrasted to ratings for significant others.

Memory

Attempts to account for traumatic memory processing must consider the "interplay between social and cognitive mechanisms" (Wright & Gaskell, 1992, p. 277). Freyd's theory of shareability argues that certain characteristics and properties of a memory change just through the process of sharing information. As a person intends to share a memory with someone else, the memory is recoded to be less continuous and dynamic and more categorical and easier to communicate (Freyd, 1996). The social context actually changes the qualities of the memory. Thus remembering involves not only accessing available information, but also reconstructing the past in the present to meet desired psychosocial uses, and reconstructing with others through collective remembering of personal and historical events. In the proposed model, social cognitions are hypothesized to directly influence the characteristics of the reconstructed rape memory. This conceptualization represents an expansion of our earlier findings that the retrospective construal of an unwanted sexual act influenced several dimensions of memory (Koss, Figueredo, Bell, Tharan, & Tromp, 1996).

Intrusive memories of trauma accompanied by cyclic attempts to avoid triggers of memories are the central feature of PTSD (American Psychiatric Association, 1994). Thus, memory phenomena are central to our understanding of PTSD. Traumatic memories, however, have many other characteristics beyond the extent to which they intrude involuntarily into consciousness. Traumatic memories are said to be retrieved in the form of sensory and affective elements that include visual, olfactory, affective, auditory, and kinesthetic experiences (van der Kolk, 1996). We hypothesized that several dimensions of recall assessed by the Memory Characteristics Questionnaire (Suengas & Johnson, 1988) may increase the likelihood of PTSD. These dimensions of voluntary recall include affective intensity, vivid/lifelike detail, extensive sensory components, and thoughts, feelings, and bodily sensations reminiscent of the original experience during memory encoding.

METHOD

Participants

Participants were recruited by a postal survey that screened for rape and requested volunteers for a paid, private interview (see Koss et al., 1996). Surveys were mailed to 5,411 female medical center and university employees. Responses were received from 2,142 (40% response rate). Of these women, 618 (29%) met selection criteria for rape, and 279 (45%) consented for interviews. Subsequently, 267 (95%) were interviewed. The present study focused on the last 139 of these interviews where supplemental qualitative assessment was added to the standard quantitative measures.

Demographic characteristics of the survey respondents (mean age 40 years), the full interview sample (mean age 38 years), and the subsample examined here (mean age 39 years) are presented in Table 1. Statistical comparison is precluded because the three samples are subsets of each other. Inspection, however, revealed minimal differences in the demographic makeup of these groups. The present sample, compared to survey respondents, contained slightly fewer Asians, more people with no religious affiliation, more people with some college but fewer with graduate degrees, and more women with incomes lower than $7,500 but fewer with incomes over $50,000. Overall, the participants in the present study can be characterized as urban working women who were predominately white (89%), Protestant (39%), educated (6% with less than high school education), married/living with a partner (48%) or divorced (30%) with middle to lower income (only 14% had household incomes over $50,000, 19% reported incomes of less than $15,000).

Although this was a "non-clinical" sample and the mean time since the rape was slightly over 15 years, 23% of the survivors in the current study still met diagnostic criteria for current PTSD according to DSM-IV criteria (American Psychiatric Association, 1994). Thus, clinically significant levels of pathology were reflected in the sample.

TABLE 1. Demographic Frequencies in Percentages

Variable	Subsample (N = 137)	Full Sample (N = 253)	Survey Data (N = 2141)
Race			
African American	0.7	1.2	1.2
American Indian	0.7	0.4	0.9
Asian	0.7	0.4	2.2
Hispanic	7.1	9.4	7.9
White	89.3	87.9	87.7
Religion			
Catholic	27.1	31.6	30.7
Protestant	38.6	30.1	37.7
Jewish	2.1	3.1	4.3
Christian	12.9	17.6	14.8
Other	5.7	5.9	4.7
None	12.9	11.3	7.8
Education – completed			
Grades 7-12	1.4	1.6	1.1
High School Graduate (or GED)	4.3	5.9	4.7
Business/tech school	4.3	7.0	3.8
Some college	29.3	29.7	22.7
College degree	26.4	31.6	28.0
Graduate degree	33.6	23.8	39.6
Total Household Income – last year			
$7,500 or less	5.7	3.4	2.6
$7,501-15,000	12.9	11.7	9.2
$15,001-25,000	32.1	30.9	19.3
$25,001-35,000	15.0	17.2	17.4
$35,001-50,000	20.0	22.7	20.0
Over $50,000	13.6	13.7	31.6
Marital Status			
Single	16.4	16.0	17.1
Married	36.4	39.5	56.2
Living with Partner	12.1	14.1	7.0
Separated or Divorced	29.3	26.6	16.8
Widowed	4.3	3.1	2.8

Measures

Rape. The Sexual Experiences Survey, previously modified for use with women workers (Koss, Woodruff, & Koss, 1991) was used to screen for rape. Five questions operationalized rape, which was legally defined as vaginal, oral, or anal penetration against consent, by force, threat of force, or when the victim was intoxicated and incapable of giving consent. Penetration, no matter how slight, was sufficient to complete rape. The recall period was bounded by the participant's 14th birthday, representing the cut-off age for statutory rape. Only two states set a statutory age (the age below which sexual penetration is automatically rape) below 14 years (Searles & Berger, 1987). An example of a typical item includes: "Has a man made you have sex by using force or threatening to harm you? When we use the word 'sex' we mean a man putting his penis in your vagina even if he didn't ejaculate (come)." The word "rape" was not used in these questions, permitting a woman to be classified by researchers as a rape victim without necessarily accepting that self-label. Internal consistency reliability in the present data was .72, which is consistent with other published figures. All survivors were rescreened at interview and all endorsed one or more items consistent with rape.

Cognitive Avoidance

Given the variability in conceptualization and measurement of avoidance coping evident in the literature, we chose to build a measure from qualitative data allowing the components to emerge phenomenologically. Operating from an experiential avoidance perspective, our intention was to measure the extent to which participants avoided thoughts and emotions related to their trauma. Qualitative data for this measure were obtained by asking participants to complete a lifeline and mark and label the significant events in their lives. This technique was based on theoretical models of recovery that emphasize integrating the event into the life story (e.g., Brewin et al., 1996; Harvey, 1996). Participants then responded to follow-up questions depending on whether or not they placed the index rape, which was identified in screening as the unwanted sexual experience they remembered best, among the significant points in their lifelines. Those who placed the index rape on their lifelines were asked, "What role did or does it play in your life?" and "Why was this experience important to you?" Those who did not place the index rape on their lifelines were asked instead, "I notice that you did not list the unwanted sexual experience as a significant event on your lifeline. What role has this event played in your life?" and also "Can you tell me in what ways has it been less significant than the events you chose?" These responses were analyzed inductively (Patton, 1990). The categories of analysis were not imposed on the data prior to data collection and analysis, but instead emerged from the data. Labels used came from the language of the respondents. The coping strategies identified in the qualitative material are described below.

Blocking consisted of responses associated with not wanting, or not being able, to remember or think about the event, as well as feeling the experience was dream-like or unreal. Included were all responses suggesting that a participant attempted to block memories as a coping strategy, regardless of the effectiveness of their efforts. The term blocking was used because it appeared so frequently in the responses. Using the participants' own language was part of the qualitative approach to the data we used. It is not our intent to make connections to any technical definitions of this term. Examples of blocking responses include, " I have it pretty well blocked off . . . ," and "I have not thought about it in years," as well as, "I just don't want to think about it." Responses of this type were made by 43% of survivors. Downplaying was characterized by justifications, minimizations, rationalizations, or normalizations such as "It was just something that happens to women" or "It could have been a lot worse," or "As the sky is blue, violence against women just is." Fifty-eight percent of survivors included at least one remark of this type in their narrative. Selectivity included responses that suggested participants included only positive or rewarding experiences, rather than unhappy, or socially unacceptable events in their life narrative. "I just listed the good things, you know," and "I think the events I chose were more socially acceptable events," are examples of selectivity, which was identified among the responses of 30% of survivors. Useful Learning Experience included responses indicating something had been gained from the experience such as boundaries, awareness of rape issues and prevalence, or self-awareness, or motivation to leave an unhealthy relationship. Examples include, "It did start me on the road to making changes," and " . . . so it helped . . . in the long run to gain more self-esteem and to learn to take control of the situation rather than letting things happen to me. . . . " Statements of this type were made by 26% of survivors. Integration was scored when participants placed the index rape on their lifelines. Just 12% of survivors actually placed their rape among the events they considered most significant in the story of their lives.

Once the classification system was established, each narrative was coded by two independent readers who rated each response as 1 (for the presence) or 0 (for the absence) for each of these coping strategies. Interrater reliabilities ranged from 88% to 100%. Agreement was established on every discrepancy between the two raters. These individual strategies formed an Avoidance/Integration factor, whose development is explained in the discussion of the measurement model. Having established that the five categories formed an internally-consistent construct of cognitive coping strategies, we then engaged in the development of a more informative continuum of avoidance such that each strategy could be assigned an empirically meaningful weight. A continuum of avoidance was then established based on these empirical weights. Each participant then received a Cognitive Avoidance score that reflected the highest level of avoidance strategy that she used. A more complete description of this procedure can be found in the description of the measurement model (p. 235).

Our original qualitative analysis also identified strategies labeled Negative Attitude-Others, Negative Attitude-Self, and Negative Behavior Changes. These strategies did not load on the Avoidance/Integration factor, however, and thus were not included in the later analyses.

Social Cognitions

Causal Attributions. Causal Attributions were assessed with the Rape Attribution Questionnaire (Frazier, 1990), which consists of 21 items comprising three subscales that assess the participants' behavioral, characterological, and external attributions about rape. Ratings were made on a 5-point Likert scale ranging from Never (1) to Very Often (5). This assessment was included to determine how an actual sexual assault influenced an individual's causal attributions about rape. The Behavioral Blame scale determined the degree to which participants blamed rape on the victim's behavior. The scale included items such as, "You put yourself in a vulnerable situation." Characterological Blame assessed to what extent participants blamed their own characters or personalities for rape (e.g., "You are just the victim type."). The External Attribution scale asked questions directed at blaming societal factors or the rapist (e.g., "Men need to feel power over women."). Published reliabilities include alpha coefficients for Behavioral Blame at 3, 10, and 30 days post-rape that ranged from .87 to .89. The comparable figures for Characterological Blame and External Blame ranged from .75 to .82 and .64 to .76, respectively. Alpha coefficients in the full sample were .83, .76, and .81 for Behavioral, Characterological, and External Blame respectively. Characterological and Behavioral Blame have been associated with poorer psychological outcomes in rape populations (Arata, 1999; Frazier, 1990; Frazier et al., 1996; Frazier & Schauben, 1994).

Cognitive Schemas

Trauma-Related Beliefs. Beliefs were assessed by the McPearl Belief Scale Revision D, which was the most recent version available of the scale now known as the TSI/CAAPS Belief Scale (Pearlman, 1996). This 80-item scale measured individuals' beliefs about the self, others, and the world. A higher score indicated maladaptive changes in those cognitive schemas vulnerable to change by trauma exposure. The items ranged from specific, self-oriented statements such as "I find myself worrying a lot about my safety," to general feelings like "The world is filled with emotionally disturbed people." Responses were indicated on a 6-point Likert scale from Disagree Strongly (1) to Agree Strongly (6). The scale consisted of 10 sub-scales, with reported internal consistencies that ranged from .76 to .88. Alphas in the full sample were .55 to .88. The development of a single factor from these scales is described under the measurement model.

Personal Constructs. Personal constructs were assessed through the Family Perception Grid, based on Kelly's (1955) Role Construct Repertory Grid as modified by Harter et al. (1988). Participants rated their own characteristics in the past, the present, and the future. They were also asked about their construal of significant others including their mother, father, a male significant other, the typical man, the typical woman, close female friend, and rapist. The 10 characteristics rated on a 13-point Likert scale included: attractiveness, strength, intelligence, trustworthiness, dominance, warmth, independence, emotionality, openness, and reliance. These ratings were used to derive the following measures: (a) self-ideal discrepancy, which represented the difference between ratings of future self and present self; (b) gender polarization, which was represented by the sum of all ratings of men, subtracted from the sum of all ratings of women; and (c) rapist-self discrepancy, which was represented by the difference between participants' ratings of the rapist and themselves. It was hypothesized that rape survivors would report increased discrepancies between perceptions of the present and future self (self-ideal discrepancy), and between men in general and women in general (sex-role polarization). However, since the majority of rapes are committed by acquaintances, not stereotypical violent, deranged strangers, it was hypothesized that a rape experience would decrease the discrepancy between the self and the rapist (rapist-self discrepancy). Harter and colleagues (1988) expressed their data as Euclidean distances (sums of squared difference scores). We transformed our data by taking the square root of the Euclidean distances, giving us the Root Mean Square Differences. Because squared terms often have non-normal distributions, this transformation rendered the distributions more tractable.

Memory Characteristics

Participants were asked to recall everything possible about their rape or unpleasant experience and to make ratings of the qualities of their reconstructed memory in response to the Memory Characteristics Questionnaire (MCQ) (Suengas & Johnson, 1988). The full 43 item MCQ includes the 17 items that compose the four memory factors constructed and cross-validated by Koss et al. (1996). In the present study the additional items were assigned on a theoretical basis to these factors. The procedures used to confirm these item assignments are detailed later in the description of the measurement model. The factors as well as their internal consistency reliabilities in the full sample were the following. The first factor, called Clarity (alpha = .890), consisted of 28 questions pertaining to visual details of the event, emotional intensity felt at the time of the event, and how often the memory is thought and talked about. The Affect factor (alpha = .610) contained three ratings of valence (positivity or negativity) of feelings and the unexpectedness of the event remembered. The Reexperiencing factor (alpha = .798) contained eight items reflecting participants' subjective reexperiencing of the physical sensations, emotions, and thoughts that characterized the original event. The fourth factor, Nonvisual Sensory (alpha = .724), consisted of five questions about sensory components of memory including touch, smell, taste, or sound (vision loaded on the Clarity factor). All items were rated on a 7-point scale.

Post-Traumatic Stress Disorder

Symptoms of PTSD were assessed with the Post-Traumatic Symptoms Scale–Rater version (Foa, Riggs, Dancu, & Rothbaum, 1993), which corresponds to DSM-IV PTSD criteria. This 17-item scale allows categorical diagnosis of PTSD, dimensional scores for each sub-scale (avoidance, intrusion, and hyperarousal), as well as a global severity score. Internal consistency reliability for the re-experiencing, avoidance, and arousal sub-scales in the full-sample were .76, .72, and .71 respectively. These reliabilities are similar to reported figures (.78, .80, and .82; Foa et al., 1993). Test-retest reliability across one month was .74. The inter-rater reliability was kappa = .97 for the severity score (Foa et al., 1993). The estimation of the relationships of the subscales to a higher order factor representing global PTSD severity is described in the measurement model. We could not assume that PTSD was a single factor in a non-clinical population.

Data Analyses

Univariate Analyses

Missing Data. Scores on multi-item factors were imputed for respondents with one or more of the item scores missing based on the nonmissing values for the same person on all the other items comprising the factor. A respondent was only deleted when all indicators were missing. Only two respondents were lost using this multivariate imputation procedure (Figueredo, McKnight, & McKnight, 1996).

Residualization on Demographics. Demographic variables might have been correlated with some of the variables used in the model. To determine the amount of variance accounted for by demographics, they were entered into regression equations to predict each of the 289 items to be included in the multivariate model. Overall, seven of 289 regressions resulted in R squared's significant at the Bonferonni corrected probability of p < .0002. None of these effects involved ethnicity, marital status, or income. Five effects involved age and two involved education. These effects accounted for between three and 22 percent of the variance in study variables. Given the small number of significant effects, we chose to residualize the variables prior to multivariate analysis. Residualization subtracts any deviation systematically predicted by demographic variables from each score (Cohen & Cohen, 1983). This procedure statistically controls for the influence of demographics without explicitly including demographics in the multivariate model (P. M. Bentler, personal communication, October 1989). The adjusted scores, or regression residuals, were then used for multivariate modeling.

Effects of Time. The passage of time is well documented to ameliorate the effects of trauma, specifically as demonstrated by the reduced rate of PTSD observed in longitudinal studies. Most of this natural recovery appears to occur within the first few months after the trauma and then levels off to a slow, gradual improvement over time (Creamer et al., 1992; Rothbaum et al., 1992). No participants in this study were interviewed during that initial period of nonlinear recovery. We examined whether time constituted a threat to the internal validity of the present data. Specifically, did time significantly moderate the effect of rape on PTSD, thus violating the assumptions of a linear and additive model? To examine this question, a hierarchical regression model was run on the present participants and a group of 50 nonraped women selected from among survey respondents. The results revealed main effects for rape on PTSD, $F(1,297) = 4.89$, $p = .028$, and for time on PTSD, $F(1,297) = 4.49$, $p = .0\,35$, but no significant interaction between them in the prediction of PTSD, $F(1,297) = 0.26$, $p = .604$. Thus, PTSD symptom severity decreased linearly over time since rape. We did not residualize the effects of time as was done with demographic variables because any mediating processes must occur during the time elapsed. Residualizing the effects of time would have removed the effects of the hypothesized mediators (see Pedhazur & Kerlinger, 1982).

Multivariate Analyses

A factor analytic structural equations model consists of two major components: (1) a measurement model, and (2) a structural model.

The Measurement Model. The measurement model is the component of the model where a number of directly measured items are related to a smaller set of hypothetical constructs (called latent variables or common factors) presumed to be underlying the correlations among them. Although the present sample was not small in absolute terms, the items were too numerous with respect to the sample size to support item factor analytic procedures for lower-order scales. Instead, lower-order factor scores were estimated as unit-weighted factor scales. Items were assigned to factor scales based on the standard scoring of the measures. To examine internal consistency, item-factor correlations were computed and tested for statistical significance. This procedure generated tables of bivariate correlations that provide more detailed information on the factor loadings of the individual items than the simple Cronbach's alphas reported earlier. The results reproduced the original authors' scoring for the scales, with the exception of the TSI, which was found to be adequately represented by a single higher order factor rather than by eight subscale scores. This higher-order factor was also estimated using unit weighting. The bivariate correlations between individual items and factor scores are found in Table 2 (Avoidance/Integration factor), Table 3 (Behavioral Self-Blame, Characterological Self-Blame, and External Blame), Table 4 (the Gender Polarization factor), and Table 5 (four cross-validated memory factors). A higher order Belief factor was found to adequately represent the lower order factors obtained using the scales' recommended scoring. The bivariate correlations between each lower order factor and the higher order Belief factor are summarized in Table 6.

One hypothesis, whether there is a general PTSD factor in a nonclinical population, was considered of sufficient theoretical interest to perform Confirmatory Factor Analysis using Bentler's (1989) structural equations modeling program (EQS). The higher order factor was then incorporated as an explicit component of the structural equation model.

TABLE 2. Avoidance/Integration Factor: Bivariate Correlations of Item Scores to Unit-Weighted Factor Scores

Item description	Blocking
Blocking Cognitive Strategy	.482*
Downplaying Cognitive Strategy	.556*
Selectivity	.491*
Integration	−.740*
Useful Learning Experience	−.492*

*$p < .05$.

TABLE 3. Causal Factors: Bivariate Correlations of Item Scores to Unit-Weighted Factor Scores

	Causal Factors		
Item	Behavioral	Characterological	External
You are a poor judge of character.	.675*	.566*	.154
You made a bad decision.	.762*	.445*	.018
You should have been more careful.	.812*	.487*	.025
You didn't resist.	.641*	.437*	.005
You didn't know how to defend yourself.	.533*	.352*	.287*
You put yourself in a vulnerable position.	.778*	.434*	.035
You sent the wrong message.	.641*	.460*	−.021
You can't take care of yourself.	.520*	.639*	.227*
You are just the victim type.	.286*	.554*	.306*
You have bad luck.	.393*	.555*	.170*
You are a careless person.	.502*	.730*	.169*
You are a bad person.	.314*	.688*	.148
Attract men who hurt women.	.326*	.596*	.410*
You trust people too much.	.519*	.590*	.050
Never help around when you need it.	.147	.240*	.581*
Men don't respect women.	.183*	.395*	.745*
Perpetrators get off too easy.	.100	.241*	.693*
Men need to feel power over women.	.091	.313*	.773*
The perpetrator was sick.	.063	.088	.592*
Men are angry at women.	.107	.285*	.790*

*$p < .05$

Constructing the Cognitive Avoidance Continuum. Item Response Theory (IRT) was used to assign weights to the dichotomously coded coping strategies so an avoidance continuum could be constructed from the indicators of the Avoidance/Integration factor. Useful Learning Experience and Integration were first reverse scored and relabeled *Non-Learning Experience* and *Non-Integration* to ensure that their scores indicated avoidance. A one parameter logistic (Rasch) model was then used to assess item difficulty according to IRT. In general, IRT is thought to have advantages over classical test theory for providing item characteristics that are not group dependent (see

TABLE 4. Personal Constructs: Bivariate Correlations of Item Scores to Unit-Weighted Factor Scores

Euclidian Differences	Gender Polarization
Present mother and father	.804*
Typical man and typical woman	.676*
Male friend and female friend	.747*

*p < .05

Hambleton, Swaminathan, & Rogers, 1991, for a thorough discussion of these advantages and of IRT in general). The one parameter logistic model

was calculated with the equation $P_i(\theta) = \dfrac{e^{\left(\theta - b_i\right)}}{1 + e^{\left(\theta - b_i\right)}}$ using the IRT

program BIGSTEPS (Linacre & Wright, 1994). In this model, θ represents the propensity for avoidance or the avoidance score, $P_i(\theta)$ represents the probability that a randomly selected participant with a propensity for avoidance equal to θ endorses item i, and b_i represents the propensity for avoidance at which $P_i(\theta) = 0.5$, or 50%. Thus, the item difficulty parameter, and the parameter of greatest interest in this weighting procedure, is b_i. Because θ (in this case, avoidance propensity) is a standardized continuum, the b_i parameter can be negative or positive, with b_i parameters that are more negative indicating items requiring relatively low levels of θ to be coded and b_i parameters that are more positive indicating items requiring relatively high levels of θ to be coded.

The b_i parameters assigned to the avoidance codes were − 2.19 for Non-Integration (indicating that a very low avoidance propensity is required to achieve this code), − .84 for Non-Learning Experience (indicating that relatively more avoidance propensity is required to achieve this code), .71 for Downplay, 1.06 for Blocking, and 1.81 for Selectivity (indicating that a very high propensity for avoidance is required to achieve this code; see Table 7). For the purposes of this analysis, these b_i parameters were converted such that the lowest b_i (Non-Integration) was set to 1, and the relative distances between the b_i parameters for each code were preserved. With this conversion, weights were assigned to the codes as follows: 1 for Non-Integration, 2.35 for Non-Learning, 3.36 for Downplay, 4.25 for Blocking, and 5 for Selectivity (see Table 7). This scheme also allowed for a possible score of zero (no codes).

TABLE 5. Memory Factors: Bivariate Correlations of Item Scores to Unit-Weighted Factor Scores

Item	Memory Factor			
	Clarity	Affect	Reexpr	Sensory
Your memory of the event is little/clear	.746*	.115	.396*	.635*
Your memory involves VISUAL DETAIL a little/lot	.607*	−.037	.234*	.478*
Your memory of the event is in black & white/color	.407*	−.012	.072	.366*
The overall vividness of the memory is vague/vivid	.810*	.157	.475*	.650*
Order of events in your memory is confusing/orderly	.526*	.023	.121	.352*
The incident in your memory is simple/complicated	.284*	.154	.310*	.236*
The story in your memory seems unreal/realistic	.413*	−.016	−.025	.212*
The memory for the location is hazy/clear	.390*	−.022	−.022	.238*
The incident...occurs somewhere unknown/familiar	.288*	.028	.034	.098
The arrangements of the objects vague/clear	.593*	.025	.148	.342*
The arrangements of the people vague/clear	.551*	.017	.046	.372*
For the period in your life of event vague/clear	.567*	−.042	.049	.272*
Your memory for the YEAR is vague/clear	.569*	−.101	.023	.308*
Your memory for the SEASON is vague/clear	.421*	−.140	.208*	.348*
Your memory for the DAY is vague/clear	.498*	−.196*	.258*	.332*
Your memory for the HOUR is vague/clear	.673*	−.027	.345*	.474*
Time in your memory seems shortened/leng-thened	.388*	.186	.213*	.325*
At time... had serious implications not at all/def-initely	.545*	.152	.477*	.292*
Remember how you felt at the time not at all/def-initely	.521*	.115	.431*	.272*
Your feelings at the time were not intense/intense	.388*	.280*	.195*	.212*
Overall, you remember this event hardly/very well	.766*	.142	.489*	.563*
Memory for events before this event not at all/clearly	.506*	−.068	.304*	.245*
Memory for events after this event not at all/clearly	.505*	.033	.312*	.299*
Doubts of accuracy of the memory great deal/no doubt	.465*	.163	.125*	.243*
Since happened, thought about not at all/many times	.308*	.026	.536*	.090
Since happened, talked about not at all/many times	.275*	−.092	.311*	−.027
The completeness of the memory is sketchy/com-plete	.752*	.089	.311*	.661*
Your memory involves SOUND little/a lot	.475*	−.059	.221*	.681*
Your memory involves SMELL little/a lot	.290*	.046	.245*	.701*
Your memory involves TOUCH little/a lot	.408*	.105	.294*	.643*
Your memory involves TASTE little/a lot	.349*	.052	.151	.696*
Overall tone of the memory is negative/positive	−.051	.778*	.067	.016
Your feelings at the time were positive/negative	.032	.719*	.064	.015
Remembering now, feelings are positive/negative	−.077	.735*	.191*	−.008

TABLE 5 (continued)

Item	Memory Factor			
	Clarity	Affect	Reexpr	Sensory
Event was surprising or unexpected not at all/extremely	.258*	**.340***	.035	.154
Looking back, serious implications not at all/definitely	.324*	.207*	**.657***	.220*
Now, feelings are intense/not intense	.256*	.209*	**.729***	.246*
Re-experiencing physical sensations no/complete	.376*	.038	**.741***	.355*
Now, re-experiencing emotions no/complete	.228*	.071	**.701***	.172
Now, re-experiencing thoughts no/complete	.402*	−.048	**.685***	.357*
Memory reveals something of you not much/a lot	.192*	.155	**.588***	.186*
Felt would affect me a long time none/extremely	.289*	.055	**.492***	.225*
In memory...you are in control/just happening to you	−.176	−.005	−.053	−.064

Note. Bold text indicates items scored on each factor. *$p < .05$.

TABLE 6. Traumatic Beliefs: Bivariate Correlations of Subscale Scores to Higher Order Belief Factor

Subscales	Belief Factor
Safety	.687*
Self Trust	.771*
Other Trust	.795*
Independent	.700*
Power High	.460*
Power Low	.776*
Other Esteem	.735*
Self Esteem	.828*
Self Intimacy	.656*
Other Intimacy	.799*

*$p < .05$.

Infit and outfit mean square statistics were also calculated to provide additional information about the coping indicators as scale items. The infit is a mean square statistic sensitive to unexpected responses to items whose b_i is near an individual's own level of θ (in this case, θ being propensity for avoidance). The outfit is a mean square statistic sensitive to unexpected responses to items whose b_i is far from an individual's level of θ (Linacre and

TABLE 7. IRT Scaling Procedure Outcomes for Cognitive Avoidance Continuum

Code	Original b_i	Transformed weight	Infit	Outfit
Non-Integration	-2.19	1	.61	.27
Non-Learning	-0.84	2.35	1.07	.96
Downplay	0.71	3.36	1.01	.99
Blocking	1.06	4.25	.97	1.28
Selectivity	1.81	5	1.17	1.21

Wright, 1994). In general, infit and outfit statistics lower than .5 indicate dependency in the data, while those higher than 1.5 indicate noise in the data. Of all the codes, only one (Non-Integration) showed signs of dependency in the data, with an outfit of .27.

For these analyses, the five individual coping items were lined up on a continuum by weight. Given the assumption of IRT, that b_i indicates the level of θ required to be endorsed by a given individual, it was decided that an individual's total avoidance score would be indicated by the most strongly weighted code she received. That is, a participant's total avoidance score reflected the most strongly weighted coping strategy she used. So for example, if a participant was coded Non-Learning Experience, Downplay and Blocking, but not Non-Integration or Selectivity, that individual received a total avoidance score of 4.25, reflecting the weight of the Blocking strategy code. An alternative scoring option would have been to sum the weighted codes for a new scale score. Given the assumptions of IRT, however, we thought it prudent to avoid exaggerating the effects of these empirically derived weights.

Another alternative would have been to use estimates of participant or person θ instead of the estimates of item θ we described above. When conducting an IRT analysis, one derives both item estimates of θ (here, avoidance) and also person estimates of θ (the level of θ the model predicts an individual to possess). We chose to use the individual's highest scoring avoidance code item θ for calibration purposes because it was more interpretable. As it turns out, the estimates of person θ correlated at .7 (p < .001) with the level of θ assigned by an individuals highest scoring avoidance code. Thus, the distinction between the two types of estimates is only a theoretical, not an empirical one.

The Structural Model. The structural component of the model is essentially a path analysis between the factors. Path analysis, or structural equations modeling, consists of imposing a restricted set of causal relationships (or pathways), specified a priori, and testing them against the observed correlations. Any structural model that can adequately reproduce that pattern of intercorrelations with a reduced set of hypothesized causal pathways is judged superior by the principle of parsimony. Here model parsimony was produced primarily by the restriction of the direct causal pathways between non-successive categories of mediators in our theoretically derived hypothesized sequence (see Figure 1). Although it was not possible to wholly omit all of these residual direct effects, priority of inclusion was given to those additional pathways that both (1) bypassed fewer stages in the temporal sequence, and (2) could be associated with plausible alternative hypotheses consistent with prior research. Thus, some respecification was required of the strictly sequential causal model we initially hypothesized, but these were done in a systematic way according to predetermined, hierarchial rules of inclusion.

The only residual effects that were specified were the residual correlations among the memory factors. Residualized correlations represent those portions of the correlations between factors that remain unexplained by the model because they are not attributable to any effects of the model predictors. In contrast to the causal attribution variables, there was no theoretical justification for hypothesizing any particular causal sequence between the four memory factors. Nevertheless, these memory factors had been found significantly correlated in samples of both raped and nonraped women. That is, their "residual" correlations were the naturally occurring correlations between these factors that were not attributable to the spurious effects of the rape experience (serving as a common causal influence on all of them within raped women). Thus, they were left as unexplained or "residual" correlations for that reason. It would be unreasonable to model their total covariances with our restricted structural model of the effects of rape. Table 8 presents the residual correlations below the diagonal and the unresidualized correlations above the diagonal for the memory factors. Residual correlations probably represent more generalizable estimates of the correlations that other investigators will find if they extend this work to populations other than rape survivors. No other residual correlations were specified.

TABLE 8. Memory Factor Intercorrelation Matrix

Memory factor	1	2	3	4
1. Clarity Overall		.063	.463*	.672*
2. Affect	.058		.139*	.069
3. Re-experiencing	.570*	.048		.361*
4. Sensory nonvisual	.686*	.038	.367*	

Note: The numbers above the diagonal are unresidualized correlations; those below the diagonal are residualized. See text for discussion of each type of correlation.
* *p* < .05.

Structural equations models were evaluated by use of chi-square, the Bentler-Bonnett Comparative Fit Index (CFI), the Bentler-Bonnett Normed Fit Index (NFI), and the Bentler-Bonnett NonNormed Fit Index (NNFI) (Bentler, 1989; Bentler & Bonnett, 1980). Chi-square measures the statistical goodness-of-fit of the covariance matrix observed to that reproduced by the model. A significant chi-square is therefore grounds for rejection of the model specified. The Bentler-Bonnett indices are measures of practical goodness-of-fit for large sample sizes. Index values greater than 0.90 are considered satisfactory levels of practical goodness-of-fit, even if significant chi-square values are obtained (Bentler, 1989; Bentler & Bonnett, 1980).

RESULTS

Figure 2 depicts the final results of the restricted structural equations model. The path coefficients are standardized regression weights obtained by Maximum Likelihood estimation. The correlated residuals among endogenous factors are not represented graphically to avoid visual clutter, but they are presented in Table 8 and discussed later. Although the chi-square value was statistically significant, X^2 (88) = 114.225, p = .011, indicating that the model did not perfectly predict the covariances among the constructs, the

FIGURE 2. Structural Equations Model of the Cognitive Mediators of the Experiential Avoidance-PTSD Relationship

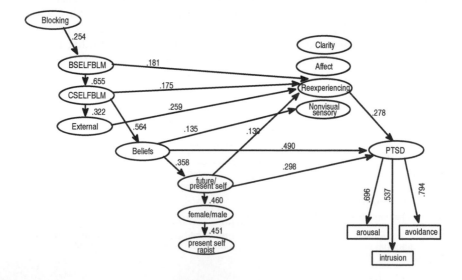

practical indices of fit were acceptable (NFI = .832, NNFI = .928, CFI = .944). The following description of the findings begins with the measurement component of the model, and then proceeds to the direct effects of each construct in the hypothesized temporal sequence. Finally, the indirect pathways by which PTSD was influenced are described.

The Measurement Model

The latent construct representing overall PTSD severity had large factor loadings on the subscales of Arousal (.696), Intrusion (.537), and Avoidance (.794). This finding demonstrated that there was strong convergent validity among the symptoms of PTSD even in this non-clinical population.

The Structural Model

Direct Effects

Cognitive Avoidance ("Blocking"). Cognitive Avoidance had a direct positive effect on Behavioral Self-Blame (.254). Those women who used cognitive strategies to try to avoid thoughts of the experience were more likely to blame themselves for the event. Cognitive Avoidance did not directly influence any other causal attributions, nor did it directly influence any cognitive schemas, memory characteristics, or PTSD.

Causal Attributions. All three types of attributions had direct effects on the Reexperiencing component of Memory: Behavioral Blame (.181), Characterological Blame (.175), and External Blame (.259). Engaging in any type of blame was associated with recall richer in re-experiencing of sensation, thoughts, and feelings associated with the original incident. Only Characterological Blame directly influenced Beliefs (.564), suggesting it may have a distinct capacity to cause more psychological disruption than does Behavioral Blame or External Blame. However, the distinctiveness of Characterological Blame should be interpreted with caution due to the high residual intercorrelation between Characterological and Behavioral Blame (.655). Causal attributions did not directly influence any other memory characteristics, any other cognitive schemas, or PTSD.

Cognitive Schemas

Beliefs. Beliefs had a strong direct effect (.497) on PTSD. Disruption in beliefs was associated with increased PTSD severity. Beliefs also had direct effects on the size of the Future/Present Self discrepancy (.358) that suggested disrupted beliefs were associated with finding oneself falling short on many character dimensions. No other direct pathways to personal constructs were supported. Beliefs contributed directly only to the Nonvisual Sensory aspect of Memory (.135).

Personal Constructs. The Future/Present Self discrepancy directly influenced PTSD (.298). Those women with a larger discrepancy were more likely to suffer symptoms of PTSD. The gender polarization construct representing discrepant views of men and women failed to predict negative psychological outcome.

Memory. Memory had a direct effect on PTSD through the Reexperiencing factor of Memory (.278). None of the other memory factors (Clarity, Affect, or Nonvisual Sensory) exhibited any influence on PTSD.

Mediated Effects

The social cognition factors, including causal attributions about rape and cognitive schemas, played an important role in mediating the influence of experiential avoidance on PTSD through two distinct sets of pathways. The social cognition factors exerted their influence by: (1) indirectly influencing PTSD through the qualities of reconstructed memory, specifically through the Reexperiencing factor; and (2) directly influencing PTSD mainly through the Beliefs factor.

Influence of Social Cognitions Mediated by Memory. Behavioral Blame, Characterological Blame, and External Blame all indirectly influenced PTSD through their effects on the Reexperiencing memory factor. Rape survivors who engaged in any of these forms of blame experienced more thoughts and feelings reminiscent of the original event during voluntary memory reconstruction and reported more symptoms of PTSD.

Direct Influence of Social Cognitions. Beliefs had the strongest direct effect of all the mediators on PTSD (.497). Women whose beliefs were most disrupted were the most likely to experience symptoms of PTSD. Beliefs also indirectly influenced PTSD through personal constructs. Those women with disrupted belief systems were most likely to experience a large discrepancy between their present and future self (.358), and in turn to suffer from more PTSD symptoms. The only direct influence on disruption of beliefs was exerted by Characterological Blame (.564). Characterological Blame played a role in both sets of pathways that influenced PTSD and was the only mediator to directly influence Beliefs, the strongest predictor of PTSD severity.

Summary of Effects

The structural model as a whole accounted for 60% of the variance in PTSD. The main effect of Cognitive Avoidance on PTSD must be attributed entirely to the collective action of the hypothesized mediators because there was no significant direct effect of Avoidance remaining in the model. The total effect of Cognitive Avoidance on PTSD was .08, which indicated that it only accounted for 1% of the variance. Thus, the remaining 59% of the explained variance in PTSD was predicted by social cognitions and memory characteristics. The bivariate correlation between Avoidance and PTSD was also virtually zero ($r = -.01$). We had originally thought that Avoidance would play a larger indirect role in predicting PTSD. Contrary to the strong avoidance theory, however, cognitive avoidance had very little influence, direct or indirect, on PTSD.

DISCUSSION

What does explaining 60% of the variance in PTSD mean in this context? Because the level of analysis used in this model is the individual survivor, it means that 60% of the variance in individual recovery (or lack thereof) from rape-induced PTSD was explained by the cognitive mediators. Our model shows what those mediating mechanisms might be, as well as some cognitive risk factors that may prolong recovery. An understanding of these processes will inform the assessment of survivors seeking care and contribute to our theoretical understanding of treatment effects.

The results of this study suggest that cognitive avoidance strategies were detrimental in terms of PTSD severity for a sample of survivors interviewed an average of 15 years post-rape. These findings are consistent with the bulk of the sexual assault coping literature, and specifically support the approach avoidance theory that hypothesizes experiential avoidance to be a maladaptive long-term coping strategy. Because downward social comparison strategies were included in our continuum of cognitive avoidance (coded as downplaying strategies), the effect on symptoms might have been expected to be negative. Making downward social comparisons through minimization and rationalization has been referred to as a strategy of positive illusion, a concept that has been found to maintain mental health (Taylor & Brown, 1988; Taylor, Wood, & Lichtman, 1983).

The social comparison strategies in this study (down-playing) did not earn as much statistical weight as indicators of avoidance compared to strategies directed at completely blocking out thoughts of the rape specifically (blocking) or thoughts of negative life events generally (selectivity). Thus the social comparison strategies may not have had much influence in this model. It is possible that a homogeneous measure of positive illusion would play a more adaptive role in mediating psychological distress. For example, Positive Distancing strategies, which are a combination of cognitive distancing, optimism, and acceptance statements from the Abbreviated Version of the Ways of Coping Inventory (Parkes, 1984), have been associated with less psychological distress in a population of sexual assault survivors (Valentiner, Foa, Riggs, & Gershuny, 1996). Future research projects that separate and investigate the unique influence of each individual cognitive coping strategy on psychological symptoms will further refine theory in this area. Finally, since this study only investigated the influence of cognitive coping strategies on PTSD, future studies also need to systematically investigate whether purely behavioral or purely emotional avoidance strategies are more adaptive coping mechanisms.

The findings of this study expanded the existing literature by using a statistically weighted qualitative measure that isolated the cognitive strategies involved in experiential avoidance. Even more importantly, though, the findings estimated the magnitude of their effect on PTSD, not as an isolated process, but in the context of other components of recovery. The results of this study suggest that cognitive avoidance exhibited only a very small effect on psychological outcomes compared to the role of social cognitions. Such a finding has important clinical implications. Although survivors will not be harmed by therapeutic approaches that strive to replace survivors' avoidance coping strategies with more adaptive approach ones, clinicians are likely to make a larger impact by focusing on their clients' disrupted belief systems instead. Our results suggest that in terms of predicting psychological symptoms, it is relatively unimportant whether or not a survivor uses cognitive avoidance strategies to cope with her rape experience.

Several of the effects were mediated through the Reexperiencing memory factor. This construct captured the extent to which feelings, physical sensations, emotions, and thoughts from the original trauma were reexperienced in voluntary recall. The results suggested, however, that these meta-memory ratings of rape recall played a limited role in the prediction of PTSD. There is a concern about possible bias in this relationship as well. We were conceptually clear about the distinctions between voluntary reexperiencing and intrusive memory, and the questions to indicate each were different. An example of the reexperiencing items is "As you are remembering now, to what extent are you reexperiencing in your mind or body the EMOTIONS or FEELINGS that you had during the event?" Whereas, typical content of an intrusive memory items was the following, "Have you had recurrent or intrusive distressing thoughts or recollections about the incident?" Although conceptually distinct, we cannot reject with the present data the alternate hypothesis that the relationship between the two is explained by conceptual, semantic, or measurement overlap with the content of intrusive memory component of PTSD assessment.

The results also replicated in a third independent sample of survivors the lack of predictive power for health outcomes demonstrated for the remaining memory characteristics of Clarity, Affect, and Nonvisual Memory (Koss et al.,

1996). The bulk of our hypotheses about the effects of social cognitions on how memory is reconstructed in a social setting failed to receive support. Although there was a small effect of belief disruption to increase the nonvisual sensory components in recall, this effect was a dead end that failed to have any relationship with PTSD. None of the social cognitions had an influence on vividness or emotional intensity, nor did these memory characteristics predict the severity of PTSD.

Although some may disagree with how we chose to assess memory characteristics, we used a standardized and cross-validated measure that duplicated the range of phenomena across which memory is known to vary. Critics of our measure may suggest that individuals are just not very good at making meta-memory ratings. It should be noted, though, that the diagnosis of the PTSD intrusion criteria depend on a similar introspection and memory rating process. It is currently difficult or impossible to reconcile studies of memory among rape or other trauma survivors because measurement has been so varied. For example, Mechanic, Resick, and Griffin (1998) reported that 82% of rape survivors had a clear memory of the assault at 3 months postrape, whereas we have reported that rape memories are more vague and hazy than memories for other emotionally intense experiences. Mechanic and colleagues (1998) used single clinician ratings to represent memory clarity. We encourage future research to explore alternative methods of measuring memory. Memory phenomena are central to theories of the etiology and treatment of PTSD. It is incumbent on those who promote these conceptualizations to devote attention to their measurement with the same precision that is evident in assessment of PTSD.

With the exception of Reexperiencing, the experiential avoidance-PTSD relationship was mediated entirely by social cognitions. The present findings extend existing literature (e.g., Frazier, 1990; Frazier et al., 1996; Frazier & Schauben, 1994) demonstrating that behavioral blame has a negative impact on PTSD. Even more interesting was the finding that characterological blame appeared to play a unique role in predicting PTSD severity through its large, deleterious effect on maladaptive belief change. It is still debatable, however, whether or not characterological self-blame is distinct from behavioral self-blame as Janoff-Bulman (1979) originally hypothesized. The conceptual distinction is questioned by the sizable empirical relationship between measures of behavioral and characterological self-blame. The distinction is not successfully defended empirically.

Trauma-related alterations in core beliefs proved to be the most potent predictors of PTSD symptomotology. They influenced PTSD both directly, and indirectly through the tendency of shattered beliefs to translate into a large discrepancy between how survivors actually viewed themselves and how they would ideally like to be. The finding that the future/present self-discrepancy was associated with increased symptoms of PTSD is consistent with Strauman's and his colleagues' theory that such self-discrepancies are markers of cognitive vulnerability that contribute to the onset and maintenance of emotional disorders (Strauman, 1994). Experimental studies have found discrepancies between the present and ideal self to be associated with depression (Strauman, 1994). In the present study, this future/present self-discrepancy appeared to capture the sense of permanent damage and irremediable shame that has been historically associated with raped women. The discrepancy may also reflect rape survivors' negative self-perceptions related to their perceived powerlessness to alter the course of their assault. By implication, therapeutic attempts to reverse or mollify some of these cognitions should result in lowered PTSD severity. Cognitive Behavioral Therapy (CBT) has been found to be effective in reducing self-discrepancies and symptoms of clinically depressed patients (Strauman, 1994). And, CBT has been found effective in treating PTSD among rape survivors (e.g., Resick & Schnicke, 1992). Future treatment studies could address whether the self-ideal discrepancy mediates clinical recovery in rape survivors with PTSD.

Our results strongly advocate for future research that focuses on the disruption of these belief systems and treatments that restore them. The findings of this study clearly suggest that a disruption in beliefs is the most important cognitive factor in predicting PTSD. Thus, we are now encouraged to focus our attention on these belief systems in an effort to pinpoint the precise components that are responsible for such psychological distress. A fine-grained, in-depth assessment of belief systems is critical to our understanding of the process by which beliefs are disrupted, and furthermore to our development of effective therapeutic interventions for rape-induced PTSD. For example, the importance of blaming highlighted by the present study leads us to interest in survivors' ideas about justice, need for revenge, and how these ends are served or hindered by current social responses to rape.

Several strengths of the present study must be highlighted. First is the community sample. Clinical populations generally consist of women whose coping strategies have failed to protect them from distressing symptoms, so the negative effects of traumas such as rape are magnified. By studying a community sample, we were able to see the full range of responses that women have to rape. Although some women did suffer from the various symptoms of PTSD, most of the women continued without symptoms that exceeded threshold. Unfortunately, our model does not identify any protective or resiliency factors, except as suggested by the absence of the factors that exacerbated symptoms. A second strength was our integrated, systemic analysis of cognitive mediators. We did not treat each mediator as an isolated variable. Only through a systemic outlook can we understand how the breakdown of one mechanism will affect another, and identify those mechanisms that cause the most damage to the system when they are disrupted. Third, the inclusion of qualitative data provided a construct that did not share the same self-report method bias of the other measurement tools. Although the measure used in the present study is admittedly unvalidated, it was based on reliable dual coded ratings of the narratives.

These strengths balance certain limitations. The structural model is based on cross-sectional data that was not cross-validated. However, all of the elements of the model except for the cognitive coping measure (which was available only on a subset of the sample) have been cross-validated in a longitudinal study of these same mediators (Koss, Figueredo, & Prince, 2000). The longitudinal study recruited rape survivors within three months of their assault and followed them for two years.

Also, because the current study was not comprised of any survivors who had been interviewed within the first three months post-rape, we were limited in our ability to assess whether or how the relationship between experiential avoidance and PTSD changes over time. Given our finding that experiential avoidance does not play such an important role in predicting psychological distress, however, this does not appear to be as pressing a research question.

Another limitation of the study is that the causal order of the mediators was theoretically based. Some may disagree with our a priori order. No theoretical model can be considered the conclusive representation of any observed phenomenon, and hypothetical constructs must be refined with the progress of psychological science. This study also only looked at mediators of experiential avoidance and PTSD. We did not measure pre-trauma influences on experiential avoidance, such as childhood abuse, nor were characteristics of the rape included that could help explain why some survivors engaged in avoidance coping. We did, however, find solid empirical support for our conceptualization. The present results suggest that many of the critical variables mediating rape and PTSD dwell somewhere within the domain of core beliefs about the self and others, the attribution of blame and responsibility, and especially social cognitions concerning control, safety, vulnerability, power, trust, and intimacy. Contrary to our expectation that experiential avoidance would play a key role in predicting PTSD, we found that avoidance coping had very little influence on psychological distress. Instead, the results reinforce the oft-cited conclusion that the impact of sexual violence is primarily an assault on the survivor's world of meaning.

REFERENCES

Abbey, A. (1987). Perceptions of personal avoidability versus responsibility: How do they differ? *Basic and Applied Social Psychology, 8*, 3-19.

American Psychiatric Association (1994). *The diagnostic and statistical manual of mental disorders* (4th Ed.). Washington, DC: American Psychiatric Association.

Arata, C. M. (1999). Coping with rape. *Journal of Interpersonal Violence, 14*, 62-78.

Bentler, P.M. (1989). *EQS: Structural equations program manual.* Los Angeles: BMDP Statistical Software.

Bentler, P.M., & Bonnett, D.G. (1980). Significance tests and goodness of fit in the analysis of covariance structures. *Psychological Bulletin, 88*, 588-606.

Brewin, C.R., Dalgleish, T., & Joseph, S. (1996). A dual representation theory of posttraumatic stress disorder. *Psychological Review, 103*, 670-686.

Christianson, S. (1997). Remembering and forgetting traumatic experiences: A matter of survival. In M.A. Conway (Ed.), *Recovered memories and false memories. Debates in psychology* (pp. 230-250). Oxford, England: Oxford University Press.

Coffey, P., Leitenberg, H., Henning, K., Turner, T., & Bennett, R.T. (1996). The relation between methods of coping during adulthood with a history of childhood sexual abuse and current psychological adjustment. *Journal of Consulting and Clinical Psychology, 64*, 1090-1093.

Cohen, J., & Cohen, P. (1983). *Applied multiple regression /correlation analysis for the behavioral sciences.* Hillsdale, NJ: Erlbaum.

Creamer, M., Burgess, P., & Pattison, P. (1992). Reaction to trauma: A cognitive processing model. *Journal of Abnormal Psychology, 101*, 452-459.

Figueredo, A.J., McKnight, K.M., & McKnight, P. (1996, November). *Structural equations modeling of small data sets.* Paper presented at the American Evaluation Association Annual Meeting, Atlanta, Georgia.

Foa, E. B., & Riggs, D. S. (1995). Posttraumatic stress disorder following assault: Theoretical considerations and empirical findings. *Current Directions in Psychological Science, 4*, 61-65.

Foa, E.B., Riggs, D.S., Dancu, C.V., & Rothbaum, B.O. (1993). Reliability and validity of a brief instrument for assessing post-traumatic stress disorder. *Journal of Traumatic Stress, 6*, 459-473.

Frazier, P. (1990). Victim attributions and postrape trauma. *Journal of Personality and Social Psychology, 59*, 298-304.

Frazier, P.A, & Burnett, J. W. (1994). Immediate coping strategies among rape victims. *Journal of Counseling & Development, 72*, 633-639.

Frazier, P., Klein, C., & Seales, L. (1996). *A longitudinal study of causal attributions, perceived control, coping strategies, and postrape symptoms.* Manuscript submitted for publication.

Frazier, P., & Schauben, L. (1994). Causal attributions and recovery from rape and other stressful life events. *Journal of Social and Clinical Psychology, 14*, 1-14.

Frazier, P., & Searles, P.A. (1997). Acquaintance rape is real rape. In M.D. Schwartz (Ed.), *Researching sexual violence against women: Methodological and personal perspectives* (pp. 54-64). Thousand Oaks, CA: Sage.

Freyd, J.J. (1996). *Betrayal trauma: The logic of forgetting childhood abuse.* Harvard University Press: Cambridge, Massachusetts.

Hambleton, R.K., Swaminathan, H., & Rogers, H. J. (1991). *Fundamentals of item response theory.* Newbury Park, CA: Sage Publications.

Harter, S., Alexander, P.C., & Neimeyer, R.A. (1988). Long-term effects of incestuous child abuse in college women: Social adjustment, social cognition, and family characteristics. *Journal of Consulting and Clinical Psychology, 56*, 5-8.

Harvey, M.R. (1996). An ecological view of psychological trauma and trauma recovery. *Journal of Traumatic Stress, 9*, 3-23.

Hayes, S.C., Wilson, K.G., Gifford, E.V., Follette, V.M., & Strosahl, K. (1996). Experiential avoidance and behavioral disorders: A functional dimensional approach to diagnosis and treatment. *Journal of Consulting and Clinical Psychology, 64*, 1152-1168.

Hill, J., & Zautra, A. (1989). Self-blame attributions and unique vulnerability as predictors of postrape demoralization. *Journal of Social and Clinical Psychology, 8*, 368-375.

Horowitz, J.J. (1986). *Stress response syndromes* (2nd Ed.). Northvale, NJ: Jason Aronson.

Horowitz, J.J., Wilner, N., & Alvarez, W. (1979). The Impact of Events Scale: A measure of subjective stress. *Psychosomatic Medicine, 41*, 209-218.

Janoff-Bulman, R. (1979). Characterological versus behavioral self-blame: Inquiries into depression and rape. *Journal of Personality and Social Psychology, 37*, 1798-1809.

Janoff-Bulman, R. (1992). *Shattered assumptions: Towards a new psychology of trauma*. New York: Free Press.

Joseph, S., Yule, W., & Williams, R. (1994). The Herald of Free Enterprise disaster: The relationship of intrusion and avoidance to subsequent depression and anxiety. *Behaviour Research and Therapy, 32*, 115-117.

Joseph, S., Yule, W., & Willliams, R. (1995). Emotional processing in survivors of the Jupiter cruise ship disaster. *Behaviour Research and Therapy, 33*, 187-192.

Kelly, G.A. (1955). *The psychology of personal constructs*. New York: Norton.

Kilpatrick, D.G., Saunders, B., Amick-McMullan, A.E., Best, C.L., Veronen, L.J., & Resnick, H. (1989). Victim and crime factors associated with the development of posttraumatic stress disorder. *Behavior Therapy, 20*, 199-214.

Koss, M.P., Figueredo, A.J., Bell, I., Tharan, M., & Tromp, S. (1996). Traumatic memory characteristics: A cross-validated mediational model of response to rape among employed women. *Journal of Abnormal Psychology, 105*, 421-432.

Koss, M.P., Figueredo, A.J., & Prince, R.J. (2000). A cognitive mediational model of rape recovery: Preliminary specification and evaluation in cross-sectional data. Manuscript under review.

Koss, M.P., Woodruff, W.J., & Koss, P.G. (1991). Relation of criminal victimization to health perceptions among women medical patients. *Journal of Consulting and Clinical Psychology, 58*, 147-152.

Kushner, M., Riggs, D., Foa, E., & Miller, S. (1992). Perceived controllability and the development of posttraumatic stress disorder (PTSD) in crime victims. *Behavior Research and Therapy, 31*, 105-110.

Lazarus, R.S., & Folkman, S. (1984). *Stress, appraisal, and coping*. New York: Springer.

Linacre, J.M., & Wright, B.D. (1994). *A user's guide to bigsteps: Rasch-model computer program*. Chicago, IL: Mesa Press.

McCann, I.L., & Pearlman, L.A. (1990). *Psychological trauma and the adult survivor: Theory, therapy, and transformation*. New York, NY: Brunner/Mazel.

Mechanic, M.B., Resick, P.A., & Griffin, M.G. (1998). A comparison of normal forgetting, psychopathology, and information-processing models of reported amnesia for recent sexual trauma. *Journal of Consulting and Clinical Psychology, 66*, 948-967.

Meyer, C., & Taylor, S. (1986). Adjustment to rape. *Journal of Personality and Social Psychology, 50*, 1226-1234.

Norris, F.H. (1992). Epidemiology of trauma: Frequency and impact of different potentially traumatic events on different demographic groups. *Journal of Consulting and Clinical Psychology, 60* 409-418.

Norris, F., & Kaniasty, K. (1991). The psychological experience of crime: A test of the mediating role. *Journal of Social and Clinical Psychology, 10*, 239-261.

Parkes, K. R. (1984). Locus of control, cognitive appraisal, and coping in stressful episodes. *Journal of Personality and Social Psychology, 46*, 655-668.

Patton, M.Q. (1990). *Qualitative evaluation and research methods* (2nd ed.). Thousand Oaks, CA: Sage.

Pearlman, L.A. (1996). Review of the TSI/CAPP Belief Scale. In B.H. Stamm (Ed.), *Measurement of stress, trauma, and adaptation* (pp. 415-417). Lutherville, MD: Sidran Press.

Pedhazur, E.J., & Kerlinger, F.N. (1982). *Multiple regression in behavioral research: Explanation and prediction* (2nd ed.). New York: Holt, Rinehart, & Winston.

Resick, P.A., & Schnicke, M.K. (1992). Cognitive processing therapy for sexual assault victims. *Journal of Consulting and Clinical Psychology, 60*, 748-756.

Resnick, H.S., Kilpatrick, D.G., Dansky, B.S., Saunders, B.E., & Best, C.L. (1993). Prevalence of civilian trauma and posttraumatic stress disorder in a representative national sample of women. *Journal of Consulting and Clinical Psychology, 61*, 984-991.

Roth, S., & Cohen, L.J. (1986). Approach, avoidance, and coping with stress. *American Psychologist, 41*, 813-819.

Rothbaum, B.O., Foa, E.B., Riggs, D.S., Murdock, T., & Walsh, W. (1992). A prospective examination of post-traumatic stress disorder in rape victims. *Journal of Traumatic Stress, 5*, 455-475.

Santello, M.D., & Leitenberg, H. (1993). Sexual aggression by an acquaintance: Methods of coping and later psychological adjustment. *Violence and Victims, 8*, 91-104.

Searles, P., & Berger, R.J. (1987). The current status of rape reform legislation: An examination of state statutes. *Women's Rights Law Reporter, 10*, 25-43.

Solomon, S.D., & Davidson, J.R.T. (1997). Trauma: Prevalence, impairment, service, use, and cost. Repairing the shattered self: Recovering from trauma. *Journal of Clinical Psychiatry, 58*, 5-11.

Strauman, T.J. (1994). Self-representations and the nature of cognitive change in psychotherapy. *Journal of Psychotherapy, 4*, 291-316.

Suengas, A.G., & Johnson, M.K. (1988). Qualitative effects of rehearsal on memories for perceived and imagined complex events. *Journal of Experimental Psychology: General, 117*, 377-389.

Taylor, S., & Brown, J. (1988). Illusion and well-being: A social psychological perspective on. *Psychological Bulletin, 103*, 193-210.

Taylor, S., Wood, J., & Lichtman, R. (1983). It could be worse: Selective evaluation as a response to victimization. *Journal of Social Issues, 39*, 19-40.

Tobin, D.L., Holroyd, K.A., Reynolds, R.V., & Wigal, J.K. (1989). The hierarchical structure of the Coping Strategies Inventory. *Cognitive Therapy and Research, 13*, 343-361.

Ullman, S. E. (1996). Social reactions, coping strategies, and self-blame attributions in adjustment to sexual assault. *Psychology of Women Quarterly, 20*, 505-526.

Valentiner, D.P., Foa, E.B., Riggs, D.S., & Gershuny, B.S. (1996). Coping strategies and posttraumatic stress disorder in female victims of sexual and nonsexual assault. *Journal of Abnormal Psychology, 105*, 455-458.

van der Kolk, B.A. (1996). Trauma and memory. In B.A. van der Kolk, A.C. McFarlane, & L. Weisaeth (Eds.), *Traumatic stress: The effects of overwhelming experience on mind, body, and society* (pp. 279-302). New York, NY: The Guilford Press.

Wright, D., & Gaskell, G. (1992). The construction and function of vivid memories. In M.A. Conway, D.C. Rubin, H. Spinnler, & W.A. Wagenaar (Eds.), *Theoretical perspectives on autobiographical memory* (pp. 275-292). Dordrecht: Kluwer Academic Publishers.

Autobiographical Memory Disturbances in Childhood Abuse Survivors

Valerie J. Edwards
Robyn Fivush
Robert F. Anda
Vincent J. Felitti
Dale F. Nordenberg

SUMMARY. Clinicians have noted that childhood abuse survivors frequently report that they have forgotten large parts of their childhood. While memory for abusive experiences has attracted a great deal of attention from researchers, other types of memory disturbances may also accompany a history of childhood trauma. Many clinicians report that certain types of sexual abuse, and abuse at certain developmental stages, is more likely to result in reports of gaps in memory for the abuse. However, because information has been mainly collected in clinical populations, the possibility of confounding between abusive experiences and psychological disturbances cannot be ruled out. This article reports on data gathered from a large, epidemiologic study conducted within a health maintenance organization. A history of childhood physical or sexual abuse doubled the prevalence of general autobiographical memory loss for women, while for men, the rate increased 1.5 times over those with no abuse history. Higher rates of autobiographical memory loss were noted where both types of abuse were reported. Further, multiple incidents of sexual abuse, sexual abuse by a relative, and more severe sexual abuse increased reports of autobiographical memory loss. Theoretical perspectives on changes in the memory

Address correspondence to: Valerie J. Edwards, Centers for Disease Control and Prevention, Mailstop K-47, 4770 Buford Highway, NE, Atlanta, GA 30341.

[Haworth co-indexing entry note]: "Autobiographical Memory Disturbances in Childhood Abuse Survivors." Edwards, Valerie J. et al. Co-published simultaneously in *Journal of Aggression, Maltreatment & Trauma* (The Haworth Maltreatment & Trauma Press, an imprint of The Haworth Press, Inc.) Vol. 4, No. 2, (#8), 2001, pp. 247-263; and: *Trauma and Cognitive Science: A Meeting of Minds, Science, and Human Experience* (ed: Jennifer J. Freyd, and Anne P. DePrince) The Haworth Maltreatment & Trauma Press, an imprint of The Haworth Press, Inc., 2001, pp. 247-263. Single or multiple copies of this article are available for a fee from The Haworth Document Delivery Service [1-800-342-9678, 9:00 a.m. - 5:00 p.m. (EST). E-mail address: getinfo@haworthpressinc.com].

system that may affect trauma survivors are discussed. *[Article copies available for a fee from The Haworth Document Delivery Service: 1-800-342-9678. E-mail address: <getinfo@haworthpressinc.com> Website: <http://www.Haworth Press.com> © 2001 by The Haworth Press, Inc. All rights reserved.]*

KEYWORDS. Childhood abuse, autobiographical memory, sexual abuse, physical abuse, amnesia, survivors, trauma

Autobiographical memory forms the core of who we are. It is the narrative of our life story. Most of us have access to autobiographical memories from as early as three to four years of age, although this may be influenced by various factors, including how frequently and how elaborately parents reminisce about the past (Fivush, 1997; Nelson, 1993; Pillemer, 1997). Moreover, this narrative has a seamless feel to it, although details may be lost over time. For most of us, our autobiographical life story helps provide a sense of identity and continuity over time (Bruner, 1987; Fivush, 1988, 1997). Yet intriguingly, many survivors of trauma seem to suffer disturbances of autobiographical memory (e.g., Herman & Schatzow, 1987). In particular, the clinical literature is rife with descriptions of childhood sexual abuse (CSA) survivors who report large gaps in their memories of childhood. Not only may memory for the trauma itself be fragmented and/or vague, but CSA survivors often report fewer memories for more mundane events that comprise most individuals' autobiographical self. To date, there has been little systematic investigation of this issue. Virtually no comparison of abused and non-abused individuals on childhood memories has been performed. We were in a unique position to address this issue as part of a large, epidemiologic study of the long-term effects of childhood abuse on adult health. Thus, in this article we examine the association between a reported history of childhood abuse and autobiographical memory loss in a non-clinical adult population.

REMEMBERING ABUSE

The study of memory in trauma survivors, and in particular those who have experienced childhood sexual abuse, has largely concentrated on the retention and accuracy of memory for the trauma itself. There are contradictory predictions in the literature concerning memory for a traumatic event. Some theorists have argued that trauma is so overwhelming that the individual will dissociate, or distance themselves from the experience, leading to an unintegrated, incoherent memory (e.g., Putnam, 1997; van der Kolk, 1996). Others have argued that trauma leads to a narrowing of attention to the core details of the event, leading to an enhanced, more highly elaborated memory of the experience (e.g., Christianson, 1992; Easterbrook, 1959). With more recent advances in neuropsychobiology, several theorists are now arguing that the emotional and sensory aspects of the traumatic event may be encoded, stored, and retrieved separately from the consciously available narrative or linguistic representation (Brewin, 1989; LeDoux, 1996). That is, one could remember an event emotionally but have no conscious recollection of it. Intriguingly, there is empirical evidence supporting all of these views, suggesting that memory of trauma is complex and quite likely multiply determined.

Questions specific to childhood abuse include whether adults can recall their abuse experiences and whether recollection of these experiences is continuous. Three studies have directly interviewed documented childhood abuse survivors to determine the rate of "forgetting" of abuse. Williams (1994) reported that 38% of women with verified histories of childhood sexual abuse failed to report the target incident when interviewed almost twenty years later, despite their willingness to disclose other personally intimate life experiences. Widom and Shepard (1996) related that 40% of adults physically abused as children could not be classified as abused by their responses to the Conflict Tactics Scale (CTS) (Straus, 1979). Similarly, Della Femina, Yeager, and Lewis (1990) found that 28 of 69 adults (40.6%) gave accounts of childhood physical abuse discrepant with court records. However, in follow-up interviews, when confronted with evidence of their abuse, all admitted being aware of it. Varying reasons for disavowing the experience were put forth by the participants, including a conscious desire to forget the past, or a lack of rapport with the interviewer. Thus, we must be extremely cautious in confusing lack of reporting with lack of memory.

Other studies have simply asked respondents who now recall childhood abuse if there were periods of time during which they were unable to remember the abuse. Feldman-Summers and Pope's (1994) survey of psychologists revealed that 40.5% of the respondents who had experienced childhood abuse reported a period of time during which they could not remember some or all of the abuse. Briere and Conte (1993) recruited adult sexual abuse survivors through therapists and found that 59% reported that they were unable to remember their first molestation experience for some time. Elliott and Briere's (1995) national probability sample found that 42% of those who had been sexually abused reported periods of partial to total amnesia for the abuse. In Herman and Schatzow's (1987) therapy group for women incest survivors, 28% reported severe memory deficits for their childhood, including the abuse they were ostensibly working through. Loftus, Polonsky, and Fullilove (1994) interviewed women in substance abuse treatment and found that, of the 54% who reported experiencing childhood sexual abuse, 19%

reported that they completely forgot the abuse occurred for a time, while 12% claimed partial memory of the abuse. Although it is unclear how to interpret individuals' retrospective reporting of periods of forgetting, the data converge on the conclusion that many survivors of childhood sexual abuse claim periods of amnesia for the traumatic experience.

Moreover, certain aspects of childhood abuse appear to be more strongly associated with a period of forgetting, specifically incestuous sexual abuse involving some violence or threat, and an onset of abuse before adolescence. For instance, of the four categories of abuse studied (sexual abuse by a relative or nonrelative, and physical abuse by a relative or nonrelative) in Feldman-Summers and Pope's (1994) sample of psychologists, sexual abuse by a relative resulted in the highest proportion of reported forgetting (56.2%). Similarly, Williams (1994) found that the closer the relationship between the perpetrator and the victim, the more likely that the abuse was not reported in her sample. Briere and Conte (1993) and Elliott and Briere (1995) both found that those abused subjects who had at some time been amnestic for the abuse were more likely to have been threatened with harm and to have been more distressed by the experience. Williams also reported that the degree of force was related to failure to report the abuse, although this trend did not reach statistical significance. Herman and Schatzow (1987) stated that 75% of group therapy patients who described violent abuse were amnestic for these experiences for "a prolonged period of time" (p. 5). Only Loftus et al. (1994) found no association between violent abuse and periods of forgetting, but they used an unusual definition of violence, namely vaginal or anal sex.

Respondents who were younger at the time of the abuse were also more likely to be amnestic for the abuse in Williams' (1994), Herman and Schatzow's (1987), and Briere and Conte's (1993) samples, but in Elliott and Briere's (1995) larger national sample no relation between age and continuous and discontinuous memory for abuse was found. Amnesia for abuse in early childhood, of course, must be interpreted within the general finding that adults have difficulty recalling events that occurred before the age of 3 to 4 years (see Fivush, Pipe, Murachver, & Reese, 1997, for a review). Because events of the first four years of life are generally not recalled, it is not surprising that traumatic or abusive events from this period are not recalled either. However, what is still unknown is the extent to which a history of abuse renders even non-abusive experiences difficult to remember after the age of 3 to 4 years, when most adults are able to recall childhood memories in a more or less continuous manner.

REMEMBERING THE PAST

Whereas most research on trauma and memory has focused on memory *for* the trauma, less is known about the effect of trauma on memory more generally. Because of the controversy over memory for trauma, the possibility of more overarching autobiographical memory disruptions in childhood abuse survivors has been largely overlooked. There are several compelling reasons to postulate general disturbances of autobiographical memory in traumatized populations. If, indeed, experiencing trauma is overwhelming and the individual dissociates (Putnam, 1997; van der Kolk, 1996), then it is quite likely that with repeated or chronic trauma, individuals would develop a dissociative style, leading to fragmented and disorganized memories in general. Related to this, Brewin (1989) has argued that a general expectation of negative life occurrences leads to the development of a negative schema, which incorporates the specific details of events into a more abstract representation. If a traumatized individual develops such a negative schema, then even more positive experiences may be assimilated into this negative worldview, and specific experiences may be difficult to recall. Both of these approaches posit less detailed, elaborated memories overall in traumatized and depressed populations. More specific to incestuous sexual abuse, Freyd (1997) has argued that the unsolvable dilemma faced by a young child who is emotionally and physically betrayed by her caregiver leads to denial and forgetting of these early experiences. As these experiences may be unavailable to consciousness, surrounding nontraumatic experiences may be blocked as well.

In addition to psychological mechanisms, there is growing evidence that trauma may cause structural changes in the brain. In particular, some traumatized individuals display reduction in hippocampal volume (Bremner, Krystal, Southwick, & Charney, 1995; Yehuda, Resnick, Kahana, & Giller, 1993). Because the hippocampus plays a major role in encoding memories, a history of trauma may adversely affect the ability to process and encode all subsequent experiences, traumatic or not.

Where data have been collected, they suggest that childhood sexual abuse is related to autobiographical memory disturbances. Herman and Schatzow's (1987) study of a therapy group for incest survivors reported that a significant proportion of participants asserted that they were unable to remember large parts of their childhood, although the actual proportion was not specified. Kuyken and Brewin (1995) compared the memory functioning of depressed female patients with and without a history of child physical and sexual abuse and found that those with a sexual abuse history retrieved less specific memories in response to both positive and negative cues than nonabused or physically abused subjects.

Other studies of depressed inpatients and PTSD sufferers have also uncovered deficiencies in autobiographical memory. Most of this research has utilized the Autobiographical Memory Test (AMT) (Robinson, 1976). In this paradigm, subjects are presented with five pleasant words and five unpleasant words and are given one minute to retrieve a specific personal memory in response to the cue. Use of this procedure has focused attention on two properties of memory: (1) response latency to a positively or negatively valenced cue; and (2) ratings of memory specificity. Williams and Broadbent (1986) found that suicidal patients were more likely to report general, rather than specific memories, particularly in response to positively valenced cues. McNally, Lasko, Macklin, and Pitman (1995) compared memory retrieval in Vietnam veterans with and without PTSD. Difficulties in retrieving specific memories, particularly in response to positive cues, were characteristic of the PTSD group, but were less pronounced in the non-PTSD combat veterans. Bremner, Steinberg, Southwick, Johnson, and Charney (1993) reported that amnestic symptoms best distinguished between Vietnam veterans with and without PTSD, with amnestic periods that varied from minutes to hours to days. Additionally, Bremner et al. (1995) have identified structural differences in neuroanatomy, wherein PTSD sufferers exhibit a significant reduction in the size of their left hippocampus relative to matched controls. One study used a variant of the AMT that analyzed written rather than verbal memories, using a standardized scoring system. Moffitt, Singer, Nelligan, Carlson, and Vyse (1994) classified undergraduates by depression status and then analyzed the text written in response to the memory cues. Depressed undergraduates provided reliably less detailed written memories than non-depressed students in response to a request for a positive self-defining memory.

This body of evidence suggests that, at least for psychiatric inpatients and others with varying psychopathology, there is a relation between traumatic experiences and less specificity in autobiographical memory. However, whether these results may be due to some comorbid condition, in particular, depression or PTSD, or whether trauma itself is responsible for these findings is unclear. To better understand this phenomenon, data from a non-clinical population should be analyzed in order to gather baseline information on the extent of autobiographical memory loss where no severe psychopathology exists. Further, demographic characteristics such as age and gender, as well as characteristics of the abuse, need to be considered when examining these types of data in order to disentangle possible theoretical interpretations.

In this research, we examined the relation between reported childhood sexual or physical abuse and autobiographical amnesia. In addition, we assessed whether specific characteristics of childhood sexual abuse, such as repeated abuse, incestuous abuse, and abuse that involved force are more likely to result in general amnesia for childhood periods. The role of depression as an intervening or modifying variable was also explored.

METHODS

These data were collected as part of a larger study on adverse childhood experiences and their relation to adult chronic disease and health behavior. A more complete description of the methods and preliminary findings is available elsewhere (Felitti et al., 1998). A large sample (13,494) of consecutive patients visiting a preventive health clinic in a metropolitan health maintenance organization (HMO) was mailed a questionnaire titled the Family Health History. This instrument was developed to mirror other large, nationally normed questionnaires in this topic area. The survey requested detailed information on childhood experiences related to physical, emotional, and sexual abuse, family alcoholism and violence, as well as current lifestyle questions concerning smoking, drinking behavior, and reproductive history. The response rate to the questionnaire was 70.5%.

As part of this survey, participants were asked: "Are there any large parts of your childhood after age 4 which you can't remember?" (Yes/No). The respondent was then asked to check off each period (in two year increments) between ages 4 and 18 for which they had memory deficits. Subjects were classified as amnestic if they responded affirmatively to the amnesia-screening question, or if they checked off any of the amnestic periods.

Depression was assessed with a modified version of the Diagnostic Interview Schedule (DIS) (Robins, Helzer, Croughan, & Ratcliff, 1981), which consisted of two items enquiring whether the respondents had experienced two weeks or more of depressed mood in the last year, and a second item asking whether they had experienced two years or more of depressed mood in adulthood. Childhood sexual abuse was assessed with four questions that progressed in severity, from fondling to attempted intercourse to actual intercourse (see Appendix). Subjects were classified as sexually abused if they responded affirmatively to any one of the four sexual abuse screeners, and were less than 18 years of age when the incident occurred. For each sexual abuse question answered affirmatively, the number of times the abuse occurred was requested. Additional information was requested concerning the relationship between the abuser and the participant, and whether force was used in the abuse from those who indicated that they had been sexually abused.

Physical abuse was judged as present in those individuals who responded "often" or "very often" to either of the following two questions, adapted from Straus (1979): "Did a parent, stepparent or adult living in your home (a) actually push, grab, shove, slap, or throw something at you?" or (b) "hit you so hard that you had marks or were injured?"

We analyzed the data separately by gender, because of the known association between childhood abuse and gender. Moreover, there is growing evidence that women generally have more elaborated and detailed memories of their past experiences than men (Fivush, 1998). We used chi-square tests of significance to detect group differences.

RESULTS

The findings are organized into three sections. In the first section, analysis of the rate of reported general amnesia for the entire population is described. Next, information about rates of childhood physical and sexual abuse is reported. Lastly, the relation between reports of childhood abuse and autobiographical amnesia is analyzed, as well as the moderating effects of depression and characteristics of reported abuse on this relation.

General Amnesia

Overall, 18.9% of the sample reported experiencing amnesia for some portion of their childhood after age 4. The frequency of reported amnestic periods by age of respondent is detailed in Table 1. Age 4-6 was the most frequently selected amnestic period, with frequencies decreasing as a function of age. For those who indicated the presence of amnestic periods, the average number of periods of amnesia was 1.89 (SD = 1.37). As indicated in Table 1, older subjects reported a reliably lower frequency of amnesia than did the youngest respondents: 16.6% in ages 60 and older vs. 23.9% in 19 to 29-year-olds, $X^2(4, N = 9115) = 35.1, p < .001$.

Childhood Physical and Sexual Abuse

Rates of reported childhood sexual and physical abuse by age group and gender are reported in Table 2. Among women, 26.8% reported some type of sexual abuse in childhood. Among men, the rate was 15.8%. These resemble

TABLE 1. Number and Percentage of Respondents Reporting Specific Periods of Autobiographical Amnesia[1]

Current age	Amnestic Period											
	4 – 6		7 - 9		10 - 12		13 - 15		16 - 18		18+	
	N	%	N	%	N	%	N	%	N	%	N	%
19 - 29	90	37.34	72	29.88	39	16.18	21	8.71	12	4.98	7	2.91
30 - 39	168	37.92	131	29.57	75	16.93	40	9.03	18	4.06	11	2.48
40 - 49	277	37.13	215	28.82	129	17.29	59	7.91	38	5.09	28	3.75
50 - 59	281	40.67	194	28.08	114	16.50	47	6.80	28	4.05	27	3.91
60+	512	45.15	298	26.28	152	13.40	80	7.06	46	4.06	46	4.06
Total	1328	40.78	910	27.96	509	15.64	247	7.59	142	4.36	119	3.66

[1] Respondents could choose multiple time periods.

TABLE 2. Percentage of Respondents Reporting Sexual and Physical Abuse by Age and Gender

Age	Sexual abuse		Physical abuse	
	Men	Women	Men	Women
19-29	17.97	31.84	12.12	9.84
30-39	18.95	30.15	10.71	15.86
40-49	16.36	30.31	15.20	15.91
50-59	19.42	28.38	11.88	13.98
60+	16.25	22.43	7.93	7.51
Overall	15.84	26.75	10.47	11.49

prevalence estimates obtained in other samples. A recent nationally representative telephone survey of adults estimated that 27% of women and 16% of men had been sexually abused (Finkelhor, Hotaling, Lewis, & Smith, 1990). Among women, reports of sexual abuse were significantly related to respondent's age, X^2 (4, N = 4662) = 33.6, p < .001, although the only large difference was between the oldest subjects, who reported sexual abuse at a markedly lower rate, and all other age groups. For men, no significant difference by age group was found, X^2 (4, N = 4128) = 6.2, p > .05. Physical abuse was reported by 11% of the study population overall, with women having a slightly, but not significantly higher prevalence, X^2 (1, N = 9401) = 2.5, p > .1. No discernable pattern of differences in physical abuse reports by age was noted.

Relation Between Abuse and General Amnesia

Tests of association between the presence of sexual abuse and general amnesia were performed for each gender separately. For women, the rate of reported amnesia in the sexually abused group was roughly double that of the nonabused group (31.5% vs. 16.4%, X^2 (1, N = 4524) = 127.3, p < .001). Among men, the sexually abused group reported a rate of amnesia 1.5 times greater than the nonabused group (20.7% vs. 15.3, X^2 (1, N = 3993) = 11.50, p < .001).

The relation between physical abuse and amnesia was also analyzed by gender. As with sexual abuse, the presence of childhood physical abuse significantly elevated reports of amnesia. Again, women were about twice as likely to report amnesia if they also reported physical abuse (37.8% versus 18.5%, X^2 (1, N = 4877) = 113.0, p < .001). Results obtained among physically abused men mirrored those obtained among sexually abused men, with men in the affected group reporting about 1.5 times the prevalence of general amnesia than those who reported no physical abuse (22.5% vs. 16.0%, X^2 (1, N = 4204) = 12.3, p < .001).

Subjects were then re-classified into four groups. Those who reported both physical and sexual abuse were designated as "multiply abused," while those who reported only one type of abuse remained within the respective physically or sexually abused group. The nonabused group consisted of those respondents who did not indicate either type of abuse. Table 3 details the results of this analysis by gender. When abuse was analyzed separately for men and women, physical abuse and sexual abuse had approximately the same association with reports of amnesia. Those who indicated that they had experienced both types of abuse, regardless of gender, showed a considerably greater level of endorsement of general amnesia than those who had experienced only one form of abuse, X^2 (1, N = 8496) = 211.3, $p < .001$.

Because more detailed information on childhood sexual abuse was available from the Family Health History than for physical abuse, more extensive analyses of the sexual abuse data were possible. The effects of three characteristics of sexual abuse on reported rates of amnesia were assessed: the severity of abuse, the frequency of abuse, and the relationship between the victim and the perpetrator. For these analyses, those individuals who indicated that they had experienced only sexual abuse were included.

Severity of abuse. Three classes of severity were created from the four sexual abuse items: abuse involving intercourse, attempted intercourse, and fondling. These three categories were contrasted with individuals who indicated no sexual abuse (Table 4). Among women, there was an overall significant difference in general amnesia by abuse severity, X^2 (3, N = 4308) = 137.1, $p < .001$. A graded relation between severity of abuse and amnesia was noted, with reports of general amnesia rising from 25.9% in the group who experienced fondling only through 41.0% in those who indicated abuse involving penetration. For men, the overall chi-square was also significant, X^2 (3, N = 3926) = 14.5, $p < .002$, but a less linear relation between severity and general amnesia was noted, with those men who indicated attempted inter-

TABLE 3. Percentage of Respondents Reporting Autobiographical Amnesia by Abuse Type

| | Gender | |
| | Men | Women |
Abuse type		
No abuse	15.28%	15.20%
Physical abuse only	19.73%	31.33%
Sexual abuse only	19.60%	28.13%
Both physical and sexual abuse	27.82%	44.20%

TABLE 4. Percentage of Respondents Reporting Autobiographical Amnesia by Severity of Sexual Abuse

	Gender	
Abuse severity	Men	Women
Type of Abuse		
No abuse	15.65	16.48
Fondling	17.83	25.85
Attempted intercourse	27.69	35.00
Intercourse	22.07	41.01
Violence of Abuse		
Abuse not involving violence	20.57	24.37
Abuse involving violence	18.18	34.78

course having a higher prevalence of general amnesia than those who indicated that their abuse involved penetration (27.7% vs. 22.1%).

Another way of characterizing severity is by whether the respondent indicated that threat of force or being physically forced or overpowered was involved in the abuse. Among women reporting violent abuse, 34.8% also reported general amnesia, as opposed to 24.4% of those who did not describe their abuse as violent, X^2 (1, N = 890) = 10.7, p < .001. However, violent abuse did not differentiate amnesia rates for men, X^2 (1, N = 462) = .14, p > .05.

Frequency of abuse. Sexual abuse victims who indicated that the abusive experience had occurred only once were then contrasted with those who reported multiple (more than one) episodes of abuse. Among women, 29.8% of those who experienced multiple abusive experiences also reported general amnesia, as opposed to 22.0% of single incident victims, X^2 (1, N = 764) = 6.1, p < .02. Among men, a similar nonsignificant trend was noted, with 23.5% of multiple incident male victims reporting general amnesia, as contrasted with 16.5% of single incident victims, X^2 (1, N = 411) = 3.1, p < .08.

Relationship of perpetrator. For each sexual abuse victim, the abuse experience was classified as incestuous if the abuser was described as a family member living in the home. All other relationships were treated as non-incestuous. Again, separate analyses were performed for men and women. Among women, 39.83% who reported incestuous abuse also reported amnesia, as opposed to 28.54% of women who did not describe an incestuous abuse experience, X^2 (1, N = 928) = 8.8, p < .003. Among men, there was a similar nonsignificant trend, X^2 (1, N = 495) = 3.23 p < .08. Of those men who described their perpetrator as a relative living in the home, 28.6% reported general amnesia, as contrasted to 18.5% whose abuser was not so closely related to them.

The Role of Depression

The presence of elevated levels of reported amnesia in both physically and sexually abused adults prompted the examination of the relation between reported amnesia and depression. It was theorized that depression might be the common link between childhood experiences and memory loss. Among both men and women who answered affirmatively to having had two weeks or more of depressed mood in the last year, the rate of reported amnesia was 30.4% vs. 15.1% in nondepressed individuals, X^2 (1, N = 8956) = 246.6, p < .001). Depression was related to reports of childhood sexual abuse: 34.6% of CSA victims versus 21.0% of nonabused subjects reported being depressed. Next, subjects were stratified by gender and depression status. Analyses of amnesia by sexual abuse were conducted within each stratum. These results are presented in Table 5. Women CSA survivors with two weeks or more of depressed mood reported general amnesia at almost twice the rate of depressed women who did not report childhood sexual abuse. Among men, the increase in general amnesia was about 1.5 times that of nonabused depressed men. However, even among the nondepressed abuse survivors, reported amnesia for each gender separately significantly exceeded that of nonabused subjects, X^2 (1, N = 3170) = 3.7, p < .055 for men, and X^2 (1, N = 3217) = 46.7, p < .001 for women. Therefore, elevated depression levels alone cannot account for a higher rate of amnesia within sexual abuse victims.

DISCUSSION

We examined the relation between autobiographical amnesia and a self-reported history of childhood abuse in a non-clinical population. Among respondents who indicated that they had experienced childhood abuse (physi-

TABLE 5. Percentage of Respondents Reporting Autobiographical Amnesia by Sexual Abuse and Depression

	Men		Women	
	Depressed	Not Depressed	Depressed	Not Depressed
	Amnestic	Amnestic	Amnestic	Amnestic
Sexual abuse status				
No sexual abuse	22.55	14.08	26.77	12.91
Sexual abuse	31.25	17.51	45.47	23.26

cal, sexual, or both), the rate of autobiographical amnesia was roughly double that reported by those with no history of abuse. These findings, derived from a large-scale epidemiologic study, demonstrate the powerful long-term effects of childhood abuse on subjective memory experiences.

Before discussing these findings in greater depth, it should also be noted that these data represent the first estimates of perceived autobiographical amnesia base rates in a non-clinical population. Approximately 15% of the sample with no trauma history agreed with the statement that there were large parts of their childhood that they did not remember. Little normative information about people's beliefs about autobiographical memory has been collected; therefore, it is not possible to determine whether this sample, drawn from a population of health maintenance organization participants, is representative of the public at large.

Surprisingly, the oldest participants were the least likely to agree to autobiographical memory loss. This may be a "reminiscence" effect, wherein the eldest respondents may be more likely to think about and discuss the past. On the other hand, older respondents may be more sensitive to the issue of memory loss and therefore less willing to describe themselves in a stereotypically elderly way.

However, the most intriguing findings concern the association between a reported history of childhood abuse and agreement with the notion of having forgotten large parts of one's childhood. These results extend the findings of previous studies detailing the presence of generalized memory disturbance associated with depression and a history of childhood abuse to a non-clinical population. Unlike Kuyken and Brewin (1995) however, elevated reports of amnesia were found in adults physically abused as children, well as those who were victims of childhood sexual abuse at roughly similar levels. Experiencing multiple types of abuse greatly increased reports of autobiographical amnesia. Although depression appears to play a major role, and is related to reports of abuse, depression alone cannot explain these results. Rather, these findings make a strong case for the disruptive power of sexually and physically abusive experiences on memorial processes.

While some researchers have argued that trauma memories are different from other memory types (e.g., van der Kolk & Fisler, 1995) what these findings suggest is that trauma may affect memory in total. In other words, it may not be that individuals remember trauma differently from other types of events, but rather that the experience of trauma itself changes the memory system, rendering even non-traumatic events more difficult to recall. Certainly, this view is substantiated by the morphological changes that have been noted in trauma survivors by Yehuda et al. (1993), Bremner et al. (1995), and others. Recent research by Freyd and her associates (DePrince & Freyd, 1999; Freyd, Martorello, Alvarado, Hayes, & Christman, 1998) has demonstrated that individuals high in dissociation, which often accompanies a history of trauma, indeed process information differently from those with low dissociative tendencies. High dissociators showed more interference in the Stroop task (Stroop, 1935), a standard measure of attentional processing, and poorer memory for emotionally charged words than did low dissociators. These findings suggest that trauma history may lead to a qualitatively different cognitive style, at least in some individuals. Our research further suggests that one aspect of this cognitive style is impoverished autobiographical memories. What cannot be determined from this study, however, is the source of memory loss, in other words, whether trauma affects encoding, processing, or retrieval, or perhaps some combination of these memory operations.

Moreover, the question used to classify individuals as amnestic or non-amnestic is somewhat vague and subjective. It is not possible to determine whether participants who responded positively to the item truly have autobiographical deficits or if they simply *feel* as if they do. Further work on normative expectations for autobiographical memory, along with more objective measures of autobiographical recall, need to be collected to better understand these results. Research currently underway in our laboratory is probing the phenomenological experience associated with remembering and forgetting childhood sexual abuse survivors.

Importantly, this is the first study in the literature to systematically document relations between abuse and autobiographical memory loss. Of course, some caution must be exercised when interpreting these results. This survey relied on retrospective reports of childhood abuse, which may be subject to both false positives and false negatives, although the rates of abuse obtained are consistent with other, nationally normed surveys. Further, severity and frequency of abuse appear to drastically increase the prevalence of reported autobiographical memory loss, as does sexual abuse by a family member.

A loss of autobiographical memory is not simply a cognitive deficit but lies at the heart of a disruption of self-understanding. To lose our memories is tantamount to losing our selves. Childhood abuse survivors who suffer from a lack of childhood memories are not anchored by a sense of self in time, a continuous self that defines who they are and how they fit with others in an interwoven web of shared memories. Without this anchor, childhood abuse survivors may feel a sense of isolation and a lack of social support. One of our interview study participants, who indicated that she believed that she had forgotten much of her childhood, said, "I need to remember in order to forget." As feminist theorists have argued, to be able to tell one's story, to have voice, gives power and memory to events (Belenky, Clinchy, Goldberger & Tarule, 1986). With the diminution of memory, childhood abuse survivors have lost their voice, their reality. Without their memory, they are silenced.

AUTHORS' NOTE

The authors wish to thank Naomi Howard, Laura Gamble, and Matthew Sydney for their assistance in the collection and preparation of the data used in this study. Parts of this study were reported at the meetings of the International Society for Traumatic Stress Studies, October 1998, Washington, D.C., and the American Psychology and Law Conference, April 1998, Redondo Beach, CA. This research was funded by cooperative agreement #TS-44-10/11 between the Centers for Disease Control and Prevention and the Association of Teachers of Preventive Medicine.

REFERENCES

Belenky, M. F., Clinchy, R. M., Goldberger, N. R., & Tarule, J. M. (1986). *Women's way of knowing.* New York: Basic Books.

Bremner, J. D., Krystal, J. H., Southwick, S. M., & Charney, D. S. (1995). Functional neuroanatomical correlates of the effects of stress on memory. *Journal of Traumatic Stress, 8,* 527-53.

Bremner, J. D., Steinberg, M., Southwick, S. M., Johnson, D. R., & Charney, D. S. (1993). Use of the Structured Clinical Interview for DSM-IV Dissociative Disorders for systematic assessment of dissociative symptoms in posttraumatic stress disorder. *American Journal of Psychiatry, 150,* 1011-1014.

Brewin, C. R. (1989). Cognitive change processes in psychotherapy. *Psychological Review, 96,* 379-394.

Briere, J., & Conte, J. R. (1993). Self-reported amnesia for abuse in adults molested as children. *Journal of Traumatic Stress, 6,* 21-31.

Bruner, J. (1987). Life as narrative. *Social Research, 54,* 11-32.

Christianson, S. A. (1992). Remembering emotional events: Potential mechanisms. In S.A. Christianson (Ed.), *Handbook of emotion and memory: Research and theory* (pp. 307-340). Hillsdale, NJ: Lawrence Erlbaum.

Della Femina, D., Yeager, C. A., & Lewis, D. O. (1990). Child abuse: Adolescent records vs. adult recall. *Child Abuse and Neglect, 14,* 227-231.

DePrince, A. P., & Freyd, J. J. (1999). Dissociative tendencies, attention, and memory. *Psychological Science, 10,* 449-452.

Easterbrook, S. A. (1959). The effect of emotion on the utilization and the organization of behavior. *Psychological Review, 66,* 153-201.

Elliott, D. M., & Briere, J. (1995). Posttraumatic stress associated with delayed recall of sexual abuse: A general population study. *Journal of Interpersonal Violence, 8,* 628-647.

Feldman-Summers, S., & Pope, K. S. (1994). The experience of "forgetting" childhood abuse: A national survey of psychologists. *Journal of Consulting and Clinical Psychology, 62,* 636-639.

Felitti, V. J., Anda, R. F., Nordenberg, D., Williamson, D. F., Spitz, A. M., Edwards, V.A., Koss, M. P., & Marks, J.S. (1998). Relationship of childhood abuse and household dysfunction to many of the leading causes of death in adults: The Adverse Childhood Experiences (ACE) Study. *American Journal of Preventive Medicine, 14,* 245-58.

Finkelhor, D., Hotaling, G., Lewis, I. A., & Smith, C. (1990). Sexual abuse in a national survey of adult men and women: Prevalence, characteristics, and risk factors. *Child Abuse and Neglect, 14*, 19-28.

Fivush, R. (1988). The functions of event memory: Some comments on Nelson and Barsalou. In U. Neisser & E. Winograd (Eds.), *Remembering reconsidered: Ecological and traditional approaches to the study of memory* (pp. 277-282). New York: Cambridge University Press.

Fivush, R. (1997). Event memory in early childhood. In N. Cowan (Ed.), *The development of memory in childhood* (pp. 139-162). Sussex, England: Psychology Press.

Fivush, R. (1998). Children's recollections of traumatic and nontraumatic events. *Development and Psychopathology, 10*, 699-716.

Fivush, R., Pipe, M. E., Murachver, T., & Reese, E. (1997). Events spoken and unspoken: Implications of language and memory development for the recovered memory debate. In M. A. Conway (Ed.), *Recovered memories and false memories: Debates in psychology* (pp. 34-62). Oxford, England: Oxford University Press.

Freyd, J. J. (1997). *Betrayal trauma: The logic of forgetting childhood abuse.* Cambridge, MA: Harvard University Press.

Freyd, J. J., Martorello, S. R., Alvarado, J. S., Hayes, A. E., & Christman, J. C. (1998). Cognitive environments and dissociative tendencies: Performance on the standard Stroop task for high versus low dissociators. *Applied Cognitive Psychology, 12*, 91-103.

Herman, J. L., & Schatzow, E. (1987). Recovery and verification of memories of childhood sexual trauma. *Psychoanalytic Psychology, 4*, 1-14.

Kuyken, W., & Brewin, C. R. (1995). Autobiographical memory functioning in depression and reports of early abuse. *Journal of Abnormal Psychology, 104*, 585-591.

LeDoux, J. (1996). *The emotional brain: The mysterious underpinnings of emotional life.* New York: Simon and Shuster.

Loftus, E. F., Polonsky, S., & Fullilove, M. T. (1994). Memories of childhood sexual abuse: Remembering and repressing. *Psychology of Women Quarterly, 18*, 67-84.

McNally, R. J., Lasko, N. B., Macklin, M. L., & Pitman, R. K. (1995). Autobiographical memory disturbance in combat-related post-traumatic stress disorder. *Behaviour Research and Therapy, 33*, 619-630.

Moffitt, K. H., Singer, J. A., Nelligan, D. W., Carlson, M. A., & Vyse, S. A. (1994). Depression and memory narrative type. *Journal of Abnormal Psychology, 103*, 581-583.

Nelson, K. (1993). The psychological and social origins of autobiographical memory. *Psychological Science, 4*, 7-14.

Pillemer, D. (1997). *Momentous events, vivid memories.* Cambridge, MA: Harvard University Press.

Putnam, F. W. (1997). *Dissociation in childhood and adolescents: A developmental perspective.* New York: Guilford Press.

Robins, L. N., Helzer, J. E., Croughan, J. L., & Ratcliff, K. S. (1981). National Institute of Mental Health Diagnostic Interview Schedule: Its history, characteristics, and validity. *Archives of General Psychiatry, 38*, 381-389.

Robinson, J. A. (1976). Sampling autobiographical memory. *Cognitive Psychology, 8*, 578-95.

Straus, M. A. (1979). Measuring intrafamily conflict and violence: The Conflict Tactics (CT) Scales. *Journal of Marriage and the Family, 41*, 75-88.

Stroop, J. R. (1935). Studies of interference in serial verbal reactions. *Journal of Experimental Psychology, 18*, 643-662.

van der Kolk, B. A. (1996). Trauma and memory. In B. A. van der Kolk, A. C. McFarlane, & L. Weisaeth (Eds.), *Traumatic stress: The effects of overwhelming experience on mind, body and society* (pp. 3-23). New York: Guilford Press.

van der Kolk, B. A., & Fisler, R. (1995). Dissociation and the fragmentary nature of traumatic memories: Overview and exploratory study. *Journal of Traumatic Stress, 8*, 505-525.

Widom, C. S., & Shepard, R. L. (1996). Accuracy of adult recollections of childhood victimization: Part 1. Childhood physical abuse. *Psychological Assessment, 8*, 412-21.

Williams, J. M. G., & Broadbent, K. (1986). Autobiographical memory in attempted suicide patients. *Journal of Abnormal Psychology, 95*, 144-149.

Williams, L. M. (1994). Recall of childhood trauma: A prospective study of women's memories of child sexual abuse. *Journal of Consulting and Clinical Psychology, 62*, 1167-1176.

Yehuda, R., Resnick, H., Kahana, B., & Giller, E. L. (1993). Long-lasting hormonal alterations to extreme stress in humans: Normative or maladaptive? *Psychosomatic Medicine, 55*, 287-297.

APPENDIX

Sexual Abuse Items

Some people, while growing up in their first 18 years of life, had a sexual experience with an adult or someone at least five years older than themselves. These experiences may have involved a relative, family friend, or stranger. During the first 18 years of life, did an adult or older relative, family friend, or stranger ever:

1. Touch or fondle your body in a sexual way?
2. Have you touch their body in a sexual way?
3. Attempt to have any type of sexual intercourse (oral, anal, or vaginal) with you?
4. Actually have any type of sexual intercourse (oral, anal, or vaginal) with you?

A Preliminary Report Comparing Trauma-Focused and Present-Focused Group Therapy Against a Wait-Listed Condition Among Childhood Sexual Abuse Survivors with PTSD

Catherine Classen
Cheryl Koopman
Kirsten Nevill-Manning
David Spiegel

SUMMARY. Childhood sexual abuse (CSA) is a prevalent problem and the psychological and behavioral consequences are great. Despite this, we are still in the early stages of understanding how best to treat survivors of childhood sexual abuse. One fundamental question for treating CSA survivors is whether it is necessary or helpful for psychotherapists to focus on working through survivors' memories of childhood trauma in order to reduce current distress and improve function-

This research was supported by grant MH52134 from the National Institute of Mental Health. The authors wish to thank Deborah Rose, Lindsay Picard, Brian Chin, Julia Zarcone and all of the women who participated in this research, as well as Mount Zion Hospital and the Metropolitan Community Church in San Francisco for providing office space for this research.

Address correspondence to: Catherine Classen, PhD, Department of Psychiatry and Behavioral Sciences, Stanford University School of Medicine, 401 Quarry Road, Stanford, CA 94305-5718 (E-mail: classen@leland.stanford.edu).

[Haworth co-indexing entry note]: "A Preliminary Report Comparing Trauma-Focused and Present-Focused Group Therapy Against a Wait-Listed Condition Among Childhood Sexual Abuse Survivors with PTSD." Classen, Catherine et al. Co-published simultaneously in *Journal of Aggression, Maltreatment & Trauma* (The Haworth Maltreatment & Trauma Press, an imprint of The Haworth Press, Inc.) Vol. 4, No. 2, (#8), 2001, pp. 265-288; and: *Trauma and Cognitive Science: A Meeting of Minds, Science, and Human Experience* (ed: Jennifer J. Freyd, and Anne P. DePrince) The Haworth Maltreatment & Trauma Press, an imprint of The Haworth Press, Inc., 2001, pp. 265-288. Single or multiple copies of this article are available for a fee from The Haworth Document Delivery Service [1-800-342-9678, 9:00 a.m. - 5:00 p.m. (EST). E-mail address: getinfo@haworthpressinc.com].

ing, or is it better to focus on current problems in living? Consequently, a pilot study was conducted among women who have been sexually abused as children and who meet the criteria for current PTSD as a result of that abuse. CSA survivors with PTSD were randomly assigned to one of three conditions: (1) a trauma-focused group psychotherapy, (2) a present-focused group psychotherapy, and (3) a waiting list no-treatment control condition. In this article, preliminary data on the question of whether group treatment of either type is better than no treatment is presented. Those who received group therapy resulted in a significant reduction in two kinds of trauma symptoms, dissociation and a sexual trauma index, and in two types of interpersonal problems, being vindictive and being nonassertive. When those individuals in the study with a history of having been sexually revictimized in the previous six months were isolated, at post-treatment only 38% of the women who were in the treatment group were revictimized compared to 67% of women in the wait-list condition. Given the small sample size, these differences were not statistically significant. However, a 50% reduction in revictimization is clinically significant. Further research with a larger sample of women is needed to confirm these findings and to test for differential effects of trauma focused group therapy and present focused group therapy. *[Article copies available for a fee from The Haworth Document Delivery Service: 1-800-342-9678. E-mail address: <getinfo@haworthpressinc.com> Website: <http://www.HaworthPress.com> © 2001 by The Haworth Press, Inc. All rights reserved.]*

KEYWORDS. Psychotherapy, child abuse, memory, therapy efficacy, revictimization, dissociation

INTRODUCTION

The prevalence of child sexual abuse (CSA) among females in the general population is high, ranging from a low of 4.5% of girls reporting sexual abuse by a father or stepfather (Russell, 1986), to highs of around 13-27% if sexual abuse is defined more broadly (Finkelhor & Dziuba-Leatherman, 1994; Finkelhor, Hotaling, Lewis, & Smith, 1990; Koss & Dinero, 1989). Indeed there are certain communities where the majority of matched samples of white and African-American women report having been sexually abused (Wyatt, 1985). Not surprisingly, a large number of CSA survivors appear to experience later distress as well as behavioral and interpersonal problems (Chu & Dill, 1990; Gelinas, 1983; Herman, Russell, & Trocki, 1986; Westen, Ludolph, Misle, Ruffins, & Block, 1990).

Numerous studies have documented the psychological and behavioral seque-lae of CSA (Beitchman et al., 1992; Browne & Finkelhor, 1986; Polusny & Follette, 1995). The long term effects of CSA include PTSD (Rodriguez, Ryan, Kemp, & Foy, 1997; Rowan & Foy, 1993; Rowan, Foy, Rodriguez, & Ryan, 1994), major depression (Pribor & Dinwiddie, 1992), anxiety disorders (other than PTSD) (Pribor, 1992), dissociative symptoms (Briere & Runtz, 1991), borderline personality disorder (Herman & Schatzow, 1987), alcohol or substance abuse (Herman & Schatzow, 1987), and suicidality (Saunders, Villeponteaux, Lipovsky, Kilpatrick, & Veronen, 1992). Along with psychiatric symptoms, childhood sexual abuse has been shown to be related to poor social adjustment and interpersonal skills (Browne & Finkelhor, 1986; Wyatt, 1985), revictimization (Beitchman et al., 1992), sexual dysfunction (Briere, 1988; Gorcey, Santiago, & McCall-Perez, 1986; Herman et al., 1986; Hunter, 1991; Jehu, 1989; McCarthy, 1990; Mullen, Martin, Anderson, Romans, & Herbison, 1994; Talmadge & Wallace, 1991; Wyatt, 1990) relationship problems (Cahill, Lewelyn, & Pearson, 1991) and medical disorders (Felitti et al., 1998). Survivors of childhood sexual abuse report difficulties trusting their partners, often perceiving them as over-controlling and uncaring (Mullen et al., 1994). Problems in interpersonal functioning may stem not only from the sexual abuse itself, but also from the context of family dynamics in which the sexual abuse occurred, with powerful and lasting effects on the abused child's personality (Freyd, 1996; Pelletier & Handy, 1986).

The diagnosis of post-traumatic stress disorder (PTSD) has been proposed as a way to classify many of the central clinical features that are present in adult abuse survivors (Greenwald & Leitenberg, 1990; Rowan & Foy, 1993). In a recent study of 47 help-seeking CSA survivors using a standardized instrument (SCID) to assess PTSD symptomatology (Rowan et al., 1994), 69% met the full DSM-IIIR criteria for PTSD, with an additional 19% displaying partial PTSD (meeting criteria for two of the three symptom clusters). Although trauma researchers and clinicians have debated whether the criteria for the diagnosis of PTSD adequately capture the symptomatology in this population (Finkelhor, 1988; Herman, 1992b; Rowan & Foy, 1993), a syndrome specific to sexual abuse has yet to be established (Beitchman et al., 1992). There is, however, little question that trauma symptomatology is prevalent in adult survivors of childhood sexual abuse and that treatment needs to address these symptoms.

Survivors of childhood sexual abuse who also suffer from PTSD are individuals who have become psychologically immobilized by their abuse experiences because of their inability to process fully the traumatic experiences (Classen, Koopman, & Spiegel, 1993; Foa & Rothbaum, 1989; Herman, 1992a; Spiegel, Hunt, & Dondershine, 1988; van der Kolk & Kadish, 1987). The persistent re-experiencing of aspects of the trauma, the psychic numbing and avoidance of reminders of the abuse, and the persistent symptoms of hyperarousal indicate that these individuals have been unable to integrate the traumatic events. These individuals use dissociation, numbing and avoidance as a way of managing overwhelming feelings of fear, rage, shame, and guilt. Hyperarousal occurs because they are continually on the alert for danger, yet respond to it as unexpected because of their avoidant defenses.

Despite the prevalence of sexual abuse and its serious aftereffects, we are still in the early stages of understanding how to best treat survivors of childhood sexual abuse. One fundamental question regarding psychotherapy for trauma survivors is whether it is necessary or helpful for psychotherapists to focus on working through survivors' memories of childhood trauma in order to reduce current distress and improve functioning. A review of literature describing therapeutic interventions with sexual abuse survivors suggests that most clinicians specializing in this area assume that coming to terms, both affectively and cognitively, with the meaning and impact of traumatic events is a central component of recovery (Coons, Bowman, Pellow, & Schneider, 1989; Herman, 1992a; McCann & Pearlman, 1990; Paddison, Einbinder, Maker, & Strain, 1993; Roth, 1993; Spiegel, 1989). Such psychotherapy tries to help the patient to integrate memories of the trauma into a new perspective, thereby facilitating the development of a more adaptive and coherent sense of self. In contrast, a present-focused psychotherapy emphasizes learning about the link between one's symptomatology, one's present internal state and the immediate environment; whereas the trauma-focused approach emphasizes learning about the link between one's symptomatology and one's past environment. Therefore, from the present-focused viewpoint, making different choices based on a newfound awareness can attenuate distress symptoms without revisiting past traumas (Yalom, 1980, 1995). From a trauma-focused viewpoint, distress symptoms can be attenuated by retrieving and reinterpreting memories of events that led to the symptoms and construction of the self-structure (Coons et al., 1989; Herman, 1992a; McCann & Pearlman, 1990; Paddison et al., 1993; Roth, 1993; Spiegel, 1989).

The need for randomized clinical trials comparing these different treatment approaches for CSA survivors is clear. There has been much debate in the literature and society at large about childhood sexual abuse, with much of the current focus being on the veracity of abuse memories (Cicchetti & Rizley, 1981; Loftus, 1993; Loftus & Hoffman, 1989). This debate has led to a general concern regarding the appropriate method for treating women with self-reported histories of CSA. Thus, this program of research asks whether psychotherapy that focuses on working through memories of sexual abuse is helpful in ameliorating trauma-related symptoms and improving current psychosocial functioning. This question is important for several reasons. Foremost, we need to be better informed about how best to treat this troubled population. If we find that it is helpful to provide therapy that focuses on memories of trauma, it will highlight the need for clinicians to learn clinically responsible ways of working with memories. Learning appropriate ways to work with memories is important not only because of the current memory debate but also because the process of memory retrieval carries with it its own risks, including contamination with suggestion and expectancy (Loftus & Hoffman, 1989; Spiegel, 1994). Clinically, it has been recognized that the process of working with traumatic memory content may be temporarily distressing and therefore must be weighed against ultimate therapeutic gains (Spiegel, 1994). Thus, if trauma-focused therapy does not produce psychological benefits, then the risks of working with memories are not warranted.

There is limited outcome data for treatment of adult survivors of childhood sexual abuse. To date, reports of group therapy outcomes with adult survivors of childhood sexual abuse have been primarily case reports or pre- and post-treatment designs without comparison treatment or wait-list control groups (Carver, Sheier, & Weintraub, 1989; Hazzard, Rogers, & Angert, 1993; Herman & Schatzow, 1984; Paddison et al., 1993; Tsai & Wagner, 1978) or nonrandomized designs (Hall, Mullee, & Thompson, 1995; Morgan & Cummings, 1999; Richter, Snider, & Gorey, 1997).

To our knowledge, there have been only two randomized clinical studies of group therapy for women sexually abused as children (Alexander, Neimeyer, & Follette, 1991; Zlotnick et al., 1997). Neither study focused on working through the memories of the traumatic event. Alexander and colleagues compared two time-limited group formats, a process group and a more structured interpersonal transaction group, against a wait-list control condition. They found that participants in the treatment conditions experienced significant reductions in depression and distress compared to the wait-list condition. Further, participants in the interpersonal transaction group showed greater improvement in distress compared to the process group while the process group showed greater improvement in social functioning compared to the interpersonal transaction group. Zlotnick and colleagues found that participants in an affect management group improved more in PTSD symptoms and dissociation compared to a wait-list control condition.

Consequently, we conducted a pilot study testing two kinds of group therapy for women who have been sexually abused as children and who meet criteria for current PTSD for that abuse. The purpose of this study was to address the following question regarding survivors of childhood sexual abuse: Is it better to focus on survivors' memories of childhood sexual abuse (CSA) in order to reduce distress and improve functioning or is it enough to focus on current problems in living? Furthermore, is participation in a group treatment beneficial compared to no treatment? To address these questions we randomly assigned CSA survivors with PTSD to one of three conditions: (1) a trauma-focused group psychotherapy, (2) a present-focused group psychotherapy, and (3) a wait-listed no-treatment control condition. In this report, we present preliminary data on the question of whether group treatment is better than no treatment. Thus, we present data on the effectiveness of being in either of these two group therapy conditions compared to a wait-list no treatment control condition. We hypothesized that receiving group therapy would result in a greater reduction of trauma symptoms, interpersonal problems, and sexual revictimization compared to being in the wait-listed condition.

METHOD

Subjects

Subjects were recruited by placing advertisements in newspapers and distributing flyers to 20 community agencies. A press release was also issued and as a result we received free radio advertising and an article about the study appeared in a local newspaper. Three hundred and eight individuals were screened over the telephone. Of these individuals, 95 passed the initial phone screen and met with a research assistant for the face-to-face screening interview. Fifty-eight women met all inclusion/exclusion criteria and were accepted into the study. For various reasons, three of these women dropped out of the study before the group intervention began, leaving a total of 55 women who participated in the intervention trial. There were a total of three therapy groups that were conducted in the first wave of this pilot study: two were trauma-focused and one was present-focused. Seven individuals were assigned to each therapy group. We received follow-up data on 52 participants for a follow-up rate of 95%. See Table 1 for demographic characteristics of the individuals who completed baseline and 6-month follow-up questionnaires. The inclusion/exclusion criteria used in this pilot study included all of the following:

1. Female.
2. 18 years of age or older.
3. English-speaking.
4. Have at least two explicit memories of sexual abuse that involved genital contact.
5. At least two sexual abuse events occurred when the survivor was between 3-15 years of age.
6. The perpetrator was at least 5 years older than the survivor.
7. The survivor knew the perpetrator prior to the sexual abuse.
8. The survivor has discussed or attempted to discuss details of the sexual abuse previously with another person (e.g., family member, friend, or therapist) at least 6 months prior to being interviewed for the study.
9. Meets DSM-IV criteria for current PTSD.
10. Provides informed consent.

Criteria for exclusion included any of the following:

1. Diagnosed as meeting one of the following diagnostic categories: schizophrenia and other psychotic disorders; dementia and delirium and amnestic or other cognitive disorders.
2. Reports ritual abuse.
3. Is currently receiving psychotherapy (including individual or group psychotherapy).
4. Individuals who are alcohol or drug dependent.
5. Individuals who are currently suicidal (i.e., within the last month).

TABLE 1. Demographic Characteristics (N = 52)

Variable	N	%	Mean (Standard Deviation)
Age			38.4 (11.7)
Marital Status			
Single	19	37	
Married or currently living as married	27	52	
Separated or divorced	2	4	
Other	4	8	
Ethnicity			
Black/African American	4	8	
Hispanic/Latina	8	15	
Native American	2	4	
White/European American	33	64	
Other	5	10	
Sexual Orientation			
Heterosexual	43	83	
Lesbian	5	10	
Bisexual	4	8	
Education			
High School	3	6	
Some College	17	33	
College Graduate	23	44	
Graduate/Professional School	9	17	
Household Income			
Less than $20,000	9	17	
$20,000 - $39,999	20	39	
$40,000 - $59,999	11	21	
$60,000 - $79,999	3	6	
$80,000 or above	8	15	
Don't know or refuse to answer	1	2	
Employment Status			
Not employed	9	17	
Employed part-time	11	21	
Fully employed	31	60	

Informed consent. All participants solicited for participation in the study were asked to sign informed consent protocols approved by the Stanford Committee on the Use of Human Subjects in Medical Experiments. Informed consent was obtained for participating in the screening procedure and a second informed consent was obtained once participants were accepted into the study.

Randomization procedure. Each participant was randomly assigned to either the immediate treatment group or the wait-list group and then to receive either trauma-focused group therapy or present-focused group therapy. Participants were informed about whether they were in the immediate treatment group or the wait-list groups after all baseline measures were completed. If they were assigned to the immediate treatment group, they were also informed at that time about which type of intervention they would be receiving. Participants in the wait-list treatment group were told which type of intervention they would be receiving only after they completed their 6-month follow-up assessment.

Compensation and other incentives. Participants were paid a nominal fee of $25 for the baseline assessment and $50 for each of the follow-up assessments to encourage their continued participation in this study.

Intervention

Both treatment conditions involve a group intervention of 24, 90 minute, weekly sessions. Two experienced group leaders led each group and were supervised on a weekly basis by an expert in trauma. Therapists included psychologists and one licensed MFCC. All sessions were videotaped for supervision purposes.

Trauma-Focused Treatment

Aims of treatment. In trauma-focused treatment the goal is to help survivors work through and integrate their traumatic abuse experiences. This involves helping them to reconstruct their traumatic experiences, integrate the affect associated with the trauma, modify the negative views of self that arose because of the abuse, and integrate their traumatic history into their conscious awareness of self and others.

Phases of treatment. Prior to the first group meeting, the group participants were met individually by their group leaders in order to prepare them for the group intervention. This involved discussing the purpose and structure of the trauma-focused group, informing the individual of basic group rules such as attending regularly and maintaining confidentiality, answering any questions or addressing any concerns she may have, and helping the individual to identify the problems she wished to work on and to set a realistic goal for therapy.

The beginning phase of treatment had three goals: (1) establishing a basic sense of trust and safety in the group, (2) having each group member share with the group the problems she plans to work on in therapy and the goal she has set for herself, and (3) orienting the group members to the trauma-focused intervention. Establishing a rudimentary sense of trust and safety is crucial for reducing distress and bolstering their ability to tolerate and cope with the painful affect that will be stimulated by discussion of their traumatic past (Gold, 1997; Herman, 1992a). This can take anywhere from 2-9 sessions (Donaldson & Cordes-Green, 1994). The task of the treatment during this phase was to establish a therapeutic alliance and help members identify their feelings of mistrust along with the specific fears that were activated by being in the group.

An important role of the therapists during the middle phase of treatment was to begin to teach the group members about the meaning of their trauma symptoms and to link their trauma symptoms to their trauma histories. The therapists were instructed to listen closely to both the verbal and nonverbal communication. Sometimes group members talked spontaneously about their traumatic past and at other times trauma-related material arose covertly. When the trauma-related material was covertly presented, the therapist helped the survivor examine how this material was related to her abuse experiences. This typically involved having the survivor share her memories of her childhood trauma. There were several goals during this phase of treatment. One goal was to help the person who was sharing the memory to access as fully as possible the verbal, affective and imagery traces of the memory (McCann & Pearlman, 1990). This was of central importance because it addressed a main maladaptive coping strategy, which is to dissociate aspects of the traumatic experience (Classen et al., 1993; Spiegel et al., 1988). Consequently, helping survivors to fully access their cognitive, affective, visual and auditory representations of the trauma was essential for reconstructing and integrating the meanings and beliefs derived from the traumatic experiences into their conscious experience of self and others. Often the reconstructions occurred because the survivor had been able to access information that had previously been unavailable or only partially available, thereby enabling her to reconstruct these events in a more adaptive fashion (Foa & Kozak, 1986; Spiegel, 1989). A second goal was to work through the transference expectations that the survivor had in telling her story to the group. The aim was to achieve an experience in the group that disconfirmed their fears about the judgment of others in response to the trauma (Gold-Steinberg & Buttenheim, 1993). A third goal was to help the individual understand how the trauma was connected to the problems she had chosen as her focus in therapy. The traumatic experience could thereby be drawn on during the remainder of the therapy to assist the individual as she worked on her self-identified problems and towards her treatment goal (Spiegel, 1989). A fourth goal was to enhance the group's sense of shared experience as well as their differences, to decrease feelings of alienation from self and others, and to promote self-acceptance among all group members.

In the final phase of treatment the focus was on consolidating what had been learned and working through the issues that were evoked by termination. Approximately the last four weeks were spent on termination issues. Termination was a time to appreciate what had been gained but also to mourn what had been lost. This included mourning the loss of the group as well as the losses that occurred as a result of their traumatic past, such as not experiencing a "normal" and secure childhood, the failure of parental protection, the loss of innocence, and having one's psychological growth impeded because of the past. It was also a time to plan for the future. Members were helped to identify the progress they had made and to identify goals they wished to continue working towards.

Present-Focused Group

Aims of treatment. The present-focused group treatment approach is one commonly used in group therapy with many different populations (Yalom, 1995) and one that is appropriate for survivors of sexual abuse, particularly when their current functioning is problematic. If the dysfunction is severe enough, a present-focused approach may be the treatment of choice (Herman, 1992a). Survivors of childhood sexual abuse are often acutely aware of how they struggle in their daily lives. In fact, it is usually the difficulties in their daily lives that bring them to psychotherapy. The aim of this approach was to help survivors identify and modify the maladaptive patterns of behavior that had arisen as a result of their traumatic past. In the present-focused treatment the assumption is that by focusing on the here-and-now survivors can alter their current functioning and thereby address the impact of their abuse history.

Phases of treatment. Similar to the procedure in the trauma-focused group, the group participants were met with individually prior to the first meeting so that the group leaders could prepare them for the intervention. The only difference was that the therapists described the present-focused approach. Similarly, the beginning phase of treatment had the same goals as the trauma-focused group except that it involved orienting group members to the present-focused intervention rather than the trauma-focused intervention.

During the middle phase of treatment the focus shifted to participants' here-and-now experience, particularly as it related to experiencing trauma symptoms and interacting with one another in the group. The aim was to help members become aware of their own internal affective and cognitive states, to recognize the triggers for their trauma symptoms, recognize how they were affected by others, and to learn ways of managing their trauma symptoms and expressing their needs, concerns, or fears as soon as they arose. Another aspect of focusing on the here-and-now experience was to identify and utilize group process for interpersonal learning. The group examined how individuals interacted with one another and with the group leaders. This helped members step back from their subjective experiences and view them from another vantagepoint. This enabled them to recognize maladaptive ways of relating, the unconscious messages they conveyed, basic assumptions they held, or the ways in which they distorted incoming information. Occasionally, group members wanted to speak about their traumatic memories. In general, however, this was not a threat to the integrity of the present-focused approach. We attributed this to the careful manner in which the treatment modality was explained as well as the participants' overall commitment to the research study. If individual members did bring up their traumatic memories the group leaders were instructed to respond with empathy, but to not help members explore or recover memories.

As in the trauma-focused group, the focus of the final phase of treatment was on consolidating what had been learned and working through the issues that were evoked by termination.

MEASURES

Participants were given the following questionnaires at baseline and at the end of treatment.

Trauma Symptom Checklist 40 (TSC-40)

The Trauma Symptom Checklist 40 (TSC-40) (Elliott & Briere, 1991, 1992) is a 40 item, validated, self-report instrument designed to assess the impacts of sexual victimization. It yields a total score and six subscale scores. The six subscales include dissociation, anxiety, depression, sexual abuse trauma index, sleep disturbance, and sexual problems. Subjects are asked to indicate how often they have experienced each symptom in the last two months on a scale of 0-4, with "0" meaning "never" and "4" meaning "very often." This scale has been found to have good internal consistency and predictive validity regarding childhood sexual abuse (Elliott & Briere, 1992).

Inventory of Interpersonal Problems (IIP)

The Inventory of Interpersonal Problems (IIP) (Horowitz, Rosenberg, Baer, Ureno, & Villasenor, 1988) is a self-report measure that contains 127 items assessing interpersonal problems. The first 78 items begin with the phrase: "It is hard for me to. . . . " followed by such phrases as "tell a person to stop bothering me" or "stick to my own point of view and not be swayed by other people." The second 49 items are about "things that you do too much" such as "I fight with other people too much" or "I want people to admire me too much." The respondent is asked to decide whether that item describes something that has been a problem for her and to indicate how distressing it is on a scale from 0 (not at all) to 4 (extremely). There are two methods of scoring the IIP. One method is the original scoring method, which involves calculating means for six subscales. A second method developed by Alden and colleagues (Alden, Wiggins, & Pincus, 1990) uses a circumplex arrangement of interpersonal problems based on Wiggins' (Wiggins, 1979) interpersonal circle. The circumplex method was used in this analysis. Love and dominance are the two main factors that have been shown to characterize the nature of interpersonal problems (Kiesler, 1983; Wiggins, 1982). In the circumplex model, they are represented as two orthogonal factors on a two-dimensional space. Based on combinations of these two factors, eight octants were identified and include domineering, vindictive, cold, socially avoidant, nonassertive, exploitable, overly nurturant, and intrusive (Gurtman, 1992). Each octant consists of eight items that meet statistical and geometric criteria for circumplexity. The score for each octant is the mean value of the eight items. Reliabilities for the octants have ranged from .72 (intrusive) to .85 (socially avoidant and nonassertive) (Gurtman, 1992).

Sexual Experiences Survey

The Sexual Experiences Survey (Koss & Gidycz, 1985; Koss & Oros, 1982) is a 13-item scale designed to assess hidden sexual trauma, trauma that might not be identified by the victim as sexual aggression or violation. At baseline, the items were presented in a "yes or no" format and the time frame was the previous six months. At post-treatment, participants were asked to indicate how often a particular item was experienced in the previous six months. For the sake of comparability, these items were rescored into a yes/no format. The questions begin with low severity sexual experiences and proceed through a spectrum of aggressive sexual behaviors. The measure has good test-retest reliability. The mean item agreement between two administrations to a group of 71 college-aged females was shown to be 93%. Internal consistency (Cronbach's alpha) and reliability for women students (n = 305) was .74 (Koss & Gidycz, 1985). Revictimized participants were those individuals who endorsed any items that indicated sexual coercion (items 3-7), attempted rape (items 8 and 9) or rape (items 10-12).

Data Analysis

The major outcome measures at post-treatment were the Trauma Symptom Checklist 40 (TSC-40), Interpersonal Problems Inventory (IIP), and the Sexual Experiences Scale. Difference scores on these measures served as dependent variables. These difference scores were computed for each of the TSC-40 and IIP octants and the total score on the TSC-40 by subtracting each participant's post-treatment score from her baseline score. The independent variable was a two-level variable comparing the treatment groups combined to the wait-list control group. We used t-tests for independent samples to determine the statistical significance of the differences between the two conditions on the TSC-40 and IIP scores. Because we had directional hypotheses about the effects of treatment on the dependent measures, we used one-tailed tests to determine statistical significance. To examine the significance of the treatment versus wait-list difference in the proportion of the sample who reported sexual revictimization on the Sexual Experiences Scale, we used X^2 analysis.

RESULTS

The descriptive statistics on the TSC-40 and IIP measures for the combined treatment groups and the wait-list control condition are reported in Table 2. Also shown are the results of the t-tests examining the significance of the differences between the means.

Comparisons of the treatment versus wait-list control on TSC-40 scores. Participants who had been assigned to the treatment groups compared with those who had been assigned to the wait-list condition demonstrated a significantly greater decrease in two kinds of trauma symptoms assessed on the TSC-40. Women who received group therapy showed a significantly greater reduction in dissociation ($p < .05$) and on the sexual trauma index ($p = .05$). The results also showed greater decreases in the treatment condition compared to the wait-list condition for anxiety, sexual problems, and for the total TSC-40 score, although none of these differences were statistically significant.

Comparisons of the treatment versus wait-list control on IIP scores. Compared with women who had been wait-listed, those who had been assigned to receive group therapy demonstrated a significantly greater decrease in three kinds of interpersonal problems assessed on the IIP (see Table 2). Women who were offered one of the therapy groups showed a significantly greater reduction in nonassertiveness ($p < .01$), being exploitable ($p < .05$) and in vindictiveness ($p < .01$). They also showed a statistical trend ($p < .07$) toward having a greater reduction in social avoidance. The results also

TABLE 2. Mean Difference Scores from Baseline to 6-Month Follow-up Assessment on Scores on the Trauma Symptom Checklist (TSC-40) and Inventory of Personal Problems (IIP) Comparing the Treatment Condition (Combined Treatment Groups) versus the Wait-List Control Condition (N = 52)

Dependent measure	Control group Mean (SD) n = 33	Treatment group Mean (SD) n = 93	T-test value
TSC-40			
Anxiety subscale	0.2 (3.0)	1.1 (3.9)	−0.87
Depression subscale	1.5 (4.5)	1.6 (3.5)	−0.08
Dissociation subscale	0.3 (3.3)	2.1 (2.6)	−1.9*
Sexual abuse trauma index	0.8 (3.9)	2.6 (3.6)	−1.6*
Sexual problems subscale	1.0 (4.3)	2.1 (5.4)	−0.7
Sleep difficulties subscale	1.7 (3.9)	0.2 (4.0)	1.2
Total score on TSC-40	3.8 (14.1)	8.1 (17.0)	−0.9
IIP			
Vindictive	0.7 (3.0)	3.0 (2.8)	−2.5**
Cold	1.4 (3.6)	2.2 (4.0)	−0.7
Social avoidance	1.0 (3.5)	3.2 (6.0)	−1.5
Nonassertive	−0.1 (3.1)	4.0 (5.6)	−2.7**
Exploitable	−0.4 (5.4)	2.2 (4.8)	−1.6*
Overly nurturant	1.7 (3.6)	2.4 (4.1)	−0.6
Intrusive	1.5 (4.0)	2.5 (4.1)	−0.8
Domineering	1.7 (2.8)	3.1 (4.7)	−1.0

*$P \leq .05$.
**$P < .01$.

showed greater decreases in the treatment condition compared to the wait-list condition for the mean IIP scores on being cold, overly nurturant, intrusive, and domineering, but none of these differences were statistically significant.

Comparisons of the treatment versus wait-list control on sexual revictimization. The women assigned to the treatment groups did not show significantly less sexual revictimization compared to those in the wait-list control condition. Overall, 32% of those receiving treatment reported sexual revictimization at the post-treatment assessment, compared with 33% in the wait-list control, a nonsignificant difference ($X^2 = 0.2$, p = n.s.). However, when we took prior sexual revictimization into consideration and limited this analysis to those who reported sexual revictimization experiences in the six months prior to the baseline assessment, the results were in the expected direction. Among this subset of women (n = 17), 67% of the women in the wait-list condition reported sexual revictimization, compared with 38% of the women in the treatment condition, although this difference was not statistically significant (X^2 = 1.4, p = n.s.).

DISCUSSION

In this preliminary examination of trauma-focused and present-focused group psychotherapy for women with PTSD for childhood sexual abuse, our sample size was far too small to have adequate statistical power to test the differences in treatment outcome. Therefore, in order to increase our statistical power to detect whether receiving group therapy is better than not receiving group therapy, we combined participants who received either the trauma-focused or present-focused therapy into one treatment group.

We found that receiving group therapy resulted in a significant reduction in two kinds of trauma symptoms, dissociation and a sexual trauma index. Although we conducted multiple comparisons we did not do a Bonferroni correction. Given the small sample size we lacked statistical power and thus a Bonferroni correction would have greatly increased the likelihood of a Type II error. Given this limitation, the reader is urged to interpret these findings with caution. Nevertheless, it should be noted that a difference of 1/2 standard deviation represents a moderate effect size and suggests that these may be meaningful differences. In addition, combining the group therapy participants into one group for statistical analysis does not permit us to distinguish between the effects of the trauma-focused and present-focused group therapies. Nevertheless, we offer some possible interpretations based on the therapeutic strategies of each of these interventions and the items that comprise the dissociation and sexual trauma index scales. These interpretations are purely speculative and require empirical testing before any conclusions can be drawn.

The dissociation subscale includes problems related to having flashbacks, "spacing out," dizziness, memory problems, feelings that things are "unreal," and feelings of not being in your body. The reduction in dissociation suggests that participation in group therapy may have resulted in these women not needing to rely on dissociation as a coping mechanism and this might be especially true for the trauma-focused intervention. The aim of the trauma-focused intervention is to help survivors work through the consequences of the sexual abuse by focusing directly on memories of the abuse. In a safe, controlled and gradual process, survivors are invited to talk about their abuse experiences particularly as they relate to problems they are having in their current lives. Working with their memories in this way may have resulted in a reduction in flashbacks because the survivors learned how to have greater control over when and how they remember. Furthermore, having greater control over their memories may have resulted in their not needing to "space out" or "go away in your mind" as would happen when memories return unbidden. Similarly, there would be less of a need to detach from one's body or to detach in a way that makes things feel unreal. A further consequence of working directly with memories is that the survivor would learn to tolerate the intense affect associated with these memories. Consequently, there would be less need to leave one's body or to make things feel unreal in order to protect oneself from overwhelming affect. Thus, women in the trauma-focused group may have learned how to tolerate reminders of the abuse requiring less need for their dissociative defense.

In the present-focused group, individuals may have learned new strategies for managing situations that in the past would have caused distress. In the present-focused intervention survivors were helped to focus on current-day problems, particularly as they were expressed in the group process. The theory behind present-focused group therapy is that problems in living are enacted in the group context. This provides an opportunity to identify problematic responses, to enhance one's awareness of the underlying dynamics of the problem, and to try out new, more adaptive ways of responding. Thus, if individuals dissociated during the group, this would become a focus. They would be helped to identify the stimulus that triggered the dissociative reaction, to identify the overwhelming affect associated with the stimulus, to learn techniques for modulating the overwhelming affect, and to learn better ways of coping with these situations. This therapeutic approach would work towards reducing "spacing out," dizziness, feelings of unreality, and leaving one's body.

The sexual trauma index was designed to capture problems that are thought to be especially common with sexual abuse survivors, such as sexual problems, flashbacks, nightmares, sleep difficulties, fear of men, memory problems, bad thoughts or feelings during sex, and feeling that things are "unreal" (Elliott & Briere, 1992). Given that there was not a significant reduction in the sexual problems subscale or sleep difficulties subscale, it is likely that the changes on the SATI involved the other problem areas. Thus, participating in group therapy may have led to a reduction in flashbacks, nightmares, fear of men, memory problems, and feelings of things being "unreal."

Both the trauma-focused and present-focused groups may have been helpful in reducing fear of men. Consistent with the literature (Finkelhor et al., 1990; Russell, 1983), most survivors in our study experienced sexual abuse by a male. Thus, working directly on memories of abuse in the trauma-focused intervention may have helped survivors to work on issues related to their perpetrator and to men in general. Focusing on their memories of the perpetrator may have helped survivors to work through their relationship with the perpetrator and to achieve some measure of resolution regarding the nature of their past and current relationship with the perpetrator. Working on the relationship with the perpetrator may lead to a greater differentiation in their relationships with men in general so that not all men are experienced as perpetrators or potential perpetrators. In the present-focused intervention, survivors may have had the opportunity to discuss their fear of men or problems they were having in their current relationships with men. Both intervention strategies have the potential to reduce a fear of men.

A reduction in memory problems and nightmares would be most likely to occur in the trauma-focused intervention. Focusing on memories of abuse and helping CSA survivors to manage the overwhelming affect that these abuse experiences elicit may reduce the need to use repression as a defense. The lifting of repression would make memories more accessible and there would be less expression of unresolved conflicts through nightmares.

It must be noted that the present data does not enable us to conclude whether the present-focused or trauma-focused interventions have different benefits. To do so would require that we look at the each group separately against a wait-list control group and against each other. We were unable to do this because of the small sample size. Thus, the mechanisms described above as potentially underlying these symptom reductions are purely speculative. A larger sample size that permits a direct comparison of trauma-focused against present-focused group therapy is required to examine this question. Our lab is currently conducting such an investigation.

We also found that participating in group therapy resulted in a greater reduction in interpersonal problems having to do with being vindictive and nonassertive. There is no reason to assume that either the trauma-focused or present-focused groups would be more likely to lead to a change in these particular interpersonal problems. It could be argued that the trauma-focused group could lead to a change in these interpersonal problems because the survivor has worked through some of her anger towards the perpetrator, thereby leading to less vindictiveness. In addition, she may have discovered how and why she was not able to assert herself during the abuse and how she might be carrying this over into her current life. In the present-focused group, both problems of vindictiveness and nonassertion could arise in the group process and be worked through in the here-and-now. Again, a larger sample is required to determine whether one type of intervention has more of an impact on interpersonal problems than another.

There were no significant differences between the wait-list condition and the treatment condition on sexual revictimization when considering all participants. However, when we isolated those individuals who entered the study with a history of having been sexually revictimized in the previous six months, we found that at post-treatment only 38% of those women who were in the treatment group were revictimized compared to 67% of women in the wait-list condition. Given the small sample size, these differences were not statistically significant. However, a 50% reduction in revictimization is clinically significant. Further research with a larger sample of women with a recent history of sexual revictimization is needed to confirm this. Regarding which intervention might be more likely to reduce revictimization, an argument could be made for the benefits of either therapeutic approach. By working through and integrating the childhood sexual abuse in the trauma-focused intervention, survivors may be less likely to engage in forms of re-enactment that could set them up for sexual revictimization or they may be less likely to dissociate and therefore become more aware of their environment. Participants in the present-focused condition might come to identify behaviors that make them vulnerable to revictimization as well as learn ways of asserting themselves and attending to their environment.

Generic attributes of group therapy might also account for the benefits that were derived from being in a therapy group compared to being on a waiting list. Sharing experiences in a supportive and caring setting, being with individuals who have gone through similar experiences and share similar struggles, learning from each other, feeling accepted, and experiencing a renewed hope for the future may all contribute to participants learning new ways of being in the world. Simply taking the step of joining such a group may have constituted a way of facing the abuse rather than hiding from it. Finally, we cannot rule out the "Hawthorne effect" (Roethlisberger & Dickson, 1959) in accounting for the differences between the treatment and no-treatment groups. The participants in the therapy groups might have simply been responding to the attention they were receiving by virtue of being in the treatment group.

The preliminary results of this pilot study suggest that group therapy is beneficial for women survivors of childhood sexual abuse with PTSD. These findings have clinical and social implications. As noted earlier, the debate in academic literature and society about childhood sexual abuse has led to concern about methods of treatment for women with self-reported CSA histories. The findings of statistically significant reductions in some trauma symptomology (e.g., lowering the score on sexual trauma index) show that trauma- or present-focused group psychotherapy is better than no therapy. In the current climate of uncertainty around therapy for adult CSA survivors, this has implications for making survivors feel more comfortable and confident about seeking treatment, knowing that they will receive some psychological benefits and for clinicians in choosing what treatment to provide. Reducing symptoms like dissociation has added importance because of the prevalence of PTSD symptoms in CSA survivors (Rodriguez et al., 1997).

This study has methodological limitations related to its sample size. As previously mentioned, the sample size is too small to have adequate statistical power to compare the trauma-against the present-focused treatment groups. Thus, these two treatment modalities were combined to compare with the wait-list control group. Therefore we could not analyze the differences and similarities between to the two treatment methods. Even though we combined the treatment modalities we still lacked sufficient statistical power to rigorously test our hypotheses. Therefore, these results must be interpreted with great caution. A further limitation is that the sample was limited to adult women who were sexual abuse survivors with current PTSD and were seeking treatment. Thus, it is unclear whether the findings are generalizable to other CSA populations such as women without PTSD. Despite the small sample size, differences between the trauma and present focused groups were found and future studies with a larger sample size may be able to detect statistically significant differences between trauma- and present-focused group psychotherapy.

Future Research

Further research with a larger sample is required to test the hypothesis that trauma-focused group psychotherapy is superior to present-focused group psychotherapy and that both interventions are superior to no treatment in reducing trauma symptoms and improving interpersonal functioning. A dismantling design could be used where there are three conditions: a case management plus no group treatment condition, case management plus present-focused therapy, and case management plus trauma-focused therapy. Such a study would be using a dismantling design (Borkovec, 1993) because trauma-focused therapy builds on present-focused therapy by adding the additional component of working with the memories of abuse. Both present-focused and trauma-focused group therapy address current problems in living and use here-and-now group processes to facilitate the group work. Our laboratory is currently beginning such a trial. Examining potential mediators of treatment effectiveness might provide information useful for further refining the optimal treatment strategy and determining who most benefits from each intervention. For example, future studies with a larger sample size could also compare ethnic and cultural differences within and between treatment types. Patient preference for treatment type also deserves exploration. A match could shorten overall treatment time and increase effectiveness. By design, randomized trials such as this ignore such preferences. Future research should also assess the effectiveness of these interventions for adult survivors of CSA without PTSD symptoms. This would contribute to our understanding of the generalizability of these treatment methods to other CSA populations.

From a cognitive science perspective, an examination of trauma-focused compared to present-focused intervention for trauma survivors has the potential to address some interesting questions. What effect does working with memories in therapy have on the memories themselves? Do the memories of abuse become better elaborated and more accessible compared to pre-therapy and compared to present-focused therapy where memories are not the focus? Given that trauma-focused therapy works with both memories and the affects associated with the memories, does this linkage of affect to memory lead to less dissociation of these internal sources of knowledge about the abuse and hence greater integration of that information? One type of evidence for this would be a reduction in alterations of consciousness such as dissociative experiences (Freyd, 1996). Another form of evidence would be greater differentiation and integration of the self structure (Classen, Field, Atkinson, & Spiegel, 1998). Does working with affect and linking it to memories lead to greater accessibility of memories and even the uncovering of repressed memories? Does working with affect but linking it to current problems in living have any effect on the accessibility of memories in the present-focused group? These are just some of the many questions that could be addressed in a study comparing trauma-focused and present-focused group therapy for CSA survivors.

REFERENCES

Alden, L. E., Wiggins, J. S., & Pincus, A. L. (1990). Construction of circumplex scales for the Inventory of Interpersonal Problems. *Journal of Personality Assessment, 55,* 521-536.

Alexander, P. C., Neimeyer, R. A., & Follette, V. M. (1991). Group therapy for women sexually abused as children: A controlled study and investigation of individual differences. *Journal of Interpersonal Violence, 6*(2), 218-231.

Beitchman, J. H., Zucker, K. J., Hood, J. E., daCosta, G. A., Akman, D., & Cassavia, E. (1992). A review of the long-term effects of child sexual abuse. *Child Abuse & Neglect, 16*(1), 101-18.

Borkovec, T. D. (1993). Between-group therapy outcome research: Design and methodology. *NIDA Research Monographs, 137,* 249-289.

Briere, J. (1988). The long-term clinical correlates of childhood sexual victimization. *Annals of the New York Academy of Sciences, 528,* 327-34.

Briere, J., & Runtz, M. (1991). The long-term effects of sexual abuse: A review and synthesis. In J. Briere (Ed.), *Treating victims of child sexual abuse* (pp. 3-14). San Francisco: Jossey-Bass.

Browne, A., & Finkelhor, D. (1986). Impact of child sexual abuse: A review of the research. *Psychological Bulletin, 99*(1), 66-77.

Cahill, C., Lewelyn, S. P., & Pearson S. (1991). Long-term effects of sexual abuse which occurred in childhood: A review. *British Journal of Clinical Psychology, 30,* 117-130.

Carver, C. S., Sheier, M. F., & Weintraub, J. K. (1989). Assessing coping strategies: A theoretically based approach. *Journal of Personality and Social Psychology, 56*(2), 267-283.

Chu, J. A., & Dill, D. L. (1990). Dissociative symptoms in relation to childhood physical and sexual abuse [see comments]. *American Journal of Psychiatry, 147*(7), 887-892.

Cicchetti, D., & Rizley, R. (1981). *Developmental perspectives on the etiology, intergenerational transmission, and sequelae of childhood maltreatment.* San Francisco: Jossey-Bass.

Classen, C., Field, N. P., Atkinson, A., & Spiegel, D. (1998). Representations of self in women sexually abused in childhood. *Child Abuse & Neglect, 22*(10), 997-1004.

Classen, C., Koopman, C., & Spiegel, D. (1993). Trauma and dissociation. *Bulletin of the Menninger Clinic, 57*(2), 178-194.

Coons, P. M., Bowman, E. S., Pellow, T. A., & Schneider, P. (1989). Post-traumatic aspects of the treatment of victims of sexual abuse and incest. *Psychiatric Clinics of North America, 12*(2), 325-335.

Donaldson, M. A., & Cordes-Green, S. (1994). *Group treatment of adult incest survivors.* Thousand Oaks: Sage.

Elliott, D., & Briere, J. (1992). Sexual abuse trauma among professional women: Validating the Trauma Symptom Checklist-40 (TSC-40). *Child Abuse & Neglect, 16*, 391-398.

Felitti, V. J., Anda, R. F., Nordenberg, D., Williamson, D. F., Spita, A. M., Edwards, V., Koss, M. P., & Marks, J. S. (1998). Relationship of childhood abuse and household dysfunction to many of the leading causes of death in adults: The Adverse Childhood Experiences (ACE) Study. *American Journal of Preventive Medicine, 14*(4), 245-258.

Finkelhor, D. (1988). The trauma of child sexual abuse: Two models. *Journal of Interpersonal Violence, 2*(4), 348-366.

Finkelhor, D., & Dziuba-Leatherman, J. (1994). Victimization of children. *American Psychologist, 49*(3), 173-183.

Finkelhor, D., Hotaling, G., Lewis, I. A., & Smith, C. (1990). Sexual abuse in a national survey of adult men and women: Prevalence, characteristics, and risk factors. *Child Abuse & Neglect, 14*(1), 19-28.

Foa, E., & Kozak, M. (1986). Emotional processing of fear: Exposure to corrective information. *Psychological Bulletin, 99*, 20-35.

Foa, E. B., & Rothbaum, B. O. (1989). Behavioral psychotherapy for posttraumatic stress disorder. *International Review of Psychiatry, 1*, 219-226.

Freyd, J. J. (1996). *Betrayal trauma: The logic of forgetting abuse.* Cambridge, MA: Harvard University Press.

Gelinas, D. J. (1983). The persisting negative effects of incest. *Psychiatry, 46*(4), 312-32.

Gold, S. (1997). Training professional psychologists to treat survivors of childhood sexual abuse. *Psychotherapy, 4*(34), 365-374.

Gold-Steinberg, S., & Buttenheim, M. (1993). "Telling one's story" in an incest survivors group. *International Journal of Group Psychotherapy, 43*(2), 173-189.

Gorcey, M., Santiago, J., & McCall-Perez, F. (1986). Psychological consequences for women sexually abused in childhood. *Social Psychiatry, 21*, 129-133.

Greenwald, E. L., & Leitenberg, H. (1990). Posttraumatic stress disorder in a non-clinical and nonstudent sample of adult women sexually abused as children. *Journal of Interpersonal Violence, 5*(2), 217-228.

Gurtman, M. B. (1992). Trust, distrust and interpersonal problems: A circumplex analysis. *Journal of Personality and Social Psychology, 62*(6), 989-1002.

Hazzard, A., Rogers, J. H., & Angert, L. (1993). Factors affecting group therapy outcome for adult sexual abuse survivors. *International Journal of Group Psychotherapy, 43,* 453-468.

Herman, J. L. (1992a). *Trauma and recovery.* New York: Harper Collins.

Herman, J. L., Russell, D., & Trocki, K. (1986). Long-term effects of incestuous abuse in childhood. *American Journal of Psychiatry, 143*(10), 1293-1296.

Herman, J. L., & Schatzow, E. (1984). Time-limited group therapy for women with a history of incest. *International Journal of Group Psychotherapy, 34*(4), 605-616.

Herman, J. L. (1992b). Complex PTSD: A syndrome in survivors of prolonged and repeated trauma. *Journal of Traumatic Stress, 5,* 377-391.

Herman, J. L., & Schatzow, E. (1987). Recovery and verification of memories of childhood sexual trauma. *Psychoanalytic Psychology, 4*(1), 1-14.

Horowitz, L., Rosenberg, S., Baer, B., Ureno, G., & Villasenor, V. (1988). Inventory of interpersonal problems: Psychometric properties and clinical applications. *Journal of Consulting and Clinical Psychology, 56,* 885-892.

Hunter, J. A. (1991). A comparison of the psychosocial maladjustment of adult males and females sexually molested as children. *Journal of Interpersonal Violence, 6,* 205-217.

Jehu, D. (1989). Sexual dysfunctions among women clients who were sexually abused in childhood. *Behavioral Psychotherapy, 17*(1), 53-70.

Kiesler, D. J. (1983). The 1982 Interpersonal Circle: A taxonomy for complementarity in human transactions. *Psychological Review, 90,* 185-214.

Koss, M., & Gidycz, C. (1985). Sexual experiences survey: Reliability and validity. *Journal of Consulting and Clinical Psychology, 53,* 422-423.

Koss, M., & Oros, C. (1982). Sexual experiences survey: A research instrument investigating sexual aggression and victimization. *Journal of Consulting and Clinical Psychology, 50,* 455-457.

Koss, M. P., & Dinero, T. E. (1989). Discriminant analysis of risk factors for sexual victimization among a national sample of college women. *Journal of Consulting and Clinical Psychology, 57*(2), 242-250.

Loftus, E. F. (1993). The reality of repressed memories. *American Psychologist, 48*(5), 518-37.

Loftus, E. F., & Hoffman, H. G. (1989). Misinformation and memory: The creation of new memories. *Journal of Experimental Psychology: General, 118*(1), 100-104.

McCann, I., & Pearlman, L. (1990). *Psychological trauma and the adult survivor: Therapy, theory and transformation.* New York: Brunner/Mazel.

McCarthy, B. (1990). Treating sexual dysfunction associated with prior sexual trauma. *Journal of Sex and Marital Therapy, 16*(3), 142-146.

Morgan, T., & Cummings, A. L. (1999). Change experienced during group therapy by female survivors of childhood sexual abuse. *Journal of Consulting and Clinical Psychology, 67*(1), 28-36.

Mullen, P. E., Martin, J. L., Anderson, J. C., Romans, S. E., & Herbison, G. P. (1994). The effect of child sexual abuse on social, interpersonal and sexual function in adult life. *British Journal of Psychiatry, 165*, 35-47.

Paddison, P. L., Einbinder, R. G., Maker, E., & Strain, J. J. (1993). Group treatment with incest survivors. In P. L. Paddison (Ed.), *Treatment of adult survivors of incest* (pp. 35-54). Washington, DC: American Psychiatric Press.

Pelletier, G., & Handy, L. (1986). Family dysfunction and the psychological impact of child sexual abuse. *Canadian Journal of Psychiatry, 31*, 407-412.

Polusny, M. A., & Follette, V. M. (1995). Long term correlates of child sexual abuse: Theory and review of the empirical literature. *Applied & Preventive Psychology, 4*, 143-166.

Pribor, E. D., & Dinwiddie, S. H. (1992). Psychiatric correlates of incest in childhood. *American Journal of Psychiatry, 149*, 52-56.

Richter, N. L., Snider, E., & Gorey, K. M. (1997). Group work intervention with female survivors of childhood sexual abuse. *Research on Social Work Practice, 60*, 53-69.

Rodriguez, N., Ryan, S. W., Kemp, H. V., & Foy, D. W. (1997). Posttraumatic stress disorder in adult female survivors of childhood sexual abuse: A comparison study. *Journal of Consulting and Clinical Psychology, 65*(1), 53-59.

Roethlisberger, F. J., & Dickson, W. (1959). *Management and the worker.* Cambridge, MA: Harvard University Press.

Roth, N. (1993). *Integrating the shattered self: Psychotherapy with adult incest survivors.* Northvale, NJ: Jason Aronson.

Rowan, A. B., & Foy, D. W. (1993). Post-traumatic stress disorder in child sexual abuse survivors: A literature review. *Journal of Traumatic Stress, 6*(1), 3-20.

Rowan, A. B., Foy, D. W., Rodriguez, N., & Ryan, S. (1994). Posttraumatic stress disorder in a clinical sample of adults sexually abused as children. *Child Abuse & Neglect, 18*(1), 51-61.

Russell, D. (1986). *The secret trauma: Incest in the lives of girls and women.* New York: Basic Books.

Russell, D. E. H. (1983). The incidence and prevalence of intrafamilial and extrafamilial sexual abuse of female children. *Child Abuse & Neglect, 7*, 133-146.

Saunders, B., Villeponteaux, L., Lipovsky, J., Kilpatrick, D., & Veronen, L. (1992). Child sexual assault as a risk factor for mental disorder among women: A community survey. *Journal of Interpersonal Violence, 7*(2), 189-204.

Spiegel, D. (1989). Hypnosis in the treatment of victims of sexual abuse. *Psychiatric Clinics of North America, 12*(2), 295-305.

Spiegel, D. (1994). Hypnosis and Suggestion. In D. L. Schacter, J. T. Coyle, G. Fischback, M. M. Mesulam, & L. E. Sullivan (Eds.), *Memory distortion* (pp. 129-149). Cambridge: Harvard University Press.

Spiegel, D., Hunt, T., & Dondershine, H. E. (1988). Dissociation and hypnotizability in posttraumatic stress disorder. *American Journal of Psychiatry, 145*(3), 301-5.

Talmadge, L., & Wallace, S. (1991). Reclaiming sexuality in female incest survivors. *Journal of Sex and Marital Therapy, 17*(3), 163-182.

Tsai, M., & Wagner, N. (1978). Therapy groups for women sexually molested as children. *Archives of Sexual Behavior, 7*(5), 417-427.

van der Kolk, B. A., & Kadish, W. (1987). Amnesia, dissociation, and the return of the repressed. In B. A. van der Kolk (Ed.), *Psychological trauma* (pp. 173-190). Washington, DC: American Psychiatric Press.

Westen, D., Ludolph, P., Misle, B., Ruffins, S., & Block, J. (1990). Physical and sexual abuse in adolescent girls with borderline personality disorder. *American Journal of Orthopsychiatry, 60*(1), 55-66.

Wiggins, J. (1979). A psychological taxonomy of trait-descriptive terms: The interpersonal domain. *Journal of Personality and Social Psychology, 37*, 395-412.

Wiggins, J. S. (1982). Circumplex models of interpersonal behavior in clinical psychology. In P. C. Kendall & J. N. Butcher (Eds.), *Handbook of research methods in clinical psychology* (pp. 183-221). New York: Wiley.

Wyatt, G. E. (1985). The sexual abuse of Afro-American and white-American women in childhood. *Child Abuse & Neglect, 9*(4), 507-519.

Wyatt, G. E. (1990). The aftermath of child sexual abuse of African American and White American women: The victim's experience. *Journal of Family Violence, 5*(1), 61-81.

Yalom, I. (1995). *The theory and practice of group psychotherapy* (4th ed.). New York: Basic Books.

Yalom, I. D. (1980). *Existential psychotherapy.* New York: Basic Books.

Zlotnick, C., Shea, T., Rosen, K., Simpson, E., Mulrenin, K., Begin, A. & Pearlstein, T. (1997). An affect-management group for women with Posttraumatic Stress Disorder and histories of childhood sexual abuse. *Journal of Traumatic Stress, 10*(3), 425-436.

Dialogue Between Speakers and Attendees at the 1998 Meeting on Trauma and Cognitive Science: Questions and Answers About Traumatic Memory

Chris R. Brewin
Bernice Andrews

SUMMARY. Various issues of central importance to the field of trauma were continually raised and debated at the 1998 Meeting on Trauma and Cognitive Science. These included the representation of traumatic events in memory, the psychological and biological theories available to explain amnesia for traumatic events, the role of therapeutic suggestion in recovered memory experiences, the ways in which memories are recovered and the context in which this occurs, and the implications of our current knowledge about trauma and memory for therapy. This article details these discussions and in some cases provides a more general context from the literature on psychological trauma. *[Article copies available for a fee from The Haworth Document Delivery Service: 1-800-342-9678. E-mail address: <getinfo@haworthpressinc.com> Website: <http://www.HaworthPress. com> © 2001 by The Haworth Press, Inc. All rights reserved.]*

The authors gratefully acknowledge the assistance of Lia Biederman in providing a transcript of the question and answer sessions.

Address correspondence to: Chris R. Brewin, Subdepartment of Clinical Health Psychology, University College London, Gower Street, London WC1E 6BT, England.

[Haworth co-indexing entry note]: "Dialogue Between Speakers and Attendees at the 1998 Meeting on Trauma and Cognitive Science: Questions and Answers About Traumatic Memory." Brewin, Chris R., and Bernice Andrews. Co-published simultaneously in *Journal of Aggression, Maltreatment & Trauma* (The Haworth Maltreatment & Trauma Press, an imprint of The Haworth Press, Inc.) Vol. 4, No. 2 (#8), 2001, pp. 289-304; and: *Trauma and Cognitive Science: A Meeting of Minds, Science, and Human Experience* (ed: Jennifer J. Freyd, and Anne P. DePrince) The Haworth Maltreatment & Trauma Press, an imprint of The Haworth Press, Inc., 2001, pp. 289-304. Single or multiple copies of this article are available for a fee from The Haworth Document Delivery Service [1-800-342-9678, 9:00 a.m. - 5:00 p.m. (EST). E-mail address: getinfo@haworthpressinc.com].

KEYWORDS. Trauma, memory, amnesia, suggestion, therapy

At the present time, there are a number of key questions about trauma and memory that preoccupy scientists and practitioners alike. Contributions relevant to these questions arose from the discussions between attendees and presenters which formed a major part of the 1998 Meeting on Trauma and Cognitive Science, held in Eugene, Oregon. The purpose of this article is to document some of this dialogue. The authors were present during all presentations and discussion periods and were able to draw on a full transcript of the meeting.[1] In this article, the major questions will be summarized under five headings. In addition to material presented during the conference and transcribed from the question and answer sessions, this article draws on perspectives from the wider traumatic stress literature in order to provide a context for some of the questions raised.

The five headings, and the conference presenters who chiefly addressed them during their presentations or in the question and answer sessions, are as follows: (1) Are memories for traumatic experiences processed in an ordinary way or by special-purpose memory systems (Brewin, Fivush, Morton, van der Kolk)? (2) What existing psychological or biological theories can explain amnesia for traumatic events (Anderson, Bremner, Brewin, Freyd, Schooler, van der Kolk)? (3) How plausible is it that recovered memory experiences may arise from therapeutic suggestion (Hyman, Pezdek)? (4) What data exists on the nature of recovered memory experiences (Andrews)? (5) What are the implications of current knowledge about trauma and memory for therapy (Andrews, Brewin, Classen, Hyman, Keane, Koss, Pezdek, van der Kolk)?

ARE MEMORIES FOR TRAUMATIC EXPERIENCES PROCESSED IN AN ORDINARY WAY OR BY SPECIAL-PURPOSE MEMORY SYSTEMS?

Presenters and attendees referred frequently to different types of traumatic memory, predominantly contrasting "narrative memories" with "behavioral" or "bodily" memories, and "flashbacks." Although not always clearly defined in the literature on PTSD, the term "narrative memory" seems to refer to a consciously accessible language-based construction of the events surrounding a trauma, which can be discussed and modified through social interaction. In contrast, the term "flashback" seems to refer to an involuntary reliving of the trauma in the present, typically accompanied by vivid imagery and strong emotion. The experience is sometimes fragmented, consisting of brief images, sounds, smells, and bodily sensations, and may be hard to make into a coherent whole or to talk about in words. "Behavioral memories" or "bodily memories" also imply some reliving or reenactment of the trauma at a perceptual, physiological, or motor level, rather than at a linguistic level, and do not require that the person is consciously aware of the event which is being reenacted. What basis do these observations have in research?

From studying ordinary individuals in laboratory and real-life settings, many cognitive psychologists have claimed that memories for highly emotional events, and traumatic memories in particular, have different properties compared to those of other memories. There is now a consensus that memory for the central facts of emotional events tends to be accurate and persistent, whereas memory for peripheral details of such events is less consistent and may be impaired (Christianson, 1992; Koss, Tromp, & Tharan, 1995). In some cases, individuals retain clear detailed images for long periods ("flashbulb memories"; Brown & Kulik, 1977), although this is not invariably the case, and is related to several factors, including the personal significance of the event (Conway, 1995). For example, one study found that rape memories, compared to other unpleasant memories, were less clear and vivid, involved less visual detail, and were less well-remembered (Tromp, Koss, Figueredo, & Tharan, 1995).

Research on individuals with PTSD, reported by van der Kolk, has revealed that the intrusive memories of PTSD sufferers are often characterized by even greater clarity and persistence, are accompanied by high levels of emotional arousal, and contain strong sensory and perceptual features. However, some of these memories (the "flashbacks") appear to differ from memories of trauma reported by nonclinical samples in several ways. They often consist of parts or fragments of events rather than whole memories, they are often experienced as a reliving of the event in the present moment, and their content cannot be deliberately retrieved (Brewin, Dalgleish, & Joseph, 1996; van der Kolk & Fisler, 1995). It has been argued by several authors that the characteristics of these "flashback" memories are caused by the fact that the individuals are in a dissociative state at the time of the trauma, which prevents them from adequately encoding and processing the information (van der Kolk & Fisler, 1995). As discussed later, it is not uncommon for individuals to report being numb, in a daze, or having the sensation of leaving their body while the trauma is occurring.

In his presentation, Brewin noted that not all the memories reported by PTSD patients have the characteristics of "flashbacks," and that patients are usually able to give a narrative account of their trauma that appears to be based on ordinary language. These observations about the varying properties of emotional memories are quite consistent with recent theories, which propose that individuals store two different kinds of memory of emotion-laden events: one, an ordinary autobiographical memory, and the other, based on lower-level perceptual processing (Brewin et al., 1996).

According to Brewin et al.'s (1996) dual representation theory of PTSD, "verbally accessible" representations of trauma form part of ordinary autobiographical memory and support narrative accounts of the trauma. "Situationally accessible" representations are based on lower-level processing of the traumatic event, and although they are unavailable to direct conscious inspection, they may be triggered by internal or external trauma-related cues. These representations support the involuntary, affect-laden, and often fragmented types of trauma-related cognition, such as repetitive flashbacks, nightmares, and unconscious bodily or motor reenactments.

Other presenters and attendees noted that smell and taste seem to have a unique relationship to memory, perhaps because there are close neuroanatomical connections between the olfactory system and the limbic system. These connections may support perceptual or situationally accessible memories. Olfactory cues were thought to be particularly likely to cue affective components of memories.

A large part of the discussion at the meeting was concerned with describing these different types of memory processes from a developmental perspective. Morton described the headed records theory of memory (Morton, Hammersley, & Bekerian, 1985), which suggests that, in a young child experiencing a rapid onset of amnesia for a trauma, the trauma memory would be available in relatively small records all linked together. During therapy all these individual records could be accessed and stitched together into a larger, secondary record containing a fuller and more coherent account, and including some of the same affective components.

Fivush reported that language is often an inadequate medium for a young child to comprehend a traumatic experience (see Fivush, Pipe, Murachver, & Reese, 1997). Attendees and presenters also pointed out that sexually abused children often have difficulty developing narrative memories. This difficulty is often aggravated by perpetrators' use of language that is a distortion of the actual events. It was suggested that when children are told something inaccurate about their experiences, they may be more prone to having fragmentary memories.

WHAT EXISTING PSYCHOLOGICAL OR BIOLOGICAL THEORIES CAN EXPLAIN AMNESIA FOR TRAUMATIC EVENTS?

Dissociation

A major focus of van der Kolk's presentation, and a process much discussed during the meeting was dissociation. The process of dissociation is prominently associated with traumatic forgetting, and was the focus of theorizing by Janet in the last century (Janet, 1889). As noted by Cardeña (1994), this term "simply means that two or more mental processes or contents are not associated or integrated. It is usually assumed that these dissociated elements would be integrated in conscious awareness, memory, or identity" (p. 15). A dissociative state is an altered state of consciousness in which ordinary perceptual, cognitive, and/or motor functioning are impaired. For example, there appears to be a spectrum of dissociative states involving greater and lesser degrees of awareness of the current environment. Thus, in therapy sessions, dissociative states may range from a reduced ability to hear or see the therapist, a transient sense of depersonalization or derealization, or an out-of-body experience, to a complete loss of awareness of time and space. Other dissociative states involve what appears to be a separate personality. Although dissociation does not invariably involve amnesia, lack of memory for events experienced in different states is commonly reported.

Several trauma theorists (e.g., Alpert, Brown, & Courtois, 1996; Briere, 1992; van der Kolk & Fisler, 1995) have proposed that peri-traumatic dissociation (i.e., dissociation that occurs during the traumatic experience), is a defense that prevents the individual from experiencing the full impact of what is happening. Patients describe being temporarily detached from the situation, sometimes observing what is occurring, but without any pain or distress. Psychophysiological studies of patients who dissociate confirm that in this state there are marked bodily changes, such as reductions in heart rate and blood pressure (Griffin, Resick, & Mechanic, 1997).

What is happening in terms of the two types of traumatic memory discussed above? Because traumatic memory contains two separate, dissociable systems, Brewin suggested that the dual representation model offers a built-in explanation for these phenomena. Peri-traumatic dissociation prevents the creation of a detailed, verbally accessible or narrative memory, or creates one that cannot readily be retrieved when the trauma is over, because it is encoded as part of an alternative mental state. However, the events are encoded in situationally accessible memory, in a form that is fragmented, perceptually rich, and emotionally intense. Retrieval of a dissociated memory reflects the fact that little if any conscious processing took place at encoding. Thus, as was also argued by van der Kolk, retrieval is characterized by vivid and intense sensory and perceptual elements, by fragmentation, and by a stereotyped, repetitive quality that endures over multiple retrievals.

There was also discussion of the circumstances under which people employ dissociation. Freyd (see also Freyd, 1996) suggested that when the trauma is of human design, particularly in the paradigm case of child sexual abuse, then the experience of betrayal is particularly important in triggering a dissociative response. The question, then, is whether the dissociation observed in other traumatic circumstances, such as car accidents, terrorist bombings, or waking up in the middle of surgery, could also be viewed as being due to betrayal. It was proposed that dissociation was a strategy learned in childhood, in the context of traumatic experiences characterized by betrayal, and that the dissociative responses are automatically reinvoked when a person is exposed to trauma as an adult. This would explain why adult trauma that leads to PTSD is not necessarily linked to betrayal. Freyd responded that people might dissociate for a number of reasons, but noted that betrayal seems to be a particularly important factor, and it predicts a considerable amount of variance in the data currently available.

Other attendees noted that, in addition to its role during trauma itself, betrayal might also be experienced in the recovery period, and might contribute to prolonging symptoms. People who feel betrayed may not be able to gather sufficient resources, either in themselves or in the environment, to recover. It was also noted that betrayal trauma is not just relevant to childhood abuse, but that it is also relevant to Vietnam veterans who felt betrayed, both by society and their leaders. It was suggested that, in the military, inability to trust one's leader can lead to severe psychological damage.

Dissatisfaction was expressed by presenters and attendees with the current methods of measuring dissociation. It was noted that the most commonly used measure, the Dissociative Experiences Questionnaire (Bernstein & Putnam, 1986) is a broad measure that includes a number of aspects of dissociation, such as memory loss, absorption, and depersonalization. Bremner commented that some of these experiences are found in the normal population, such as brief periods of absorption while driving on the highway, and that these should be distinguished from pathological experiences, such as finding oneself dressed in clothes one has no memory of putting on. Absorption and hypnotizability appear to be normally distributed in the general population, and are highly correlated. In contrast, Bremner noted that the relation between dissociation and hypnotizability is less clear. High hypnotizability has not consistently been found in all traumatized populations (see Bremner & Marmar, 1998, for a detailed discussion). Attendees remarked that pathological dissociation can be measured with a subset of DES items known as a "taxon" (Waller, Putnam, & Carlson, 1996).

Repression

Apart from dissociation, the most frequently mentioned explanation for forgetting relies on the psychoanalytic concept of repression. In 1895 Breuer and Freud noted "It was a question of things which the patient wished to forget, and therefore intentionally repressed from his conscious thought and inhibited and suppressed" (p. 61). There are many indications that Freud was uncertain about whether repression should be thought of as a process that is unconscious from the outset ("primary repression"), as contrasted with a conscious act of suppression, or whether repression should be considered an unconscious process that only develops following a period of deliberate suppression ("repression proper" or "after-expulsion").

Although psychoanalytic discussion of repression has advanced considerably since Freud, Brewin noted that, theoretically, these two forms of repression have very different implications. Primary repression implies the need for preconscious or unconscious mechanisms that block any conscious processing being accorded to the traumatic scene. Thus, as with dissociation, forgetting is seen as arising from a failure to encode information. After-expulsion operates on material that has already received fairly extensive conscious processing. Therefore, the focus is on a failure of storage or retrieval, rather than on a failure to encode. Many examples of this process may be found in textbooks on cognitive psychology under the heading of "motivated forgetting" (Freyd, 1996). Because material subject to repression (in the after-expulsion sense) has been encoded normally, repressed material should be able to return as ordinary autobiographical memories and not in the fragmented, disorganized form typical of dissociated material (Brewin & Andrews, 1998).

Inhibitory Cognitive Processes

Brewin also noted that the idea that people can choose not to attend to unwanted thoughts and memories, and can learn to forget them, is consistent with a great deal of recent research in cognitive psychology (see Brewin & Andrews, 1998, for a review). Many prominent cognitive psychologists propose that selective attention is a highly flexible, goal-based system consisting of facilitating and inhibitory processes that operate in concert to produce effective and efficient thought and action. The function of this system is to remove goal-irrelevant information already in working memory, and to hinder irrelevant information from gaining access to working memory.

Unwanted items can be removed relatively simply from memory by having people learn or practice retrieval of new material. Studies, mainly with student populations, using the directed forgetting paradigm (Bjork, 1989) or the retrieval-induced forgetting paradigm described by Anderson, Bjork, and Bjork (1994), have provided persuasive evidence that people possess active inhibitory mechanisms that enable them to forget. In directed forgetting experimental subjects are instructed that certain material, typically items from a word list, is irrelevant and should be forgotten. Subsequently, subjects find this material harder to recall, although they can still identify the items on a recognition test.

Presenters and attendees raised the question whether research on college students is relevant to traumatized populations. Keane responded that student populations have often experienced high levels of trauma. Other presenters remarked that the experimental research has interesting analogues in real-life situations. For example, research on directed forgetting suggests that the inhibition preventing forgotten material from being recalled might be undone after many years if relevant material was encountered and acted as a recognition cue. This appears similar to observations of memory recovery in which an individual hears someone else describing their abuse. This line of research is also consistent with the idea that forgetting could be instituted by trauma victims instructing themselves to forget, or being instructed to forget by another person.

In retrieval-induced forgetting, practicing the retrieval of one item from a set inhibits the recall of related items from the same set. Anderson suggested that these "related items" could be alternative roles played by an abusive parent who was sometimes kind and sometimes cruel. In this case, rehearsal of "good parent" material might be effective in inhibiting the recall of information about the "bad parent." Attendees at the meeting suggested that these processes could be enhanced by a perpetrator encouraging an abused child to rehearse positive messages, such as, "Daddy loves me; Daddy's doing this because he's trying to teach me something; I'm Daddy's favorite little girl."

Relevant to Freyd's (1996) betrayal trauma hypothesis, it was also noted by attendees that currently abused children often actively suppress the representation of a known perpetrator as bad. They will cling to the person who is abusing them, talk about how they love them, and how they want to see them. In other words, there are interesting links between developmental observations of disturbed attachment behavior and the suppression of unwanted information about those attachment figures.

The forgetting observed in these paradigms is clearly analogous to the Freudian notion of repression (in the after-expulsion sense), which suggests that clinical phenomena may be at least partly accounted for by processes observable in the laboratory. Discussion focused on an example presented by Schooler of a person forgetting a court case s/he had been involved in, a situation which would clearly have received a considerable amount of encoding. It was noted that the person had subsequently left the area, and that in this case, forgetting might have been facilitated by the removal of many environmental cues to recall or recognize the events.

Biological Processes

Several questions and observations were raised in the discussion concerning the biological effects of trauma. One followed van der Kolk's report of a reduction in activation in Broca's area (the part of the brain concerned with the production of language) in traumatized individuals. Van der Kolk suggested that exposure to trauma might have the effect of both activating the amygdala (concerned with fight/flight responses), and simultaneously inhibiting Broca's area. Could the opposite happen too, so that activation of Broca's area would inhibit the amygdala? This would suggest a possible benefit of stimulating language production generally.

What about the possible different biological effects of trauma in childhood and adulthood? In reply, Bremner noted that adult combat veterans tend to show a reduction in the size of the right hippocampus, and to have deficits on both verbal and visual memory tasks. In contrast, individuals with childhood abuse tend to show a reduction in the size of the left hippocampus and have verbal memory deficits, but perform better on some of the visual memory tasks.

Bremner also noted that his findings indicating reduced hippocampal size with trauma were not unequivocal signs of atrophy brought about by trauma. At present, the literature is also consistent with the possibility that a smaller hippocampus is a risk factor for developing PTSD. This could be investigated using twin studies.

HOW PLAUSIBLE IS IT THAT
RECOVERED MEMORY EXPERIENCES
MAY ARISE FROM THERAPEUTIC SUGGESTION?

Presenters and attendees were interested in the findings from experimental laboratory research on the suggestibility of memory that could be relevant to therapy. It was noted that suggestibility was greater when the event being suggested was more plausible, and the point was made by attendees that therapists could increase the plausibility of the idea that a client had been sexually abused by identifying symptoms as characteristic of abuse survivors, dwelling on negative memories from childhood, and introducing the client to other survivors. Other attendees suggested that people who voluntarily enter therapy are likely to be emotionally vulnerable, experience memory problems, and are open to abuse of the power differential between therapist and client. Pezdek agreed that it was difficult to decide a priori what a person would find plausible or implausible–there are likely to be large individual differences.

Several other potential influences on suggestibility were raised. Pezdek reported that there was no evidence for age or gender effects. However, the favorability of the event being suggested could be an important variable (i.e., was the event something that was pleasant or unpleasant to contemplate having happened), although this has not been systematically investigated.

Hyman observed that many of the misinformation studies rely on authoritative sources to suggest the false events. Repetition is also likely to be a crucial factor. Repetition of original, true information reduces the likelihood of people being misled, but repetition of false information increases the probability that it will be believed. Even when experimental subjects were told during debriefing that one of the suggested events was false, they were often unable to identify it. However, participants were more likely to correctly identify a suggested event that was unusual or implausible in some way.

WHAT DATA EXISTS ON THE NATURE OF RECOVERED MEMORY EXPERIENCES?

To date there have been several published surveys in the literature of self-identified abuse survivors that have focused on rates of forgetting (and by definition recovering) the experience. Some have also investigated the extent of corroboration for reported episodes of forgotten trauma, or the extent to which reported memories corresponded to documented events. Surveys of therapists have focused on their beliefs and practices concerning recovered memories, in particular the extent to which therapeutic techniques are used to aid clients' recall of traumatic material. Following from these initial studies (see Pope & Brown, 1996, or Mollon, 1998, for reviews), the next step in evaluating competing explanations for the forgetting of trauma is to conduct detailed systematic investigations which address both the nature of memories recovered during therapy, and the circumstances under which they are recovered.

A recent study, one of the largest and most detailed, was reported by Andrews (see Andrews et al., 1999; Andrews, Brewin, Ochera et al., 2000). She and her colleagues followed up on a subsample of respondents who reported having clients who had recovered traumatic memories in a previous survey of 810 practitioner members of the British Psychological Society (Andrews et al., 1995). In interviews with 108 qualified psychologists reporting in detail on 236 recovered memory clients, they investigated: (1) therapists' reports of the content and characteristics of their clients' recovered memories, (to cover the different types of trauma described, as well as the plausibility and validity of the recovered memories); and (2) therapeutic involvement in the production of recovered memories, including the context in which the clients' first memory were recovered, and whether therapeutic techniques were used.

A striking finding was the heterogeneity of the recovered memory experiences. In 69% of these detailed cases, there had been no inkling of the trauma prior to recovery, but in 31% of the cases, clients had knowledge of some related trauma, although not of the incidents recovered. Similarly, only 50% of the memories involved child sexual abuse (CSA) alone: 22% involved both CSA and some other trauma, and 27% involved only non-CSA trauma. There was also variation in how events were remembered, corresponding to the distinction between narrative and "flashback" memories. When asked whether memories came back whole or in parts, respondents reported that in the relevant cases, 42% of the clients' memories came back only in fragments, 20% recalled fragments and subsequently whole memories, and 38% recalled only whole memories. The majority of the relevant cases (60%) involved full reexperiencing; 23% involved partial reexperiencing, and the remaining 17% involved no reexperiencing.

Thirty-two percent of clients were reported to have recovered their first memory before entering any kind of therapy. The results confirmed that, contrary to popular assumption, most (78%) of the clients' initial recovered memories either preceded therapy or preceded the use of memory recovery techniques used by the respondents. Techniques seemed to be used more to help the clients elaborate the memories than to facilitate their initial recovery.

In only a very small minority of the detailed cases did the memories appear improbable, either because they concerned bizarre experiences (5%), or because the events had supposedly ended before age 3 (2%). Corroborative evidence was reported for over 40% of the memories, often from more than one source. Thus, the study described at the conference by Andrews (Andrews et al., 1999; Andrews, Brewin, Ochera et al., 2000) indicates that recovered memory experiences are far more heterogeneous than has hitherto been suggested: Rather, there is considerable variation in what is remembered, how it is remembered, and when it is remembered. Some of the data are consistent with memories being of iatrogenic origin, but other data clearly point to the need for additional explanations.

WHAT ARE THE IMPLICATIONS OF CURRENT KNOWLEDGE ABOUT TRAUMA AND MEMORY FOR THERAPY?

All the above issues have important implications for therapy. For example, if trauma is represented in two different memory systems, what happens to these memories following treatment? Van der Kolk noted that, whereas before therapy, PTSD patients describe vivid reexperiencing of the trauma with strong sensory elements, after therapy, they are more likely to describe the memory as belonging to the past and as being like an everyday experience. The intensity and precision of the memory fades, and it becomes less subjectively important. Brewin noted that, in terms of dual representation theory (Brewin et al., 1996), therapy involves two separate tasks. The first is to make it harder for internal and external cues to reactivate situationally accessible trauma memories, thereby reducing distressing flashbacks and nightmares. The second is to elaborate and make readily available a narrative or verbally accessible memory that integrates the recalled material with the person's theories about themselves and the world, and does not give rise to intense secondary emotions such as anger and guilt.

As noted by van der Kolk and other contributors to the meeting, the elaboration of a post hoc narrative memory is an unreliable and flawed process that depends on the social context, on the reinforcement provided, and on the possibility of creating a plausible story. For example, Hyman reported a study by Kheriaty, Kleinknecht, and Hyman (1999) in which they asked phobic college students and their parents to explain why the students had developed their fears. The students' accounts were often plausible and partly true, but the parents were often able to add other information, not available to the students, which provided a more complete account of phobia onset. Patients' narratives will also tend to differ with the theoretical orientation of the therapist. Pezdek commented that, in the absence of external validation, there are currently no scientifically validated ways to determine whether the events described in a narrative are true or false.

If the trauma occurred at a young age, the original narrative memory may be limited and mistaken in various ways, or even completely non-existent. This may be due to childhood amnesia, inadequate linguistic skills, or attachment processes that operate to censor information threatening to the child's sense of security. New research described by Fivush has begun to examine the association between different attachment styles and children's ways of talking about the past. The more limited, fragmented, and partial the autobiographical material available, for whatever reason, the greater the scope would be for inaccuracy when fuller narrative memories are later constructed.

Presenters and attendees noted how features of therapy, such as the power differential, the claimed authority and knowledge of the therapist, and the opportunity to make repeated suggestions, could combine with the presence of limited narratives to generate "false memories." In most cases it would not be possible to verify the objective truth of the narratives produced, and the point was made that, under some circumstances, false narratives may indeed be reassuring and therapeutic. The corollary is that therapists need to be aware of the possibility that an acceptable narrative may involve non-existent events, or a false attribution of blame or responsibility to other individuals.

The literature appears to indicate that cognitively oriented treatments, in which mistaken beliefs and assumptions arising from the trauma are corrected, are effective, particularly for rape victims (e.g., Resick & Schnicke, 1993). This is consistent with the longitudinal study of rape victims presented at the conference by Koss (see article in this issue), which revealed that negative beliefs were among the strongest predictors of a poor outcome. Koss identified discrepancies between perceptions of actual self and ideal self, as well as shame, as important predictors of poor outcome. Recent data on victims of violent crime have confirmed that shame may be uniquely important in blocking recovery from some kinds of trauma (Andrews, Brewin, Rose, & Kirk, 2000).

Other treatments involve direct reexperiencing of the trauma, particularly exposure therapy (e.g., Foa, Rothbaum, Riggs, & Murdock, 1991) and eye-movement desensitization and reprocessing (Shapiro, 1995). Van der Kolk noted the existence of therapies that attempt to evoke strong memories of the trauma and then to associate them with incompatible bodily sensations, such as feeling of security. For example, martial arts training may give assault victims a sense of power in their body that is incompatible with the weakness and helplessness associated with their traumatic memories.

Keane voiced concern that the definition of "suggestive" or "aggressive" memory recovery techniques considered to exacerbate the risk of false memories is not clearly grounded in evidence, and might include standard procedures such as guided imagery, narrative production, and perhaps even systematic desensitization or exposure therapy. This would undermine much existing effective clinical practice for treating trauma. For example, legislation in preparation in Missouri, if read in a certain way, would prohibit the use of the only techniques known to help people overcome trauma, simply because they would be viewed as overly "aggressive." Hyman noted that it was vital to distinguish between the use of techniques to help recover memories initially and the use of techniques to deal with memories that have already been recovered. Andrews responded that this distinction may not always be easy to make in practice because there are frequently partial memories preexisting the recovery of new traumatic incidents (Andrews et al., 1999).

A final issue discussed at the conference concerned treatment of severely traumatized patients suffering from complex PTSD, personality disorders, and other dissociative disorders. Van der Kolk remarked that it is as though their whole life is a continuous reliving of the trauma. Their inability to modulate affect results in a series of extreme emotional reactions to everyday experiences. Recent approaches, such as Linehan's (1993), have questioned whether it is always necessary or desirable to explore traumatic memories directly. Rather, treatment involves teaching patients to observe and understand their feelings and to learn to tolerate them better. A current study described by Classen et al. (in this issue) is directly comparing two treatments for people with dissociative disorders, one based on exploring traumatic memories and one based on developing broader coping skills for dealing with affect and solving everyday problems.

CONCLUSIONS

The question and answer discussion sessions provided ample evidence that researchers and clinicians share a common set of concerns. One concern involves the need to close the gap between current scientific theories and the complexity of the clinical phenomena shown by traumatized patients. In response to this need, theoretical approaches are becoming increasingly sophisticated, and researchers are making greater attempts to heed clinical observations both in designing experiments and in drawing conclusions from their results. Another major concern is to treat patients as ethically as possible, with due regard to the possibility of doing harm, both to them and their families, in an area where so much is unknown.

It was also clear that despite its growing importance, the field is at a comparably early stage. There was general agreement that false memories could arise in therapy, but that there was still a considerable gap between the basic laboratory research and real-life clinical activity. The other questions addressed at the meeting were, to an even greater extent, open to debate, although considerable progress in research is being made. In our view, the opportunity for debate and questioning provided by conferences such as this one and the previous NATO conference on Recollections of Trauma (Read & Lindsay, 1997), have a vital part to play in challenging scientists to improve their science and practitioners to improve their practice.

NOTE

1. The tapes are available for purchase at: http://dynamic.uoregon.edu/trauma-conf.html.

REFERENCES

Alpert, J. L., Brown, L. S., & Courtois, C. A. (1996). Symptomatic clients and memories of childhood abuse: What the trauma and child sexual abuse literature tells us. *American Psychological Association Working Group on Investigation of Memories of Childhood Abuse: Final Report.*

Anderson, M. C., Bjork, R. A., & Bjork, E. L. (1994). Remembering can cause forgetting: Retrieval dynamics in long-term memory. *Journal of Experimental Psychology: Learning, Memory and Cognition, 20,* 1063-1087.

Andrews, B., Brewin, C. R., Ochera, J., Morton, J., Bekerian, D. A., Davies, G. M., & Mollon, P. (1999). The characteristics, context, and consequences of memory recovery among adults in therapy. *British Journal of Psychiatry, 175,* 141-146.

Andrews, B., Brewin, C. R., Ochera, J., Morton, J., Bekerian, D. A., Davies, G. M., & Mollon, P. (2000). The process of memory recovery among adults in therapy. *British Journal of Clinical Psychology, 39,* 11-26.

Andrews, B., Brewin, C. R., Rose, S., & Kirk, M. (2000). Predicting PTSD symptoms in victims of violent crime: The role of shame, anger, and childhood abuse. *Journal of Abnormal Psychology, 109,* 69-73.

Andrews, B., Morton, J., Bekerian, D. A., Brewin, C. R., Davies, G. M., & Mollon, P. (1995). The recovery of memories in clinical practice: Experiences and beliefs of British Psychological Society Practitioners. *The Psychologist: Bulletin of the British Psychological Society, 8,* 209-214.

Bernstein, E. M., & Putnam, F. W. (1986). Development, reliability, and validity of a dissociation scale. *Journal of Nervous and Mental Disease, 174*, 727-735.

Bjork, R. A. (1989). Retrieval inhibition as an adaptive mechanism in human memory. In H. L. Roediger & F. I. M. Craik (Eds.), *Varieties of memory and consciousness* (pp. 309-330). Hillsdale, NJ: Lawrence Erlbaum.

Bremner, J. D., & Marmar, C. R. (1998). *Trauma, memory, and dissociation.* Washington, DC: American Psychiatric Press.

Breuer, J., & Freud, S. (1895/1974). Studies on hysteria. Volume 3 of *The Pelican Freud Library* (General Editor, A. Dickson). Harmondsworth, UK: Penguin.

Brewin, C. R. & Andrews, B. (1998). Recovered memories of trauma: Phenomenology and cognitive mechanisms. *Clinical Psychology Review, 18*, 949-970.

Brewin, C. R., Dalgleish, T. & Joseph, S. (1996). A dual representation theory of post-traumatic stress disorder. *Psychological Review, 103*, 670-686.

Briere, J. N. (1992). *Child abuse trauma.* Newbury Park, CA: Sage.

Brown, R., & Kulik, J. (1977). "Flashbulb memories." *Cognition, 5*, 73-99.

Cardeña, E. (1994). The domain of dissociation. In S. J. Lynn & J. W. Rhue (Eds.), *Dissociation: Clinical and theoretical perspectives* (pp. 15-31). New York: Guilford.

Christianson, S.-A. (1992). Emotional stress and eyewitness memory. *Psychological Bulletin, 112*, 284-309.

Conway, M. A. (1995). *Flashbulb memories.* Hove, England: Erlbaum.

Fivush, R., Pipe, M.-E., Murachver, T., & Reese, E. (1997). Events spoken and unspoken: Implications of language and memory development for the recovered memory debate. In M.A. Conway (Ed.), *Recovered memories and false memories* (pp. 34-62). Oxford: Oxford University Press.

Foa, E. B., Rothbaum, B. O., Riggs, D. S. & Murdock, T. (1991). Treatment of post-traumatic stress disorder in rape victims: A comparison between cognitive-behavioral procedures and counseling. *Journal of Consulting and Clinical Psychology, 59*, 715-723.

Freyd, J. J. (1996). *Betrayal trauma: The logic of forgetting childhood abuse.* Cambridge, MA: Harvard University Press.

Griffin, M. G., Resick, P. A., & Mechanic, M. B. (1997). Objective assessment of peritraumatic dissociation: Psycho-physiological indicators. *American Journal of Psychiatry, 154*, 1081-1088.

Janet, P. (1889). *L'automatisme psychologique.* Paris: Felix Alcan.

Kheriaty, E., Kleinknecht, R. A., & Hyman, I. E. (1999). Recall and validation of phobia origins as a function of a structured interview versus the phobia origins questionnaire. *Behavior Modification, 23*, 61-78.

Koss, M. P., Tromp, S., & Tharan, M. (1995). Traumatic memories: Empirical foundations, forensic and clinical implications. *Clinical Psychology: Science and Practice, 2*, 111-132.

Linehan, M. M. (1993). *Cognitive-behavioral treatment of borderline personality disorder.* New York: Guilford.

Mollon, P. (1998). *Remembering trauma.* Chichester, UK: Wiley.

Morton, J., Hammersley, R. H., & Bekerian, D. A. (1985). Headed records: A model for memory and its failures. *Cognition, 20*, 1-23.

Pope, K.S., & Brown, L. S. (1996). *Recovered memories of abuse*. Washington, DC: American Psychological Association.

Read, J. D., & Lindsay, D. S. (1997). *Recollections of trauma: Scientific evidence and clinical practice*. New York: Plenum.

Resick, P. A., & Schnicke, M. K. (1993). *Cognitive processing therapy for rape victims*. Newbury Park, CA: Sage.

Shapiro, F. (1995). *Eye movement desensitization and reprocessing*. New York: Guilford.

Tromp, S., Koss, M. P., Figueredo, A. J., & Tharan, M. (1995). Are rape memories different? A comparison of rape, other unpleasant, and pleasant memories among employed women. *Journal of Traumatic Stress, 8*, 607-627.

Van der Kolk, B. A., & Fisler, R. (1995). Dissociation and the fragmentary nature of traumatic memories: Overview and exploratory study. *Journal of Traumatic Stress, 4*, 505-525.

Waller, N. G., Putnam, F. W., & Carlson, E. B. (1996). Types of dissociation and dissociative types: A taxometric analysis of dissociative experiences. *Psychological Methods, 1*, 300-321.

Finding a Secret Garden
in Trauma Research

Jennifer J. Freyd
Anne P. DePrince

SUMMARY. This article briefly summarizes the diversity in perspectives and methodologies captured in the current volume. The authors discuss diversity in the context of the 1998 Meeting on Trauma and Cognitive Science, and the future of traumatic stress studies. In addition, future directions for research and collaborative approaches are discussed. *[Article copies available for a fee from The Haworth Document Delivery Service: 1-800-342-9678. E-mail address: <getinfo@haworthpressinc. com> Website: <http://www.HaworthPress.com> © 2001 by The Haworth Press, Inc. All rights reserved.]*

KEYWORDS. Trauma, multidisciplinary, cognitive science

The fields of trauma and cognitive science have the potential to influence and inform one another when boundaries between traditionally segregated domains of academic pursuit are crossed. This volume (and the 1998 Meeting which inspired the volume) sought to bring together the methods, assumptions, and interpretations of trauma researchers who crossed boundaries of traditional areas within psychology and psychiatry. In so doing, the authors contributed research and theory that differed along important dimensions,

Address correspondence to: Jennifer J. Freyd, Department of Psychology, 1227 University of Oregon, Eugene, OR 97403-1227 (E-mail: jjf@dynamic.uoregon.edu).

[Haworth co-indexing entry note]: "Finding a Secret Garden in Trauma Research." Freyd, Jennifer J., and Anne P. DePrince. Co-published simultaneously in *Journal of Aggression, Maltreatment & Trauma* (The Haworth Maltreatment & Trauma Press, an imprint of The Haworth Press, Inc.) Vol. 4, No. 2 (#8), 2001, pp. 305-309; and: *Trauma and Cognitive Science: A Meeting of Minds, Science, and Human Experience* (ed: Jennifer J. Freyd, and Anne P. DePrince) The Haworth Maltreatment & Trauma Press, an imprint of The Haworth Press, Inc., 2001, pp. 305-309. Single or multiple copies of this article are available for a fee from The Haworth Document Delivery Service [1-800-342-9678, 9:00 a.m. - 5:00 p.m. (EST). E-mail address: getinfo@haworthpressinc.com].

such as population or methodology, while sharing common themes. Across the different methodologies and perspectives represented in this volume, there is an awareness that multiple forms of assessment and multiple conceptual tools are required to understand the complex relationship of trauma and human behavior. Multiple perspectives are the essential ingredient in the study of trauma and its effects. The contributions made to this volume capture the necessary diversity in methodology, theory, and interpretation that will push our understanding of trauma and its effects forward.

While diversity in theory and methodology appears to be an important goal for researchers, diversity requires the breaking down of traditional boundaries. Breaking down boundaries is a formidable task. In his welcome remarks to the 1998 Meeting on Trauma and Cognitive Science held at the University of Oregon, University President Dave Frohnmayer recognized the importance and magnitude of this task: "I especially commend you for your willingness to cross disciplinary boundaries. Combining the rigor and precision of cognitive science with the complex worlds of trauma and Clinical Psychology. Bringing these worlds together is both a challenge and an opportunity." The 1998 Meeting on Trauma and Cognitive Science and this volume provide a model for addressing problems from different perspectives, paradigms, and intellectual traditions. Now that we have this model, we can see that such collaborative efforts are a very important and productive way to operate. This multidisciplinary approach can be applied to the trauma field more generally, and psychology as a whole. When we listen to other perspectives, the opportunities for discovery and understanding increase. Unfortunately our academic fields are often divided into separate "areas" that become isolated from one another. In contrast, we believe that areas within a field or department are most valuable when used and thought of as focal points for shared intellectual interests. Such intellectual communities intrinsically have fuzzy boundaries, are ever changing, and often have overlapping edges–they are not some set of fixed, mutually exclusive, and exhaustive categories that adequately subdivide the field.

President Dave Frohnmayer (1998) also noted: "Long-standing borders are always difficult to cross; that's the history of inquiry. They are broken down with great courage and great difficulty." This sentiment reflects similar ideas expressed elsewhere in the scientific community. Rhonda Shearer and Stephen Jay Gould published an essay in the November 5, 1999 issue of *Science* magazine, in which they urged scientists not to create disciplinary boundaries where they need not exist. Shearer and Gould (1999) note that while humans have a tendency to divide into "us versus them," humans are also capable of "mental flexibility, and our consequent potential for overcoming such innate limitations by education" (p. 1093). They wrote "The contingent and largely arbitrary nature of disciplinary boundaries has unfortunately been reinforced, and even made to seem 'natural' by our drive to construct dichotomies" (p. 1093). Perhaps their most important observation is:

> Our tendency to parse complex nature into pairings of "us versus them" should not only be judged as false in our university of shadings and continua, but also (and often) harmful, given another human propensity for judgment–so that "us versus them" easily becomes "good versus bad" or even, when zealotry fans our xenophobic flames, "chosen for martyrdom versus ripe for burning." (p. 1093)

Frohnmayer (1998), as well as Shearer and Gould (1999) speak to the importance of minimizing disciplinary boundaries. What is true for large disciplinary boundaries is also true for minimizing boundaries within a discipline. The study of trauma requires that we cross and combine traditional areas.

President Frohnmayer (1998) also drew attention to the importance of combining rigorous science with compassionate humanity: " . . . to find you here, obviously indicates the seriousness of the topic and of your intellectual devotion to understanding it more deeply. . . . This conference brings to this campus obviously not only scientists who's professional experience has immersed you in the world of research, but scientists who understand human beings as human beings and the importance of that research to science and society and indeed to human well-being." Supporting Frohnmayer's emphasis on the importance of this research to society, the local newspaper for the city of Eugene covered the conference for the lay public (Mortenson, 1998; Rojas-Burke, 1998).

The future success of traumatic stress studies, and particularly the melding of cognitive science and traumatic stress, will depend upon ever increasing collaboration between scientists, scholars, and thinkers with diverse backgrounds. Key elements are necessary to support this growing diversity and commitment to breaking down boundaries. We hope to see the field become better funded to support diversity in intellectual approach. In addition, a continued emphasis on developmental effects will be essential (see also Putnam, 1997). With the growing awareness that trauma interacts with developmental time course, developmental approaches will be critical to examining the broad range of human behaviors affected by trauma. Moreover, because the study of trauma brings us face to face with human cruelty, it is ethically imperative that we incorporate not just a scientific approach but also wisdom from the humanities. Different ways of knowing, different methodologies, and different perspectives are all essential for continued progress in understanding and ameliorating traumatic stress.

As collaborative progress continues within the fields of psychology and psychiatry, we hope that trauma researchers and clinicians will seek to broaden the audience for this research. Trauma affects humanity–not any one particular subset of people, but all of humanity. Given this, we need to also break down boundaries to education about trauma and societal denial of the existence of trauma. One critical step to doing this lies in the education of future generations of students in our classrooms, as our advisees, and supervisees. We need to train our students to evaluate and measure the role of previous and current trauma in the lives of research participants, even when trauma is not the specific focus of the research, as traumatic experiences are likely to be impacting a wide variety of aspects of human functioning (including personality, social, cognitive, and neurological functioning). Similarly, we need to include the role of trauma in our curriculum as we teach students about human functioning.

In addition, trauma research can provide a framework for questioning and understanding widespread oppression in society. As collaboration between areas of psychology and psychiatry push forward, we have the opportunity to join other fields, such as women's studies and sociology in understanding how various forms of oppression, violence, and trauma are perpetrated and maintained in society. As our understanding of mechanisms and effects increases, our ability to intervene and prevent violence and trauma will hopefully increase.

There are risks in asking questions about trauma and oppression, one of which is the effect trauma work has on the worldviews we hold as researchers. In asking about trauma, we are challenged to understand our role in a culture that can tacitly support violence against women and children, our own positions of power and accountability, as well as our responsibility to name trauma. These are powerful challenges that most likely change us in the process–our sense of self, other, and context can be transformed through this work. In this transformation, we realize that we cannot remain untouched by trauma. The study of trauma, the participants who courageously share their experiences, and the knowledge of both the limits and bounds of human resilience change us as researchers. This is not what we are taught in traditional training models; rather, we have been taught that research and science require "objectivity," not transformation. And so, in studying trauma, we face a challenge to reevaluate our assumptions, values, and views.

While traumatic events, particularly those involving interpersonal violence and betrayal, can challenge one's faith, as researchers we find hope and inspiration from studying trauma, and from sharing the study of trauma with colleagues from various perspectives. As Frohnmayer said at the 1998 conference: "Your success as it is expressed at this conference will prove to be formative. I believe in the emerging field of trauma and cognitive science helping to set the agenda by focusing on the pursuit of the important cross-disciplinary questions with a three-fold combination of scientific excellence, attention to ethics, and dedication to humanity."

REFERENCES

Frohnmayer, D. (Speaker). (1998). Opening remarks at the 1998 Meeting on Trauma and Cognitive Science [audiotape]. Eugene, OR: University of Oregon. Audiotape purchase information available at: http://dynamic.uoregon.edu/traumaconf.html

Mortenson, E. (1998, July 19). Psychologists coming together over memories. *The Register-Guard*, pp. 1D-2D.

Putnam, F. (1997). *Dissociation in children and adolescents: A developmental perspective.* New York: Guilford.

Rojas-Burke, J. (1998, July 20). Professor examines "forgotten" memories. *The Register-Guard*, pp. 1C, 4C.

Shearer, R. R., & Gould, S. J. (1999). Of two minds and one nature. *Science, 286,* 1093-1094.

Index